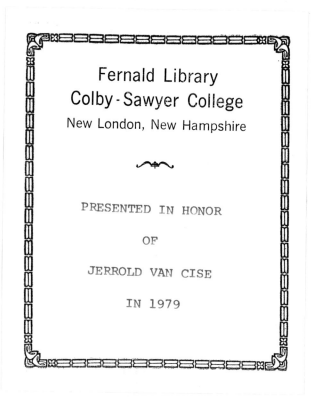

NATURAL RESISTANCE SYSTEMS
AGAINST FOREIGN CELLS, TUMORS, AND MICROBES

Perspectives in Immunology

A Series of Publications Based on Symposia

Maurice Landy and Werner Braun (Eds.)
IMMUNOLOGICAL TOLERANCE
A Reassessment of Mechanisms of the Immune Response
1969

H. Sherwood Lawrence and Maurice Landy (Eds.)
MEDIATORS OF CELLULAR IMMUNITY
1969

Richard T. Smith and Maurice Landy (Eds.)
IMMUNE SURVEILLANCE
1970

Jonathan W. Uhr and Maurice Landy (Eds.)
IMMUNOLOGIC INTERVENTION
1971

Hugh O. McDevitt and Maurice Landy (Eds.)
GENETIC CONTROL OF IMMUNE RESPONSIVENESS
Relationship to Disease Susceptibility
1972

Richard T. Smith and Maurice Landy (Eds.)
IMMUNOBIOLOGY OF THE TUMOR — HOST
   RELATIONSHIP
1974

Gustavo Cudkowicz, Maurice Landy, and
   Gene M. Shearer (Eds.)
NATURAL RESISTANCE SYSTEMS AGAINST FOREIGN
   CELLS, TUMORS, AND MICROBES
1978

NATURAL RESISTANCE SYSTEMS AGAINST FOREIGN CELLS, TUMORS, AND MICROBES

edited by

Gustavo Cudkowicz

*State University of New York
Buffalo, New York*

Maurice Landy

*Schweizerisches Forschungsinstitut
Davos, Switzerland*

Gene M. Shearer

*National Cancer Institute
Bethesda, Maryland*

Proceedings of an International Conference
Held at Timber Cove Inn
Jenner, California
October 18–22, 1976

1978

ACADEMIC PRESS   New York   San Francisco   London
A *Subsidiary of Harcourt Brace Jovanovich, Publishers*

Academic Press Rapid Manuscript Reproduction

ACADEMIC PRESS, INC.
111 Fifth Avenue, New York, New York 10003

United Kingdom Edition published by
ACADEMIC PRESS, INC. (LONDON) LTD.
24/28 Oval Road, London NW1 7DX

Library of Congress Cataloging in Publication Data

Main entry under title:

Natural resistance systems against foreign cells, tumors
and microbes.

    Includes indexes.
    1. Natural immunity—Congresses.   I. Cudkowicz,
Gustavo.   II. Landy, Maurice.   III. Shearer,
Gene M. [DNLM: 1.   Antigen-antibody reactions—
Congresses.   2.   Immunity, Natural—Congresses.
3.   Neoplasms—Immunology—Congresses. QW541 N285 1976]
QR185.2.N37   616.07'9   78-4246
ISBN 0-12-199735-9

CONTENTS

CONFEREES

Fritz H. Bach University of Wisconsin, Madison, Wisconsin
Michael Bennett Boston University School of Medicine, Boston, Massachusetts
Milivoj Boranic Ruder Boskovic Institute, Zagreb, Yugoslavia
Priscilla A. Campbell National Jewish Hospital, Denver, Colorado
Harvey Cantor Harvard University, Boston, Massachusetts
Martin J. Cline University of California, Los Angeles, California
Gustavo Cudkowicz State University of New York at Buffalo, Buffalo, New York
Jean Dausset Hôpital Saint Louis, University of Paris VII, Paris
Karel Dicke University of Texas, Houston, Texas
Bo Dupont Memorial Sloan Kettering Cancer Center, New York
Vincent P. Eijsvoogel Red Cross Blood Transfusion Service, Amsterdam, The Netherlands
William L. Elkins University of Pennsylvania, Philadelphia, Pennsylvania
Hilliard Festenstein The London Hospital Medical College, London
Robert P. Gale University of California, Los Angeles, California
Edward S. Golub Purdue University, Lafayette, Indiana
Robert Gordon Clinical Research Center, Harrow, Middlesex, England
Christopher S. Henney Johns Hopkins University, Baltimore, Maryland
John B. Hibbs, Jr. Veterans Administration Hospital, Salt Lake City, Utah
Maurice Landy Schweizerisches Forschungsinstitut, Davos, Switzerland
Daniel Meruelo New York University, New York
Donald Metcalf Walter and Eliza Hall Institute of Medical Research, Melbourne, Australia
Malcolm A. S. Moore Memorial Sloan-Kettering Cancer Center, New York

Ichiro Nakamura   State University of New York at Buffalo, Buffalo, New York

Richard J. O'Reilly   Memorial Sloan-Kettering Cancer Center, New York

Robertson Parkman   The Children's Hospital Medical Center, Boston, Massachusetts

Barbara H. Sanford   National Cancer Institute, Bethesda, Maryland

Anne-Marie Schmitt-Verhulst   National Cancer Institute, Bethesda, Maryland

Gene M. Shearer   National Cancer Institute, Bethesda, Maryland

Jonathan Sprent   University of Pennsylvania, Philadelphia, Pennsylvania

Richard Steeves   Albert Einstein College of Medicine, Bronx, New York

Rainer Storb   The Fred Hutchinson Cancer Research Center, Seattle, Washington

Osias Stutman   Memorial Sloan-Kettering Cancer Center, New York

James E. Till   The Ontario Cancer Institute, Toronto, Ontario, Canada

John J. Trentin   Baylor College of Medicine, Houston, Texas

Jonathan W. Uhr   University of Texas, Dallas, Texas

Dirk W. Van Bekkum   Institutes of the Organization for Health Research, Rijswijk, The Netherlands

Noel L. Warner   University of New Mexico, Albuquerque, New Mexico

Peter Wernet   University of Tübingen, Tübingen, West Germany

Hans Wigzell   University of Uppsala, Uppsala, Sweden

PREFACE

Natural immunity was perceived as a distinctive entity from the time of the founding of modern immunology. However, it was invariably considered to involve the same principles and mechanisms as acquired immunity. The term "natural" was appended to designate its occurrence in the absence of overt stimulation, but there was always the implication that somehow antigenic stimulation had nonetheless taken place. In retrospect, this simplistic view of natural immunity and resistance was actually more a tacit assumption than a concept resulting from coherent analysis. Remarkably enough, such an unsophisticated view has until now remained unchallenged.

During the intervening decades there have been sporadic attempts to ascertain the operational basis of natural resistance. These investigations, mostly in the 1940s and 1950s, were limited in scope, as the emphasis at that time was centered largely on humoral mechanisms. By the mid-1970s, when this conference was organized, several phenomena of natural resistance had been investigated at the cellular level and had been seen to differ from adoptive immunity with respect to cellular processes, recognition mechanisms, genetic restrictions, and regulatory influences. Some of these phenomena were of considerably more than passing interest because they involved engraftment of hemopoietic cells, tumor–host, and virus–host relationships. As this volume attests, evidence has recently emerged indicating that the mechanisms of natural resistance are indeed distinctive. As such they clearly represent a new and significant development in immunobiology.

At first glance this conference volume may give the impression that the overriding concern has been with bone marrow transplantation. This largely reflects the historic fact that the murine marrow transplantation model was the one where the relevant phenomenology was first perceived, then analyzed, and finally recognized as the prototype for a series of diverse, seemingly unrelated biologic situations. However, quite apart from the consideration of natural resistance to marrow transplantation, the conference dealt incisively with resistance to microorganisms and tumors and with the dual problems of basic immunobiology and clinical aspects of immune reconstitution, especially since the latter is influenced by natural resistance phenomena at the levels of engraftment and graft-versus-host disease.

In our view, the most meaningful contribution of the conference, as recorded in this volume, is the identification and characterization of host defense systems, endowed with specificity, yet noninduced, nonadoptive, and non-thymus dependent. These systems are clearly effective in situations generally equated with threats of host integrity and survival. At this early stage of our awareness and understanding of these systems and their operations, interpretations understandably have taken a teleologic cast. It is probable, however, that apart from surveillance, natural resistance systems could well fulfill, for example, essential physiologic roles in homeostasis by regulating cell renewal and differentiation.

Gustavo Cudkowicz
Maurice Landy
Gene M. Shearer

ACKNOWLEDGMENTS

The Conference Organizing Committee, consisting of Gustavo Cudkowicz, Maurice Landy, and Gene M. Shearer, gratefully acknowledges the encouragement and invaluable support of Dr. William D. Terry, National Cancer Institute, in planning this conference.

Funding for the conference, for the recording of discussions and retrieval by stenotypy, and for preparation of typescripts has been provided by DHEW—National Institutes of Health, National Cancer Institute, Tumor Immunology Program, under Contract No. 263-76-C-0175.

One of the editors of the volume (G. C.) especially thanks Dr. Jean Dausset for the hospitality extended at the Hôpital Saint Louis, Paris, France. The editing of this book was undertaken by G. C. during the tenure of an American Cancer Society—Eleanor Roosevelt—International Cancer Travel Fellowship awarded by the International Union against Cancer, and of a Sabbatical Fellowship awarded by the Institut National de la Santé et de la Recherche Médicale.

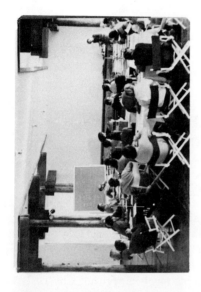
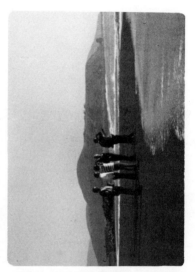
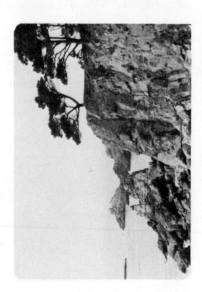
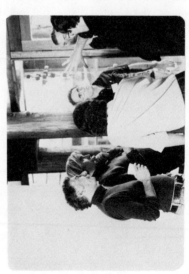

Conference scenes

NATURAL RESISTANCE TO FOREIGN HEMOPOIETIC AND LEUKEMIA GRAFTS

Discussion Introducer:

Gustavo Cudkowicz

CHAIRMAN CUDKOWICZ: It has become clear during the last decade that in mice and other mammalian species commonly used for experimental transplantation there is a natural (i.e., nonintentionally induced) resistance to the engraftment of foreign hemopoietic cells, even after heavy total-body irradiation of prospective recipients. This natural resistance manifests itself as a cytostatic effect exerted by the host environment on transplanted cells after the latter have settled into sites of hemopoiesis. In strongly resistant hosts such cells fail to proliferate and differentiate; in weakly resistant hosts the proliferation is deficient; and in susceptible hosts exponential proliferation begins about 48 hr after transplantation, with early differentiation occurring primarily in the direction of erythropoiesis, granulocytopoiesis, and megakariocytopoiesis. For a short period after transplantation, two to three days, viable transplanted stem cells can be recovered from spleens of susceptible and strongly resistant recipients. Later on, the transplanted cells disappear from the hemopoietic sites of the resistant mice.

The initial observation of graft failure in irradiated mice otherwise not pretreated led to extensive investigations. It became obvious that both the genetics and the immunobiology of hemopoietic transplants, and of lymphoma-leukemia transplants, depart quite markedly in almost every parameter considered from the familiar genetics and immunobiology of solid tissue transplants such as skin, kidney, and carcinomas. I shall describe the distinguishing features that make bone marrow transplants unique compared with other well-known types of grafts, but also a prototype model for different, less known host reactivities, which I shall refer to as "natural" to emphasize the lack of intentional induction. Other natural host responses to lymphoma, viruses, and bacteria will be discussed later in this conference and their analogies to resistance to hemopoietic cells will become evident.

It has been assumed that compatibility for all grafts rests upon multiple genetic determinants of cellular antigens inherited codominantly—the histocompatibility (H) genes. Hemopoietic transplants are subject, however, to additional restrictions by a class of *noncodominant* genes designated Hh for hemopoietic-histocompatibility. The noncodominant inheritance implies that Hh genes are not fully expressed in a heterozygote. In fact, these genes are not expressed at all in the common inbred laboratory strains of mice, unless homozygous. Should the Hh gene product be a transplantation antigen or some other kind of cell surface structure required for the take of hemopoietic grafts, one would expect that F_1 hybrid mice from inbred parents of diverse Hh type would not possess the product of one or both parental Hh alleles.

This situation is a rather convenient one to work with, since F_1 hybrids are genetically compatible for H gene products of either parent and thus are universal acceptors of parental skin and other solid tissue grafts. Since F_1 hybrids fail to express Hh alleles, they are not compatible for parental Hh gene products and thus could be resistant to parental bone marrow grafts. Most of the studies on

3

resistance were done in this convenient situation where F_1 incompatibility for parental cells could not have been due to H gene products. It should be clearly understood, however, that it is not implied that all Hh genes of mice or other species are inherited in this way. On the contrary, I think that if one were to analyze a larger number of strains or species, random bred animals, or wild mice, one would find other patterns of inheritance with less clear-cut differences of gene expression between Hh-homozygotes and heterozygotes.

Hh genes are multiple in the mouse, but most of them (all except one) are clustered on chromosome 17, the same chromosome on which the major histocompatibility complex (MHC) lies (Fig. 1). Two Hh loci, Hh-1 and Hh-3, are actually mapped within the D and K regions, respectively, of the H-2 complex. Hh-2 is 16 crossover units away from H-2D; other Hh determinants, to which a number has not yet been assigned because of incomplete genetic analysis, are scattered on the telomeric portion of the chromosome. These Hh determinants are referred to by the name of the mouse strain in which they were identified.

All of the Hh genes studied so far are inherited noncodominantly and seem to be expressed selectively in cells of the hemopoietic system. Within this heterogeneous system, the immature cells possess either more, or more effective, Hh gene product than mature cells. For example, red blood cells and granulocytes may have lost the product altogether, whereas stem cells and some of the myeloid and lymphoid precursor cells possess it. Assuming that Hh genes are the structural genes of a cell surface component of relatively immature hemopoietic cells, the gene product could be viewed as a kind of differentiation antigen recognizable *in vivo* by preexisting host cells which will exert suppressive

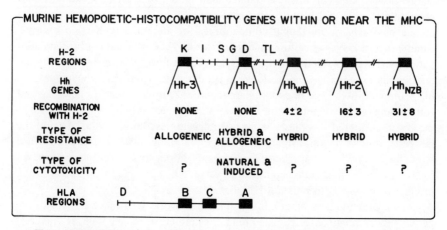

Fig. 1 Simplified map of murine chromosome 17 indicating the position of Hh genes in relation to the major histocompatibility complex. Also indicated is the effect of Hh gene products in terms of responses detected *in vivo* (resistance) and *in vitro* (cytotoxicity). Equivalent regions of the human MHC are given for comparison.

influences on target cell proliferation. Although experimental evidence for this *in vivo* effect in autologous situations is still lacking, there is strong evidence for it in parent-to-F_1 hybrid and allogeneic situations. Hh gene products are also recognized *in vitro* by preexisting cytotoxic cells (natural killer cells specific for Hh-1; Harmon, Clark, O'Toole, and Wicker, *Immunogenetics* **4**:601, 1977) and by induceable prekiller cells, which will become specifically cytotoxic within five days of culture. Figure 1 indicates the positions of Hh genes on chromosome 17 and the types of resistance *in vivo* (hybrid resistance, allogeneic resistance) and of cytotoxicity *in vitro* (natural, induced) elicited by the products of each identified MHC-associated murine Hh gene. Equivalent regions of the human MHC were included for comparison.

The genetic analysis of resistance to marrow grafts in the mouse was complicated by the existence of modifier genes that regulate the ability to recognize the Hh antigens, or the strength of host responses to Hh differences, or both. The modifier genes are similar to the well-known immune response (Ir) genes regulating humoral and cellular immunity. They ultimately determine whether resistance materializes in the face of Hh incompatibility. Ir-like genes modulating hybrid and allogeneic resistance are few in number (two for Hh-1 mediated resistance in mice), not linked to the MHC, dominant for responsiveness and additive in their effects, seemingly locus-specific. Their existence has to be remembered to correctly interpret experimental results, as will be shown later by Warner. Whether these regulator genes also influence the generation of NK cells *in vivo* and of cytotoxic cells *in vitro* is not yet known.

As to the immunobiology of *in vivo* resistance to marrow transplants, the features that distinguish it from conventional allograft reactions are several and substantial (Table 1). Mice are totally incompetent for this reactivity at birth and remain incompetent for the first three weeks of life. During the fourth week, competence is acquired rather suddenly, within 24 hr. In contrast, the compe-

TABLE 1
Resistance to Hemopoietic Grafts:
Partial or Complete Suppression of Donor Cells

Late maturation
Low sensitivity to radiation
Site dependence
Thymus independence
Marrow dependence
Macrophage dependence
Cortisone resistance
Sensitivity to antispecies sera
Immunogenetic specificity
Genetic control by structural Hh genes
Regulatory Ir genes not linked to MHC

TABLE 2

Unequal Strength of Hybrid Resistance to L5MF-22 Lymphoma Cells in Various Organs of Irradiated Mice[a]

	Uptake of ^{125}IUdR ($\% \pm$ S.E.)		
Organ	C57BL/6 (Hh-compatible)	(C57BL/6×DBA/2)F$_1$ (Hh-incompatible)	Ratio (F$_1$/C57BL/6)
Spleen	5.7 ± 0.3	1.0 ± 0.2	0.17
Femurs and tibias	1.2 ± 0.1	0.5 ± 0.1	0.42
Liver	24.9 ± 2.9	15.3 ± 1.7	0.61
Lung	1.8 ± 0.2	1.5 ± 0.2	0.83

[a] 10^6 lymphoma cells were injected i.v. into irradiated mice (800 rads of γ-rays to C57BL/6 and 950 rads to F$_1$). ^{125}IUdR was injected i.p. five days later to evaluate synthesis of DNA by transplanted cells. The ratio of uptake values in organs of resistant and genetically susceptible mice is an index of the strength of resistance. Weak resistance is reflected by a ratio of almost one, and the strongest resistance by a ratio of near zero. Data from Riccardi and Cudkowicz (unpublished).

tence for antibody formation or skin graft rejection is either present at birth or acquired within the first week. Once resistance has developed, it is relatively insensitive to radiation, so that lethal and supralethal doses of total body radiation (800–1000 rads) fail to abrogate it. Insensitivity to radiation is not absolute, however, since Trentin *et al.* have shown that doses above 2000 rads do indeed weaken resistance, and I was able to measure effects of radiation even in the dose range of 1000 rads.

By measuring the strength of resistance in different organs of an animal, one soon realizes that this activity is site-dependent. The spleen is the site in which resistance is strongest in terms of number of cells required to override it, followed by the bone cavities, as shown some years ago by Trentin *et al.* in rat-to-mouse chimeras. Since normal bone marrow cells only colonize the hemopoietic sites of an irradiated host, lymphoma cells expressing foreign Hh alleles had to be transplanted into irradiated mice to assess resistance elsewhere. The results obtained by Carlo Riccardi working in my laboratory with the H-2^b/Hh-1^b lymphoma L5MF-22 and allogeneic or F$_1$ hybrid recipients are shown in Table 2 and Fig. 2. While confirming that resistance is strongest in the spleen, followed in decreasing order by bone cavities and liver, these experiments also showed that it was weakest in the peritoneal cavity. The cytostatic effect of resistance on the leukemic cells was estimated by measuring the incorporation of IUdR in newly synthesized DNA.

It is possible that the phenotypic expression of Hh genes varies in different tumors and that cells of tumors other than L5MF-22 grow deficiently also in the peritoneum. In our opinion, what the experiment establishes is the fact that the growth of Hh-incompatible cells is restricted severely in one organ, e.g., the

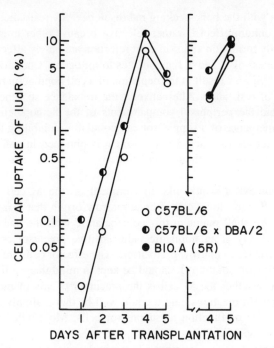

Fig. 2 Unrestricted growth of L5MF-22 lymphoma cells in the peritoneal cavity of resistant mice. C57BL/6 mice are susceptible controls; F_1 and B10.A (5R) are resistant mice, as judged by spleen colonization. 10^6 cells were injected i.p. into irradiated mice; proliferation of the transplanted cells was evaluated by measuring newly synthesized DNA by the IUdR method.

spleen of resistant mice, and still can be optimal (like in syngeneic mice) in another site. Apparently, whatever exerts cytostasis in the spleen has no influence at a distance, and the proliferation in the peritoneum has little if any influence on resistance in the spleen. The localized manifestation of resistance to bone marrow cells may account for some of the discrepancies that Van Bekkum will later point out between survival of irradiated mice given Hh-incompatible marrow and spleen colonization.

Among the features listed in Table 1, thymus independence is one that sharply distinguishes natural resistance from conventional allograft reactivity. The evidence was obtained in mice grafted 2–3 months after neonatal or 6–12 months after adult thymectomy, and in athymic nude mice. Regardless of how the athymic state comes about, resistance is not impaired. As a matter of fact, resistance is stronger in nude mice than in normal littermates, since the number of marrow cells required to override was about five times larger in the former.

The integrity of bone marrow is extremely important for natural resistance. Bennett has shown that if one selectively destroys bone marrow in mice by injecting them with the bone-seeking radioisotope ^{89}Sr, resistance is fully abrogated. The strontium effect is rather selective because other immune functions such as antibody formation and skin graft rejection are barely affected, and so are the responsiveness of B and T lymphocytes to mitogens. Continuous irradiation of marrow by ^{89}Sr may result in the depletion of a cell population required for the manifestation of resistance. Alternatively, the imbalance so generated between the marrow and the peripheral compartments of the hemopoietic system may result in the emergence of a suppressor cell population inhibiting the effectors of resistance. Evidence for such a population was obtained in collaboration with Bennett in studies of F_1 antiparent cytotoxicity induced *in vitro,* which will be discussed later.

In this context, I would like to comment on the M cell, a designation introduced by Bennett for a cell of bone marrow origin that disappears in ^{89}Sr-treated mice. We shall maintain this nomenclature with the understanding that the M cell probably is an immature radiosensitive precursor cell and not the effector of resistance to marrow grafts itself. The effector cells are expected to be rather insensitive to radiation. It should be kept in mind that no firm evidence is available as to whether the M cell is the precursor of any of the cells directly involved in anti-Hh reactions, and it could well be that it simply is the cell type regulating the size or function of suppressor cells. More will be said later by Bennett on this topic.

Now, Table 1 lists a number of manipulations aimed at weakening or abrogating resistance on the one hand, and identifying effector cells on the other.

Antimacrophage agents such as silica particles and soluble carrageenans are extremely effective in abrogating resistance *in vivo.* A single injection of relatively small amounts of these agents given shortly before or after transplantation is adequate, and it is hard to believe that the regimens employed severely deplete mice of macrophages for any length of time. I would rather say that a subpopulation of macrophages, sensitive to the cytotoxicity of these agents, plays a crucial role in the manifestation of resistance, but accessory in nature. It seems unlikely at this point that macrophages are the effector cells, since resistance is immunogenetically specific and the effectors must be capable of recognizing the products of multiple and polymorphic Hh genes.

Resistance is not weakened by administration of large doses of hydrocortisone. It is abrogated, however, by small amounts of antispecies sera (e.g., rabbit antimouse sera raised against lymphocytes, macrophages, fibroblasts, and carcinoma cells) given shortly before transplantation to irradiated mice. Though these studies have not been as informative as hoped, they provide the means of selective suppression for natural resistance without suppression of other immune responses. Rabbit antimouse tissue culture fibroblast serum, prepared by John F. Warner in my laboratory, is perhaps the best example of antiserum capable of abrogating resistance without affecting the functions of B and T lymphocytes participating in humoral immune responses.

When one tries to immunize resistant F_1 hybrids by injecting parental spleen cells before irradiation and parental marrow grafting, one easily induces unresponsiveness instead. This can be done at any age, and the duration of the unresponsive state is rather long, several months, depending on the number and size of the inoculations. Induced unresponsiveness (i.e., the conversion of genetically resistant into phenotypically susceptible hybrids) is immunogenetically specific since the animals retain resistance toward third party grafts, and third party cells fail to induce it.

This completes the description of natural resistance to hemopoietic grafts as presently seen *in vivo*. Two *in vitro* models of Hh incompatibility were recently studied as a collaborative effort with Gene M. Shearer, Rolf Kiessling, Hans Wigzell, Paula S. Hochman, Otto Haller, myself, and a few others. One model is the induction *in vitro* of specific F_1 antiparent cytotoxicity (induced CML), which Shearer will illustrate in detail later, and the other is the detection *in vitro* of natural killer cells for lymphoma targets, which Wigzell will discuss in a broader context, and Shearer as well. I would like to whet your appetite, however, by comparing in Table 3 conventional allogeneic anti-H-2 CML, F_1 antiparent CML, and noninduced CML with respect to parameters that are signif-

TABLE 3

In vitro Correlates of Natural Resistance to Hemopoietic Grafts.
Comparisons with Respect to Parameters Significant for *in vivo* Resistance[a]

Parameter investigated	Allogeneic CML	F_1 anti-P CML	Noninduced CML (NKC)
Maturation	Early	Late	Late
Radiosensitivity	High	High	Low
Site Dependence	Moderate	Moderate	High
Effectors	Thy-1(+)	Thy-1(+)	Thy-1(−)
Marrow dependence	Low	High	High
Macrophage dependence	Low	High	High
Cortisone	Resistant	Resistant	Sensitive
Antispecies sera	Slightly sensitive	Highly sensitive	Highly sensitive
Immunogenetic specificity	H-2K or H-2D	H-2D/Hh-1	H-2D/Hh-1 and other

[a]Discrepancies with *in vivo* resistance are underlined.

icant for characterizing *in vivo* resistance to marrow grafts (listed in Table 1). Noninduced CML (natural killer cells) correlates best with *in vivo* resistance to marrow grafts; the only discordant parameter is the sensitivity of NK cells to cortisone, a rather minor discrepancy. Induced F_1 antiparent CML also correlates well with *in vivo* resistance, but the effector cell line is radiosensitive and positive for the T cell marker Thy-1, two major discrepancies. As expected, induced allogeneic CML does not correlate with *in vivo* resistance.

A critical comparison is the sensitivity to radiation, since resistance is commonly observed in irradiated mice. Acute irradiation has no weakening effect on NK cell activity. I wanted to carry this observation further, and so NK cell activity as well as resistance was measured at intervals after the high sublethal dose of 700 rads of γ-rays. A normalized curve depicting the parallel changes in splenic NK cell activity and of *in vivo* resistance is given in Fig. 3. The periods of retained activities followed by rapid loss of activities and slow regeneration were quite coincidental, adding another parameter to the positive correlations.

By integrating the experimental evidence obtained *in vivo* and *in vitro* with the systems described, a comprehensive model is proposed as outlined in Fig. 4. Central to all manifestations of anti-Hh reactions is a macrophage-like cell whose properties are listed in Fig. 4 (central rectangle). This cell interacts *in vivo* with the effectors (or their precursors) of resistance to marrow grafts and lymphoma–leukemias. These *in vivo* effectors are conspicuous for lacking T cell markers and

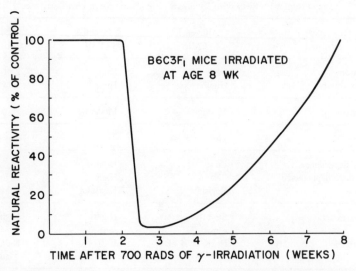

Fig. 3 Changes in the level of natural reactivities of mice after total body irradiation. Resistance to C57BL/6 marrow and splenic NK cell activity were measured and then expressed as percentage of untreated controls (data from Hochman and Cudkowicz).

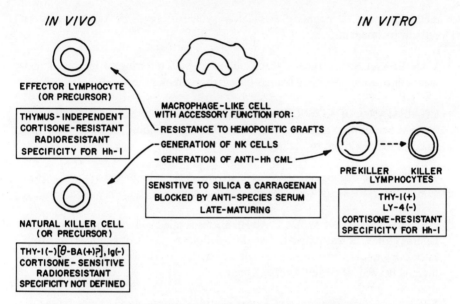

Fig. 4 Schema for the cellular deployment for accessory and effector functions in natural resistance to normal and malignant hemopoietic cells *in vivo,* and F_1 antiparent CML *in vitro.*

for low sensitivity to radiation and are viewed as subpopulations differing essentially for the target cell structure they recognize, i.e., for their specificity. *In vitro,* the same central macrophage-like cell interacts with T cells in the generation of F_1 antiparent cytotoxicity.

SANFORD: If one were to inject two different sites concurrently, can one see resistance in one and not in the other? If you inject cell sequentially, does that make a difference?

CHAIRMAN CUDKOWICZ: Concurrent injection of cells into peritoneum and spleen, for example, results in a dichotomy: resistance in spleen but not in peritoneum. The cells that grow in the peritoneum have no advantage, however, when they leave the cavity and reach the spleen.

VAN BEKKUM: It is necessary to define the end points of the measurements employed if one is going to compare different sites. What proof is there that the same phenomenon is monitored in different sites?

CHAIRMAN CUDKOWICZ: The way we evaluate cell growth is either by counting cells or by measuring one or another cell function. We prefer to measure the DNA synthesis, and we can do this in several sites, with the same methodology. Cell counting and DNA synthesis gave the same results on cells in peritoneum.

VAN BEKKUM: I assume that Cudkowicz was referring to irradiated recipients throughout. Is this a source of variation among the various strains?

CHAIRMAN CUDKOWICZ: One can view it the other way. Rather than being a source of variation, one is eliminating variation, because most host spleen cells are killed by radiation.

BACH: How certain is Cudkowicz's statement regarding recessivity of expression of the Hh genes? Are some clearly dominant?

CHAIRMAN CUDKOWICZ: All Hh alleles studied so far are not expressed in heterozygotes, at least those detected by deficient growth of parental cells in F_1 mice. One could view the alleles not generating resistance as codominant, but there is no way at present to study them.

STORB: Cudkowicz said that acute radiation does not abrogate resistance. But he then said that treatment of animals with the bone-seeking isotope ^{89}Sr does abrogate resistance. How is that explained, since in both instances one is dealing with irradiation?

CHAIRMAN CUDKOWICZ: The bone-seeking isotope provides continuing irradiation to the restricted population of cells inside bones that comprises progenitor cells, and causes their depletion. Acute irradiation does not inactivate existing mature effector cells, and so the animal maintains reactivity.

WARNER: The main point I want to stress in relation to this subject is that the genetic control operates at two levels, as Cudkowicz has shown. The H-2 region can be involved in determining the nature or expression of certain Hh antigens, and also may be involved in controlling the immune response to various cell surface antigens.

I would like to give a few illustrations using another mouse strain background to exemplify the universality of many points made by Cudkowicz, and then conclude with a hypothesis that I hope will provoke some more discussion on the point made by Bach, concerning the genetic mechanism that is operating in this apparent recessivity of Hh antigen expression.

The systems that we have studied have involved the SJL mouse strain, and we have described an Hh antigen that is associated with the H-2^s complex, and is distinct in terms of specificity from the previous Hh antigens associated with C57BL and other strains, but in all respects parallels the observations made with

TABLE 4

Deficient Growth of Parental SJL Hemopoietic Colonies in F_1 Hybrid Mice

Recipient	K	A	B	J	E	C	S	G	D	Mean CFU/10^5
SJL										20 ± 5
(SJL × C57)F_1	b	b	b	b	b	b	b	b	b	22 ± 3
(SJL × C3H.SW)F_1	b	b	b	b	b	b	b	b	b	21 ± 2
(SJL × B10.BR)F_1	k	k	k	k	k	k	k	k	k	12 ± 4
(SJL × CBA)F_1	k	k	k	k	k	k	k	k	k	9 ± 2
(SJL × B10.D2)F_1	d	d	d	d	d	d	d	d	d	<1
(SJL × NZB)F_1	d	d	d	d	d	d	d	d	d	<1
(SJL × NZC)F_1	d	d	d	d	d	d	d	d	d	<1
(SJL × B10.A)F_1	k	k	k	k	k	d	d	d	d	<1
(SJL × B10.A(2R)F_1	k	k	k	k	k	d	d	–	b	10 ± 2
(SJL × B10.A(4R)F_1	k	k	b	b	b	b	b	b	b	23 ± 2
(SJL × B10.A(5R)F_1	b	b	b	k	k	d	d	d	d	<1

MHC regions of non-SJL parent

these mouse strains. As is shown in Table 4, for example, when SJL bone marrow is inoculated into a series of SJL hybrids, wherever the H-$2D^d$ allele occurs in the recipient, the injected cells are completely rejected. The clearest comparison is between the B10.A hybrid and the B10.A(2R) hybrid, which are identical for all regions except for H-2D. The minor difference observed between the 2R and the 4R hybrids has not proved consistent in subsequent studies.

TABLE 5

The Effect of Irradiation on Hybrid Resistance: Persistence Following Acute Single Dose and Abrogation after Split-Dose

Recipient strain	Donor cells	Response 800 rads	Response 600 + 800 rads
(SJL × C3H.SW)F_1		21 ± 2[a]	24 ± 2
(SJL × B10.BR)F_1	SJL—Bone marrow	12 ± 4	22 ± 1
(SJL × B10.D2)F_1		<1	23 ± 5
(SJL × NZC)F_1		<1	24 ± 2
(SJL × C3H.SW)F_1		5.6 ± 0.2[b]	6.6 ± 0.4
(SJL × B10.BR)F_1	375 V (myeloid leuk.)	4.7 ± 0.4	7.0 ± 0.2
(SJL × B10.D2)F_1		2.4 ± 0.5	7.9 ± 0.4

[a]Mean CFU/10^5 ± S.E., seven days after injection of 2×10^5 SJL bone marrow cells.

[b]Mean ratio spleen weights (mg/g body weight), tumor cell injected/control, seven days after injection.

It might appear from Table 4 that the SJL Hh allele is in fact the same allele as is present in the C57BL strains. However, other studies to be described later using SJL tumors show that this may not be the case.

The following data stress several of the points that Cudkowicz has made concerning the mechanism of resistance to Hh incompatible cells, and I now refer only to the CFU (colony-forming units) data. The mechanism is quite radioresistant in that it is still operating in mice exposed to 800 rads of ionizing radiation (Table 5). However, using the split dose delivery of irradiation that Cudkowicz has described, with 600 rads two weeks prior to the 800-rads dose, the response is now abrogated. Presumably, the precursor of effector cells (M cell) is radiosensitive, whereas the effector cell itself is radioresistant.

It is of interest in this context that we have obtained similar results with NK (natural killer) cells, namely that the NK cell is resistant to 1000 rads delivered *in vitro*. By irradiating mice several days prior to harvesting NK cells, the precursor of NK cells also proves to be radiosensitive.

Pretreatment of mice with ^{89}Sr results in complete abrogation of resistance (Table 6), as had been shown by Bennett. Here, strongly resistant hybrids were used; nevertheless, strontium abrogated this resistance. Similarly, silica pretreatment abrogated the resistance of these hybrids (Table 6).

Thus by these diverse approaches, it becomes evident that the same mechanism is operating in resistance to SJL Hh antigen, as shown by Cudkowicz and Bennett against C57BL-associated Hh antigens.

An important point I would like to make concerns the genetic regulation of hybrid resistance, which is relevant to this general discussion.

In Table 7, it is shown in a series of different SJL hybrids that complete rejection of CFU is associated with d/s heterozygosity at the H-2D locus. How-

TABLE 6

Abrogation of Hybrid Resistance to SJL Hemopoietic Stem
Cells by Pretreatment of F_1 Mice with Silica Particles or ^{89}Sr

Recipient strain	Pretreatment of recipient (i.v.)	Splenic CFU colonies (mean ± SE)
(SJL × C57)F_1	none	12.8 ± 2.5
	2 mg silica	27.6 ± 2.3
(SJL × B10.D2)F_1	none	0.9 ± 0.5
	2 mg silica	14.8 ± 3.1
(SJL × B10.A)F_1	none	2.0 ± 0.8
	2 mg silica	17.5 ± 3.5
(SJL × C57)F_1	none	35.8 ± 2.1
(SJL × B10D2)F_1	none	2.8 ± 0.3
	^{89}Sr	38.1 ± 3.3

TABLE 7
Genetic Regulation of Hybrid Resistance to Parental
SJL Hemopoietic Grafts

Recipients	H-2D type	Cells transplanted	Response
(SJL × C57)F$_1$	s/b		7.7 ± 0.5[a]
(SJL × B10.BR)F$_1$	s/k	2 × 10^5 375V	4.0 ± 0.4
(SJL × B10.D2)F$_1$	s/d		1.6 ± 0.1
(SJL × ATH)F$_1$	s/d		4.7 ± 0.2
(SJL × C57)F$_1$	s/d		18 ± 1[b]
(SJL × B10.A)F$_1$	s/d	SJL bone marrow	0
(SJL × B10.A.5R)F$_1$	s/d		0
(SJL × ATH)F$_1$	s/d		12 ± 1

[a]Mean ratio spleen weights (mg/g body weight), tumor cell injected/
control, seven days after injection.

[b]Mean CFU/10^5 ± S.E., seven days after injection of 2 × 10^5 SJL
bone marrow cells.

ever, we have also found that when we use (SJL × ATH)F$_1$ or (SJL × ATL)F$_1$
hybrids as recipients, also d/s heterozygotes at the H-2D locus, we find essentially normal colony formation (Table 7). This has been confirmed with both SJL
CFU and tumors in a number of such experiments.

Thus, there is a second gene operating, which may be a type of immune
response gene controlling the resistance to Hh gene products. ATH and ATL
mice may lack the allele for responsiveness. One gene operates at the level of
antigen expression and the second at the level of reactivity to the Hh antigen. We
have not yet mapped the ''immune response'' gene, but considering the strain
combinations used, it probably is not linked to the I$_3$ allotype or the MHC region.
It is perhaps important to stress that other genetic factors may also be involved in
determining tumor growth in different parent into F$_1$ hybrid combinations. In
fact, if one compares tumor growth with CFU growth in various parent–hybrid
combinations, sometimes there is very good correlation, particularly where there
is a strong Hh incompatibility, and sometimes not. An example of the latter
situation is the case of NZB cells grafted into (NZB × NZW)F$_1$ hybrids, where
we find virtually no evidence of resistance to NZB tumors, but strong resistance
to NZB CFU (Table 8). Instead, it is the (NZB × C57BL)F$_1$ hybrid that resists
the tumor, while it is not resistant to CFU growth. In this case we consider that an
Ir gene confers responsiveness to the hybrid for a tumor-specific antigen.

I would like to describe now a hypothesis for the genetic mechanism of
hybrid resistance. We have to consider the possibility that one or the other of the
allelic genes is prevented from being expressed in the heterozygous state. Alter-

TABLE 8

Discordance of Hybrid Resistance to Tumor Growth and to Hemopoietic
Colony Growth

		Inhibition of growth[a]	
Donor strain	F_1 Hybrid recipient	Tumor	CFU
SJL	(SJL × C57BL)F_1	Moderate	None
	(SJL × B10.D2)F_1	Strong	Strong
B10.A (4R)	(B10.A(4R) × BALB/c)F_1	Moderate	Strong
B10.A	(B10.A × BALB/c)F_1	Moderate	None
NZB	(NZB × C57BL)F_1	Strong	Weak
	(NZB × NZW)F_1	Weak	Strong

[a]Inhibition of tumor growth or splenic colony formation in F_1 hybrids
relative to growth in syngeneic recipients.

natively, allelic interaction may occur at the posttranslational level. The blood
group systems provide a model of the latter possibility, which has been proposed
to account for the expression of Ir genes. The point to remember is that we are
dealing with Hh genes closely linked to the major histocompatibility complex,
and all the other genes in this complex show codominant inheritance.

It is postulated that Hh genes show clear codominant expression in
heterozygotes, and that gene products are enzymes (Fig. 5). Thus, in the
homozygous state, the product of the Hh^s allele is represented as one enzyme.
That particular enzyme acts on a substrate, and as a result, a series of antigenic
determinants are expressed on the substrate molecule, which occurs on a cell
membrane. In the heterozygote, a second enzyme is also present, coded for by
the alternate allele. The assumption is made that these two allelic genes determine enzymes with different active sites. When both enzymes operate on the
substrate, there may be an interaction or modification resulting in some determinants being hidden and others newly created, in contrast to the product resulting
from the action of only one enzyme. Different haplotypes may code for similar
enzymes, and thus similar surface configurations may result. Because of the
responder status determined by Ir genes, differences in growth of cells may
nevertheless be observed in heterozygotes between such two haplotypes. However (and perhaps this may apply to H-2D$^{s/d}$ mice), one could have quite different
enzyme constitutions producing completely distinct antigenic patterns and, accordingly, the potential number of antigens recognized by the hybrids given
parental cells would become greater.

CHAIRMAN CUDKOWICZ: Would Warner's model entail that the F_1 cells be
antigenic for the parent?

H-2D Hh-I

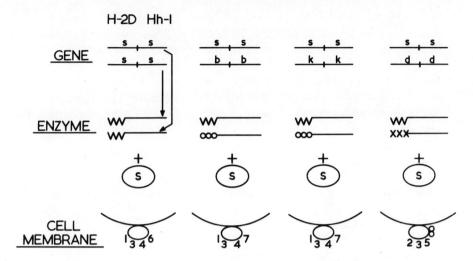

Fig. 5 Schema to account for the genetics of hybrid resistance to parental grafts.

WARNER: In some situations that would be expected.

CHAIRMAN CUDKOWICZ: In trying to secure experimental verification of models taken from molecular genetics, I was never able to find that F_1 cells were antigenic for the parent. Consequently, I regard this regretful outcome a stumbling block for any such model.

BACH: I wonder whether I could pose a model slightly different from Warner's. One possible interpretation (supported by the fact that cytotoxic T lymphocytes seem to need a certain density of presentation of antigen) is that what one is seeing in hybrid resistance is the response to a relatively weak stimulus generated by Hh, and that consequently we are dealing with threshold phenomena. If so, the heterozygote is not recognized by the parent because there is not enough phenotypic product; in the homozygous case, on the other hand, there is a higher density of the same phenotypic product. Would this in essence be a helpful variation of Warner's model?

WARNER: I don't think it is. In many of these Hh systems the resistance can be very strong. It would be unlikely that a small quantitative dosage effect could account for strong resistance.

I agree that the current data, based on the combination of F_1 cells into parent, appears incompatible with the hypothesis in Fig. 5. However, one answer to Cudkowicz's objection might relate to the importance of the Ir gene effect at the host level. It might be questioned whether or not sufficient combinations have been explored, since the F_1 may have a different determinant than would be the case in the other direction. Accordingly, there may be an important Ir control for this F_1 determinant that is not operative in the parental to F_1 situation.

BACH: I think that the threshold phenomenon can occur despite the strength of anti-Hh responses in certain hybrids. Below a given density of gene products one would not discern expression, whereas above this level the antigenicity could be very strong.

WARNER: I think it is a problem that will only be resolved when we have a clear way of identifying the "antigen" on the cell surface. To my knowledge, nobody has developed a serological reagent to these Hh cell surface components.

CHAIRMAN CUDKOWICZ: The identification of the Hh gene products is actually the major difficulty at this time. One of the reasons for not having serological reagents is the lack of congenic strains for Hh genes. Whatever combination of mouse strains is used to raise antisera, it yields potent anti-H-2D, rather than anti-Hh reagents.

I want to address myself to Warner's data. He said first that the SJL strain is sharing with the C57BL strain the Hh-1 determinant, but later he also said that this is not really so. Which is in fact the case?

WARNER: The seeming discrepancy stems from our having made reciprocal CFU studies with the allogeneic inbred strain combination of SJL and C57BL (using irradiated recipients). Rejection of SJL CFU by C57BL mice occurred. Furthermore, with many SJL tumors inoculated into inbred SJL or F_1 hybrid mice, we consistently find depressed growth in the (SJL × C57BL)F_1 hybrid. This study also relates to the earlier question of Van Bekkum, regarding the possible site of action of resistance to Hh. We are studying tumor growth in several locations such as peritoneal and skin sites. We find that silica pretreatment, which abrogates resistance in the spleen, does not necessarily weaken resistance to tumors in subcutaneous sites. One might infer that there are two different mechanisms for CFU and for tumor targets, or that the efficiency of silica in blocking resistance is different in these sites.

CHAIRMAN CUDKOWICZ: My own data on hybrid resistance to parental SJL bone marrow grafts are summarized in Table 9. They indicate that Hh-1 is the relevant gene locus. In some of our experiments seeking to cross-tolerize SJL hybrids by injecting them with SJL cells and then challenging with C57BL marrow cells, or vice versa, we concluded that the SJL and C57BL mice possess cross-reactive Hh-1 gene products. As long as one uses normal marrow cells for transplantation, there is extensive cross reactivity in both directions. In the al-

TABLE 9
The Importance of the H-2D/Hh-1 Region for Hybrid Resistance to
Parental SJL Bone Marrow Grafts[a]

Strain	H-2	Classification	Allelic substitution at subregions of the H-2[b] haplotype[b]
SJL × B10	s/b	Susceptible	—
SJL × B10.A	s/a	Resistant	K through D
SJL × B10.A(2R)	s/h2	Susceptible	K through G
SJL × B10.A(4R)	s/h4	Susceptible	K,I-A
SJL × B10.A(5R)	s/i5	Resistant	I-J through D
SJL × B10.D2	s/d	Resistant	K through D
SJL × B10.HTG	s/g	Susceptible	K through S

[a] 10^6 SJL bone marrow cells were transplanted into irradiated (1000 rad of γ-rays) recipients. Proliferation of donor-derived cells was measured by the ^{125}IUdR method five days later.

[b] Since (SJL × B10)F$_1$ hybrids were susceptible, the H-2[b] haplotype of B10 mice, or portions thereof, was substituted by employing congenic B10 strains for producing hybrids with SJL. Whenever allelic substitutions did not involve the D region, the hybrids remained susceptible, despite substitutions at all other regions of H-2. Allelic substitutions involving the D region resulted in resistant hybrids.

logeneic and tumor situations Warner may be addressing himself to an altogether different Hh specificity.

WARNER: On one point I would like clarification: is it clear that in allogeneic cell transfers using lethally irradiated recipients, conventional H-2K or H-2D gene products do not act as the antigenic stimulus for resistance to bone marrow?

CHAIRMAN CUDKOWICZ: In allogeneic transfers into heavily irradiated mice the primary response is directed to multiple Hh determinants and not to classical H-2D or H-2K alloantigens. In some strains the response is also directed to an Hh determinant linked to the K region (only demonstrable in allogeneic combinations). However, H-2D and H-2K antigens are the targets of secondary responses.

WARNER: So, Cudkowicz is saying that in allogeneic combinations, the H-2D or H-2K products themselves do not act as a stimulus when one is using irradiated recipients and yet finding resistance to bone marrow grafting.

CHAIRMAN CUDKOWICZ: That is correct, provided recipients are properly irradiated and have not been preimmunized. An additional criterion for distinguishing between anti-H-2 and anti-Hh responses is to abrogate the latter with antimacrophage agents or with heterologous antimouse sera.

MOORE: Warner presented data showing strong hybrid resistance to NZB bone marrow in the NZB/NZW F_1 mice as opposed to very weak resistance to NZB myeloma cells. Could it be that the parental tumors he selected had in their transplantation history been serially passaged in F_1 hybrids? If so, would it not be that he had in fact selected for tumors with loss of expression of Hh?

WARNER: Not for the particular tumor studied, as it had been derived from tissue culture. However, Moore's argument is certainly an important consideration.

CHAIRMAN CUDKOWICZ: Attempts by us to select normal cell lines that have lost Hh have never succeeded. However, C57BL lymphomas can in fact be adapted to grow in F_1 mice without impairment.

FESTENSTEIN: Are there any special properties of the SJL strain with respect to hybrid resistance? I ask this because Warner seems to have done most of his experiments with SJL.

WARNER: I think that SJL mice are of special interest for a number of reasons, including abnormalities of B and T lymphocyte differentiation, allotype suppression, and a high incidence of spontaneous reticular cell sarcomas. However, in the studies of hybrid resistance, we have chosen to work with this strain because of an appropriate Hh-gene and Ir-gene constitution. Indeed, analogous results were obtained in other strain combinations.

CHAIRMAN CUDKOWICZ: Hemopoietic histocompatibility has been studied extensively in mice for over a decade, and the distribution of Hh alleles seems independent of other strain properties. This experience was recently enlarged by investigations in rats and dogs and by critical analysis of bone marrow transplantation data in man. Bennett will now summarize for us his studies in rats.

BENNETT: We became interested in rat bone marrow transplantation as an outgrowth of heart transplantation in rats. In adapting to the larger animal model, one of the problems we encountered was the failure of hemopoietic cells to grow in irradiated recipients, even in syngenic host-donor combinations. This failure is not immunologic, but seems rather to be related to poor stimulation of erythropoiesis.

Even if the donor and the host are syngeneic, donor bone marrow cells simply do not grow for the first week after transplantation, requiring about two weeks to engraft and only eventually repopulate. However, if one strongly stimulates erythropoiesis by anabolic steroids (nandrolone decanoate) or commercial preparations of erythropoietin, or induction of severe iron deficiency anemia, or by cytotoxic agents such as cyclophosphamide, dimethylmyleran, or myleran, one can now follow quantitatively the growth of marrow cells.

Graded numbers of cells were transplanted and IUdR uptake was measured five days later in recipient spleens. A linear dose–response curve is obtained under these conditions. Pretreatment of recipients with dimethylmyleran causes exponential expansion of erythropoietic cells of donor origin. This can be verified microscopically.

The rat rejects bone marrow allografts (up to 8×10^7 cells) after 800 R of total body irradiation (Table 10) just as the mouse does. Also F_1 hybrid rats reject parental strain grafts, in all strain combinations tested so far. When parental cells are transferred in infant F_1 rats 17 days old, donor stem cells grow because of host immaturity. That is to say, the F_1 antiparent reactivity develops after the

TABLE 10

Demonstration of Hybrid Resistance to Parental Marrow Cell Grafts[a] in Irradiated Rats[b]:
Age Dependence and Sensitivity to Silica Particles

DONOR		HOST				
Strain	H-1 Genotype	Strain	H-1 Genotype	Age (days)	Mean splenic ^{125}IUdR uptake (%[c]	Student t-test
LEW	1/1	LEW × WF	1/2	17	1.53	
BUF	6/6	LEW × WF	1/2	17	2.06	
LEW × WF	1/2	LEW × WF	1/2	17	1.06	p < 0.01
—	—	LEW × WF	1/2	17	0.28	
WF	2/2	LEW × WF	1/2	28	0.02	p > 0.05
LEW	1/1	LEW × WF	1/2	28	0.05	
BUF	6/6	LEW × WF	1/2	28	0.02	p < 0.01
LEW	1/1	LEW × WF	1/2	28[d]	0.40	p < 0.01
BUF	6/6	LEW × WF	1/2	28[d]	0.16	
LEW × WF	1/2	LEW × WF	1/2	42	0.49	p > 0.05
LEW × WF	1/2	LEW	1/1	42	0.36	
LEW × WF	1/2	WF	2/2	42	0.61	

[a] 3×10^7 marrow cells i.v. per host

[b] Exposed to 800 R 2 hr prior to graft. Injected with 5 mg/kg nandrolone decanoate (Deca-Durabolin) one day before and on the day of irradiation.

[c] Assay performed five days after cell transfer, groups of five to seven rats.

[d] Recipients injected with 7.5 mg silica particles i.v. 24 hr prior to irradiation.

twenty-first day of life, exactly as it does in mice. Furthermore, this reactivity can also be suppressed by the injection into prospective hosts of silica particles 24 hr prior to transplantation. Thus, in our limited experience with rats, it seems that hybrid and allogeneic resistance occurs just as in the mouse, except for being somewhat stronger.

When one transplants F_1 hybrid rat cells into parental strain recipients, donor cells grew just as well as in syngeneic hybrids. Thus, it appears again that the rat is basically the same as the mouse with respect to the Hh incompatibility.

CLINE: If Bennett's thesis is that one has to stimulate erythropoiesis to favor proliferation of grafted bone marrow cells, how does the dimethylmyleran story come into that?

BENNETT: Goldwasser analyzed the serum of patients treated with dimethyl-myleran to see if erythropoietin was responsible for the stimulation of erythropoiesis, but he found no correlation. Although commercial preparations of erythropoietin from Connaught Laboratories also stimulated proliferation of syngeneic marrow grafts, a different preparation of human urinary erythropoietin did not. Accordingly, erythropoietin does not seem to be the stimulus for erythropoiesis under these conditions.

CLINE: Since Bennett is saying that the predominant proliferating cells in bone marrow chimeras are red cell precursors, then, why not use isotope incorporation method specific for erythropoiesis such as ^{59}Fe?

BENNETT: Iron incorporation is not as quantitative a method for measuring graft take as the IUdR method. One is a cytoplasmic and the other a nuclear label. However, all you see in these spleens under the microscope are erythropoietic cells. Since in the nonstimulated animal one encounters only tiny foci of hemopoiesis, seeding of the stem cells does not appear to be a problem; rather they fail to grow.

DUPONT: The issue of the lack of expression of the Hh genes in the heterozygous host could relate to the fact that several genes on the same chromosome could be involved in the control of such expression. There is the parallel situation of immune response genes where at least two genes on the same haplotype can interact in controlling a specific immune response. In man there is strong genetic linkage disequilibrium for genes within the MHC. I wonder if the absence of Hh gene products in the phenotype of heterozygotes could be due to suboptimal intergenic interaction within a haplotype. Would it be possible to select "original" mouse haplotypes, so as to test new heterozygous combinations?

CHAIRMAN CUDKOWICZ: No studies have been done with wild mice to my knowledge, the only real source of "original" haplotypes. In looking at the origin of the strains used in laboratories, one realizes that most strains can be traced to only *three* ancestor groups. That was one of the reasons for saying at the outset that Hh genes are likely to display a straight-forward recessive inheritance as long as one deals with a highly biased and selected sample of mouse strains.

BACH: The point that Dupont raised is unlikely to be the explanation in view of the number of examples Cudkowicz, Warner, and Bennett have shown us.

One of the advantages of dealing with mice as compared to man, for instance, is that one keeps a single representation of every chromosome in the F_1. Further, since we deal with inbred strains, talk about interactions between genes of the two homologous chromosomes, seems an unlikely addition to epistasis between genes represented on one chromosome unless heterozygosity per se suppresses expression or again, it comes down to a dosage effect with some kind of a threshold phenomenon. I would favor such an explanation.

CHAIRMAN CUDKOWICZ: I agree with Bach on some of his points, but the fact still remains that most of these many strains derive from an exceedingly small genetic pool.

BACH: I believe that people working with mice tend to be overconcerned with this issue. The mice we use carry recombinant chromosomes that have not been subjected to all the relative forces acting on wild mice. In rats, moreover. work by Gill *et al.* suggests that there may be as few as only *eight* AgB haplotypes. None of these arguments reflects on the basic validity of the experimental results of biological studies and I thus think that we must accept the results as Cudkowicz now has them.

SHEARER: Cudkowicz has shown that the Ir genes regulating anti-Hh reactivity are expressed both in homozygous and heterozygous mice. Moreover, they influence not only F_1 antiparent reactions but also straight allogeneic Hh incompatibility.

TRENTIN: Concerning the exchange between Cline and Bennett, I would point out that spleen colonies in the rat are quite different histologically than those in the mouse where there are four kinds of differentiated colonies. On the other hand, the rat yields only erythroid colonies, which grow very slowly. Consequently, rat spleen colonies are studied at 12 instead of 7 days as is the case with mouse spleen colonies. However, if one transfers rat stem cells into irradiated mice, then one obtains granuloid as well as erythroid colonies that grow fast. Thus, the difference is not the potential of the rat stem cell, but the microenvironment in which it grows.

I am still puzzled by dimethylmyleran speeding up the erythropoiesis in the rat. It is conceivable that the drug might activate myeloid microenvironment of the rat spleen. Has Bennett classified the growing cell types?

BENNETT: If you examine the spleen of an animal treated with dimethylmyleran under conditions that ensure erythropoiesis after transplantation, one is surprised to find that the white pulp of the spleen is almost intact. This includes the marginal zone and macrophages. However, the red pulp is empty except for a few tiny foci of hemopoiesis.

DAUSSET: Does Bennett know whether host resistance is linked to the MHC (major histocompatibility complex) in rats?

BENNETT: We have only studied AgB incompatible grafts, thus, we are assuming that resistance is linked to the AgB locus.

VAN BEKKUM: Trentin is correct in stating that colony growth is slower in the rat than in the mouse. Thus, if you measure colony growth early after transplantation very few are found. However, later on there are plenty of colonies.

We were able to repeat with the rat just about every assay done with mice in terms of spleen colonies and we have found only nominal differences. Figure 6 demonstrates measurements of regeneration of stem cells in the rat spleen done by retransplantation into secondary irradiated recipients. The so-called distribution factor f was derived by extrapolation of the straight portion of the growth curve to the ordinate. Now, the point I want to make is that the results that one finds in terms of spleen colony efficiency depend on the rat strain. I think Bennett's results reflect the strain of rats he used.

We find excellent colony formation in Sprague Dawley rats and BN rats (syngeneic); very poor, if any, colony formation in the WAG rat strain. We have not found it necessary to employ specific inhibition of erythropoiesis to condition rat recipients over and above total body X irradiation. We do find hybrid resistance, but, just as Bennett, we too have tested only a few combinations.

SHEARER: Concerning the general aspects of the Hh system genetics, I want to point out, as both Cudkowicz and Warner have done, that the immune response or Ir-like genes involved are not the H-2-linked Ir genes, the ones most extensively studied. The genes modulating marrow graft rejection are not linked to the MHC. Thus, the question can be raised whether this system of Ir genes has functional significance in immune surveillance against leukemogenesis.

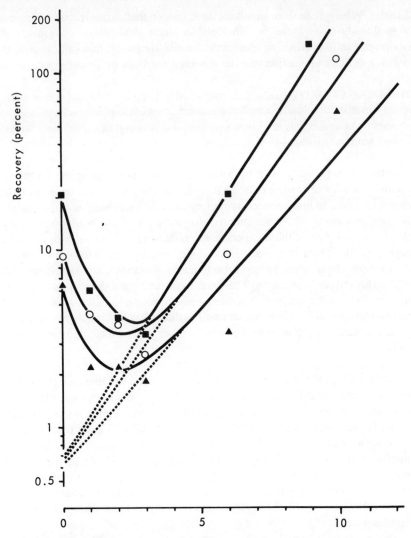

Fig. 6 CFU-s recovery curves in spleen following injection of isogeneic bone marrow cells into lethally irradiated Sprague Dawley rats. Primary recipients were given the number of bone marrow cells shown: $\bigcirc$, ♀♀, 2×10^8; $\blacksquare$, ♀♀, 1×10^8; $\blacktriangle$, ♂♂, 1×10^8. The distribution factor f as determined from the intercept of the straight part of the curves with the ordinate is 0.007 on the average. For the mouse the f factor is 0.05. Since the number of spleen colonies obtained per 10^6 rat bone marrow cells is 50 (in rat recipients) the proportion in rat bone marrow is 0.7% (mouse 0.6%).

CLINE: Would it be too simplistic to consider that these reactions are not cell-mediated, since there is considerable strain dependence of growth of hemopoietic cells in diffusion chambers as well? Therefore, many of the conclusions that cellular interaction may be involved need not be so in the rat.

CHAIRMAN CUDKOWICZ: It is important to keep in mind that one is working with irradiated animals, and that these are, moreover, phenomena that occur very rapidly after irradiation. Taken together, this makes it rather unlikely that an induced humoral mechanism is involved.

MOORE: I think we let slip by a most important point about the resistance phenomenon without really exploring it. This was the dependence on intact bone marrow function. In his introductory remarks, Cudkowicz made the point that the ^{89}Sr data in support of the requirement for integrity of the bone marrow was crucial. I would say that those experiments could be turned around to say that the integrity of the spleen is essential. One thing done by ^{89}Sr is to assure that the spleen has to take over the hemopoietic function of marrow. The same argument could go for the late maturation. The three-week time point does fit rather nicely since we find that the spleen is functioning in a bone-marrow-like manner for the first two to three weeks of life. It could well be that one is looking simply at less effective resistance of the spleen environment when it is performing bone marrow functions.

CHAIRMAN CUDKOWICZ: Bone marrow is itself a site in which Hh incompatible cells are resisted, though the resistance is weaker than in spleen. Moreover, *in vitro* experiments have shown that spleens of ^{89}Sr treated mice are incompetent for anti-Hh responses and may eventually be enriched with suppressor cells.*
        Whether this is actually the mechanism through which, *in vivo,* there is a failure to reject bone marrow grafts is not yet established. As to the cellular immunology of the anti-Hh response, it is clearly a multicellular system (effector cell, accessory cell, suppressor cell). As a result of ^{89}Sr, there could be obliteration of a cell type necessary for the response and possibly an intensified production of suppressive cells.

DICKE: Bennett described a model in which resistance can be abrogated by ^{89}Sr. I would think that in this model it should be possible to ascertain, by reconstitution, the cell type responsible for hybrid resistance. Did Bennett determine whether peritoneal macrophages could restore?

BENNETT: Short-term restoration could not be obtained in the ^{89}Sr-treated mouse or in any other analogous model. Cudkowicz and I eventually concluded

*Editors' Comment: Data supporting this statement are given subsequently in Table 27, page 111.

that the effector cells simply were not transplantable. However, if one transplants bone marrow cells and waits a few weeks, then one transfers adoptively resistance, which is taken to mean that this is a property of marrow precursor cells.

Now, with ^{89}Sr mice the problem is that even if one transplants bone marrow, this has no effect because the transferred stem cells, in order to differentiate into the effector cells, must reside in the marrow cavity, where they receive ^{89}Sr radiation and succumb.

METCALF: I want to get back to one of Cudkowicz's generalizations that mature cells do not exhibit Hh antigens. I have been wondering how that was established technically if cytostasis was one of the first endpoints. How could one observe cytostasis in a red cell or a polymorph?

CHAIRMAN CUDKOWICZ: In the case of red cells, the parameter was survival of labeled red cells. These were confirmation studies of those that Henry Kaplan did back in the 1950s. In the case of other mature cells the parameter was the ability to stimulate anti-Hh responses *in vitro*.

METCALF: Has it been determined whether these cells induce tolerance?

CHAIRMAN CUDKOWICZ: No, but one could make an educated guess that they do not. Bone marrow cells are an extremely poor source of T lymphocytes and consequently do not induce tolerance in the Hh system. This is so despite the presence in marrow of primitive cells that are Hh positive.

BORANIC: I think that we have come again to the question of differences in the growth patterns of syngeneic vs. allogeneic marrow, an issue previously taken up by Bennett, Cline, and Trentin. The question can be recast by asking which proliferating cell types are detected by the IUdR method. Presumably a variety of cell types proliferate and differentiate after syngeneic bone marrow cell transfers, whereas in allogeneic transfers some cell types may not grow as well as others. Now, we should know whether the method used measures the growth of all cell types equally well. Only if it does, can one compare syngeneic and allogeneic cell transfers.

CHAIRMAN CUDKOWICZ: The IUdR technique measures newly synthesized DNA, which is a consistent feature of dividing cells irrespective of histologic type. By labeling cells with both ^{125}IUdR and ^{59}Fe it was determined that most of the dividing cells (~95%) are erythroid in the spleen of marrow chimeras five days after transplantation.

VAN BEKKUM: We have compared the numbers of bone marrow cells required to effect 50% protection from supralethal irradiation in the mouse, dog,

TABLE 11
Bone Marrow Cell Number ($\times\ 10^{-8}$/kg Body Weight) Required for
50% Survival Rates after Supralethal Total Body Irradiation

Donor–recipient combination	Mice[a] (800 rads)	Dogs (700–800 rads)	Monkeys (800 rads)
Isologous/autologous	0.02	±0.5[b]	±0.5[c]
MHC identical	0.08	1–2	not done
MHC not identical	1.4	±20[b]	1–2[c]

[a]Equivalent conditioning in the three species.
[b]Thomas *et al.*, 1959.
[c]Crouch *et al.*, 1961.

and monkey. The data are summarized in Table 11, where it is evident that there
are major differences between the mouse and the two larger species with regard
to autologous or syngenic cells, and between mouse and monkey vs. dog for
MHC nonidentical cells. The message is that we should be careful in extrapolat-
ing experimental data from any single animal species to man. Instead, we should
look for trends that are valid in at least two species before translating it to man.

TABLE 12
CFU-s Suppression and Number of Bone Marrow Cells Needed for Radioprotection

Donor–recipient combination	BM cells needed for 50% radio-protection	CFU-S/10^5 BM cells donor to donor	CFU-S/10^5 BM cells donor to recipient
CBA/T6→CBA/T6	6×10^4	20.5	20.5
C57BL/Ka × CBA/Rij→ C57BL/Ka × CBA/Rij	5×10^4	18.1	18.1
C57BL/Ka→F1(C57BL/Ka × CBA/Rij)	8×10^4	24.3	0.9
CBA/Rij→F1(C57BL/Ka × CBA/Rij)	8×10^4	19.1	19.1
C57BL/Ka→F1(C57BL/Ka × C3H/Rij)	7×10^4	24.3	3.3
C3H/Rij→F1(C57BL/Ka × C3H/Rij)	5×10^4	28.8	27.0
CBA/T6→C3H	2×10^5	20.5	19.4
CBA/T6→AKR	2×10^5	20.5	12.2
CBA/T6→C57BL	3×10^6	20.5	13.3
CBA/T6→ND2	3×10^6	20.5	12.5
CBA/T6→RFM	3×10^6	20.5	11.2
F1→C57BL/Ka	1.5×10^6	22.4	18.5
F1→CBA/Rij	1.5×10^6	22.4	9.6
Sprague Dawley→ (C57BL/Ka × CBA/Rij)	4×10^6		5.0

We also challenge the terminology *"in vivo* rejection" on the basis that conspicuous differences in splenic resistance to repopulation by marrow grafts are contrasted by small differences, if any, in the number of marrow cells required for 50% radioprotection (Table 12).

TRENTIN: Van Bekkum questions the use of the terminology *"in vivo* rejection" on the basis that spleen colony or splenic radioactive IUdR uptake measurements do not correlate with the number of marrow cells required for an irradiated animal to survive.

I think Fig. 7 would explain why there is a seeming discrepancy. Bone marrow colony numbers, spleen colony numbers, and survival dose–response curves in mice resistant to rat bone marrow are shown. By increasing the amount of rat marrow cells, resistance is overridden both in the host cavities and in the spleen. It is especially noteworthy that marrow colonies appear at one log smaller inoculum of donor cells in host bone cavities than in host spleen. This agrees with what was brought out earlier, that resistance to marrow transplantation is stronger in spleen than in marrow or other sites.

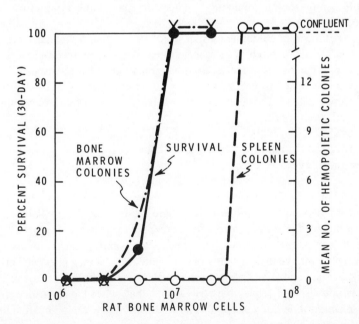

Fig. 7   Relationship of 8-day hemopoietic colonies in both the spleen and bone marrow to 30-day mouse survival following supralethal irradiation (1100 R) and infusion of Lewis rat bone marrow into resistant (C57BL/6 × A)F₁ hybrids. Note log scale for cell dose. All radiation control mice died on days 8–11.

Now, if one examines the survival curve, it is evident it is superimposed on the marrow colony curve, and not on the spleen colony curve. Thus, survival correlates very well with host bone marrow repopulation and not with early spleen repopulation.

VAN BEKKUM: We cannot restrict the argument to a few strains of mice and xenogeneic resistance to rat bone marrow. I think one has to analyze all the situations in which there is resistance in host spleen, as I would like to call it, and compare that with survival.

There are a few rat strains and rat hybrids that are extremely resistant with regard to splenic colony formation, and yet require small numbers of bone marrow cells for survival. I retain my viewpoint that there is insufficient convincing evidence that spleen resistance is related to overall reconstitution.

CHAIRMAN CUDKOWICZ: The point Van Bekkum made concerning the desirability of survival studies is well taken.

I want, however, to make a point as a comment to Table 12 of Van Bekkum, the one that pointed out that, despite resistance in the spleen, one particular parent/F_1 combination required more or less, the same number of marrow cells as syngeneic hosts.

Now, the strain combination that was listed in that particular table was, I think, CBA × C57, a hybrid of moderate resistance. This type of study, in my opinion, will have to be done in strain combinations where resistance is much stronger, where one injects 5×10^7 or 1×10^8 marrow cells and still does not see splenic repopulation. Those are the strains that will ultimately tell whether survival is affected or not.

I can only say at this point that, in those strain combinations, the mice barely survived the ten days needed to do colony assays. These, of course, are not accurate survival studies.

Now, when one looks at the relationship between resistance in the spleen and in other sites, the only site that is entirely devoid of resistance is the peritoneal cavity, but when one looks where the injected hemopoietic cells go, one sees that they go almost everywhere except in the peritoneal cavity. There is, in fact, no compelling reason why resistance should exist in the peritoneal cavity, because, after intravenous injection of hemopoietic cells, they never end up there. But in other hemopoietic sites, there is about, let us say, $1/_5$ to $1/_3$ of the resistance one sees in the spleen. Thus, one could expect that, when the resistance is strong in the spleen, proliferation of donor cells would also be severely impaired in those sites of weaker resistance.

THYMIC FUNCTIONS AND RESISTANCE TO FOREIGN HEMOPOIETIC GRAFTS

Discussion Introducer:

Osias Stutman

CHAIRMAN STUTMAN: I would like to discuss the restoration, by grafting, of T-cell function in athymic recipients. There are some observations published around 1968 that are being progressively rediscovered by those working with nude mice. We observed then that allogeneic thymus grafts produce poor immunological restoration of neonatally thymectomized mice. At the time we assumed that the allogeneic thymuses were inducing a GVH (graft vs. host) reaction in the recipient. The grafting of parental thymus into neonatally thymectomized F_1 hybrids produced chronic full-fledged GVH, eventually with death (*Transplantation* **6:**514, 1968; **7:**420, 1969).

Thymectomized C3H mice were grafted with syngeneic or allogeneic thymuses. Most of the animals that were restored with syngeneic thymus grafts were healthy and immunologically restored (Table 13). The animals grafted with the H-2 matched allogeneic thymuses did reasonably well, about half of them being restored, although this did not necessarily endure. The H-2 mismatched recipients fared very badly. The failure of the allografts in thymectomized hosts may be due to some of the Hh genes that have been described.

TABLE 13

Survival of Neonatally Thymectomized C3H/Bi Mice Grafted
Intraperitoneally with Thymus

Thymus donors[a]	Number of treated mice	Number of surviving mice[b]	
		150 days	430 days
C3H/Bi	19	18	15
C3Hf/Bi	20	18	16
C3H/He	10	7	5
CBA/H	20	16	3
C58	12	4	0
A/J	16	1	0
C57BL/6	25	6	0
NZB	12	4	0
T6 (H-2^d)	12	6	0
(C3H × A)F_1	23	18	4
(C3H × C57BL/6)F_1	20	18	3
(C3H × T6)F_1	16	11	4

[a]One thymic lobe from 10–20 day old sex-matched donors, intraperitoneal grafting, at 25 days of age (Stutman *et al., J. Immunol.* **103:** 92, 1969).

[b]Survival correlates with immunological recovery in all cases (measured mostly as capacity to produce GVH reactions).

33

TABLE 14

Acceptance of Allogeneic Skin Grafts in Neonatally
Thymectomized C3H Mice Grafted with F_1 Hybrid Thymus

Thymus donor[a]	Acceptance of skin allografts of same origin as thymus[b] (100 days after grafting)
(C3H × A)F_1	15/18 (83%)
(C3H × C57BL/6)F_1	1/18 (5%)
(C3H × T6)F_1[c]	3/12 (25%)

[a]Ip grafting of one thymus lobe (see Table 13).

[b]Skin grafting performed at 40 days of age, all animals rejected BALB/c skin (Stutman *et al.*, *J. Immunol.* **103**:92, 1969).

[c]T6 is an H-2^d strain, from which the CBA.T6T6 line was derived.

Incidentally, the functional failure correlates well with histology, which showed that the allogeneic grafts were not repopulated and only rarely acquired the appearance of normal thymus.

Related experiments were done with thymectomized CBA/HT6T6 hosts grafted with a syngeneic thymus and given bone marrow cells of different origin to examine migration patterns of marrow cells to the nonirradiated thymus (*Exp. Hematol.* **19**:12, 1969). We observed a marked histocompatibility restriction. While syngeneic CBA/H cells could enter the graft (10–25% of the dividing cells at 20–30 days after injection) allogeneic cells (including H-2 identical or F_1 hybrids of CBA with other strains) were difficult to detect (0–5% of dividing cells at 20–30 days after cell injection). Thus, there appears to be strict histocompatibility restrictions between thymus and migrating hemopoietic cells in models that study thymus traffic without irradiation of the recipients. This restriction is not absolute and is only apparent in models that do not use total body irradiation.

It became apparent that tolerance induction by a thymus graft to skin of the same origin was dependent on the strain combination used (Table 14). With (C3H × A)F_1 thymus in C3H hosts, tolerance was easily induced. On the other hand, with (C3H × C57BL/6)F_1 hybrid thymus there was no tolerance. The interesting point was that in some cases, we observed the paradoxical situation that the thymus graft restored the host, and then the host actually rejected the thymus graft, a fact that may have significance in clinical implantation. This experiment has been reproduced in nude mice.

WARNER: In the combinations Stutman described, F_1 thymus was grafted into parental strains. Does he have any similar data where a parental strain thymus was placed into a thymectomized F_1 hybrid recipient where Hh incompatibility might be involved?

CHAIRMAN STUTMAN: Yes. There have been two reports. In one we showed a clinical syndrome that was suggestive of GVH after grafting A strain thymus into (A × C57BL)F_1 mice (*Transplantation* **6:**514, 1968). At that time we thought that the wasting syndrome in these animals was GVH rather then postthymectomy wasting, primarily because the syndrome could not be reversed by injection of 2–3 × 10^8 syngeneic spleen cells (a procedure that rapidly reverses the postthymectomy syndrome).

When we tested a large number of other parent–F_1 combinations (*Transplantation* **7:**420, 1969), we found that there was GVH only in a few of them [e.g., A into (A × DBA/2)F_1], but not in others, i.e., it was a restricted event.*

WARNER: Is there any evidence of Hh gene expression on thymus cells? For example, did any of the combinations used by Stutman involve those strains that have been clearly defined by bone marrow studies to express Hh? For example, with C57BL thymus into F_1 hybrids, given the problem of potential GVH reactions, did that combination behave any differently from C3H into F_1 hybrids?

CHAIRMAN STUTMAN: No. GVH was observed in these combinations but we did not do a complete immunologic study on the restored animals since the intent was to ascertain whether the thymus could produce GVH.

ELKINS: Warner has asked about evidence for Hh gene expression in T cells. Bennett showed that this could occur. We have measured the DNA synthetic response of B10.D2 thymus cells in lethally irradiated B10.A, B10.A(2R), and B10.D2 mice. In the first two hosts there is an identical H-2K end-coded stimulus for proliferation of donor thymocytes, which is measured in terms of ^{125}IUdR incorporation in the host's spleen. This stimulus is missing the B10.D2 hosts, which are the controls.

Relatively low numbers of T cells grew much more in the B10.A than in the B10.A(2R) hosts, which offer additional disparity to the donor cells, namely, the b alleles of the H-2D locus (Fig. 8). This "D end inhibition" is overcome by injecting increased numbers of T cells, which then proliferate equally in B10.A

Afterthought by Stutman: The transplantation of parental thymus into neonatally thymectomized F_1 hybrids (Stutman *et al., Transplantation* **7:**420, 1969) showed evidence of GVH only when A thymus was grafted into (A × C57BL) or (A × C3H)F_1 hybrids. The other parental strain thymus produced only mild GVH in the (A × C57BL)F_1 system and none in the (A × C3H)F_1. There was mild GVH with C57BL thymus into (C3H × C57 BL)F_1 animals and no detectable effect in the alternate combination. Parent thymus grafts produced no GVH in (C3H × T6)F_1 combinations (T6 being the CBA.T6 H-2^k line).

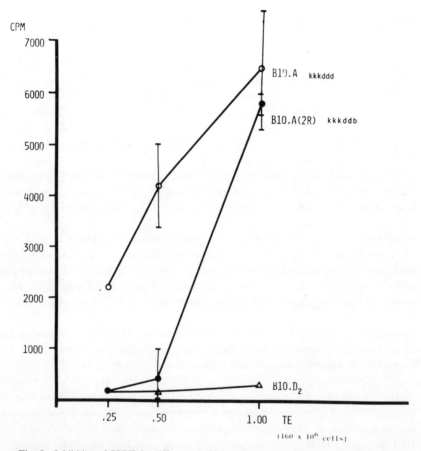

Fig. 8 Inhibition of GVHR by difference in H-2 region. Incorporation of [125]IUdR into splenic DNA of lethally irradiated B10.A(2R), B10.A, and B10.D2 hosts four days after injection of graded doses of B10.D2 thymus cells. Dose of thymus cells is expressed in donor thymus equivalents.

and B10.A(2R) hosts. Furthermore, if one injects a low number of T cells for which this D end inhibition is seen on day 4, it is lost by day 5.

I believe these data are interpretable in the light of Cudkowicz's view that there is genetic resistance to Hh incompatible cells manifested initially by cytostasis. However, in this case the antigen-driven T cell clones overcome genetic resistance because of antigenic stimulation.

I would recall for you some early experiments by Claman when he was exploring thymus and bone marrow cell interactions for production of anti-SRBC antibody in irradiated mice. He found that parental thymus and bone marrow failed to interact successfully in an irradiated F_1 in contrast to their function in syngeneic hosts. This work is consonant with the idea that genetic resistance is exerted upon T and B lymphocyte clones, which are not competent to respond to host alloantigens and thus are not "rescued" as were GVH cells.

CUDKOWICZ: We also have experiments leading to the same conclusion. When F_1 hybrids that are heterozygotes in the D region (the region closely associated with Hh-1) are grafted with parental spleen cells as an inoculum to induce GVH, pretreatment of the hosts with agents suppressing anti-Hh responses cause an acceleration and greater incidence of the GVH syndrome.

CHAIRMAN STUTMAN: I would like to describe the characteristics of the postthymic immunologically incompetent precursor cell as it is found in the periphery and compare its properties with those of mature T lymphocytes and of the prethymic stem cell. Table 15 lists these characteristics. In adults, postthymic precursors are found mainly in marrow and spleen. They are rapidly dividing, nonrecirculating, and decline rather rapidly after thymectomy. They are not present in spleen of nude mice, are insensitive to short-term treatment with ALS, and are sensitive to high doses of steroids. Thus, the thymus exports corticosteroid-sensitive precursors that eventually mature into corticosteroid-resistant cells. The main source of purified postthymic precursors (separated from competent T cells by velocity sedimentation at unit gravity in either fetal calf serum or ficoll gradients) is the neonatal spleen.

Upon injection of purified postthymic precursors with the T6 marker into animals 60 days postthymectomy, under this influence the recirculating cells that are PHA- and MLC-responsive bear the T6 marker of the postthymic precursor.

It seems reasonable that there would be an incompetent precursor in the periphery to maintain T cell homeostasis. We do not know the purpose of mature T cells within the thymus, but the essential point is that they are a resident and not an exported population, and are not needed for generating peripheral T cells. What *is* exported is a cortisone-sensitive, immunologically incompetent postthymic cell, which eventually becomes competent in the periphery, possibly under the influence of the humoral thymic factors.

SPRENT: Is the concentration of the Thy-1 on postthymic precursor cells like that of peripheral T cells or like that of cortical thymocytes?

CHAIRMAN STUTMAN: I do not have a precise answer, but based on susceptibility to cytotoxic antiserum the precursor should have low amounts of Thy-1.

GOLUB: If, as Stutman says, the cortisone-resistant population in the thymus never emerges, we are faced then with two developing systems, one of which never gets an opportunity to function in the periphery against external antigens.

TABLE 15
Comparison of Characteristics of Precursor and Mature T Cells

Biological characteristics	Prethymic	Postthymic precursor	Postthymic T cell
Tissue distribution			
adult	marrow	spleen, marrow	lymphoid tissues
newborn	liver, marrow	spleen, liver	—
embryo	yolk sac, liver, blood	liver	—
Time of appearance (days)	9 (embryo)	15 (embryo)	at birth
Traffic pattern	to spleen	to spleen	to nodes
Migration to thymus	yes	no	no
Recirculation (presence in TD)	no	no	yes
Immunological competence[a]	no	no	yes
Restoration of Tx animals			
alone	no	no	yes
with thymus graft	yes	yes	yes
with thymic factors	no	yes	yes
Effect of neonatal thymectomy	none?	depletion	depletion
Effect of adult thymectomy	none	depletion (30–40 days)	none (within 60 days)
Present in nu/nu	yes	no	no
Effect of short-term ALS	none	none	depletion
Sensitivity to high-dose steroids	none?	depletion	mostly none
Proliferative rate (^{3}H thymidine suicide)	no?	yes	no
Life span (probable)	?	30–60 days	long, usually
Density (in BSA gradients)[b]	low	low	high
Sedimentation rates (unit gravity)[c]			
adult spleen	5.0 mm/hr	5.9 mm/hr	3.7 mm/hr
adult marrow	4.6 mm/hr	5.4 mm/hr	3.6 mm/hr
newborn spleen	4.8 mm/hr	5.8 mm/hr	3.5 mm/hr[d]
liver (15-day embryo)	8.0 & 10.5 mm/hr	5.9 mm/hr	—
Adherence to nylon wool (45 min)	no	yes	no
Surface markers			
Thy.1	no	yes	yes
TL	no	no?	no
Ly 1, 2, 3[e]	none	1,2,3+	1+,2,3+,1,2,3+
Ig	no	no	no
Fc	no	no	no, usually

[a]Measured as mitogen responses (PHA, ConA), GVH reactivity, MLC, helper activity (primary antibody response to SRBC).

CHAIRMAN STUTMAN: Well, I would not go as far as that. We still have to find a role for those cortisone-resistant cells within the thymus.

BENNETT: I did not see the cortisone-sensitive thymocyte in Stutman's table. Where does it fit?

CHAIRMAN STUTMAN: We are comparing the postthymic precursor in the periphery with subsets of T cells within the thymus. By velocity sedimentation the cortisone-sensitive cell is analogous to Shortman's intrathymic cell. This is in fact the cell to be exported.

ELKINS: How does this all tie in with Stutman's earlier findings that parental thymic grafts fail to restore F_1 mice?

CHAIRMAN STUTMAN: There are two considerations: (1) an animal can be restored by a thymus graft only by generation of a postthymic population; (2) traffic into and stationing within the thymus of prethymic precursors is H-2 dependent. In allogeneic combinations, no matter how weak the differences, traffic is restricted.

SANFORD: I do not understand how Stutman distinguished between the alternatives that cortisone-resistant cells are not exported, and their export followed by destruction, for example, by natural reactivity against the sugars that are exposed only on cortisone-resistant cells.

CHAIRMAN STUTMAN: If cortisone-resistant cells were to emerge, they would be easy to detect by chromosomal markers and mitogenic response to PHA.

SANFORD: But if they were *destroyed,* there would be nothing to detect. The sugars I am referring to are the *N*-acetylgalactosamine residues that become exposed in cortisone-resistant cells.

O'REILLY: There are two issues we should now consider. One concerns the relationship between hybrid resistance and the capacity of thymic grafts to re-

---

[b]BSA discontinuous gradients, low density (A-B layers, 10–26% BSA), high density (C-D layers, 26–35% BSA).

[c]Velocity sedimentation in fetal calf serum gradients (lower values when separated in ficoll gradients). Data for "prethymic" actually apply to hemopoietic stem cells and are in accordance with values obtained by Haskill and Moore (*Nature* **226:**853, 1970).

[d]Con A reactivity only, negative to PHA or MLC. Low reactivity in GVH.

[e]Similar results for postthymic precursor cells whether tested in CBA/H, C3H, or DBA/2 (Ly.1.1; Ly.2.1; Ly.3.2) and BALB/c or C57BL/6 strains (Ly.1.2; Ly.2.2; Ly.3.2).

store. Could Cudkowicz' observation be relevant, that Hh-1 is expressed better in immature than in mature cells?

Full T cell reconstitution after allogeneic fetal liver transplants in man implies stem cell differentiation within the host thymus. This finding would not be expected if Hh incompatibility determined the outcome of stem cells interacting with host thymus. However, while fetal liver engraftment occurs in certain instances, not every fetal liver transplant reconstitutes. Consequently Hh incompatibility and the expression of Hh in immature cells may be relevant.

The second issue concerns Stutman's concept of a postthymic precursor cell. We have evidence that would suggest a similar scheme in man. If one takes fetal liver cells from 12–16 week human fetuses and exposes them to thymic extracts or thymopoietin, both T cell surface markers and PHA responsiveness appear.

In contrast, if one takes liver cells from 10 week old fetuses, i.e., prior to thymic differentiation, differentiation does not occur in the presence of the factors. Thymic epithelium is essential for this *in vitro* differentiation, and this observation is consistent with Stutman's concept of prethymic and posthymic differentiation.

CHAIRMAN STUTMAN: I think that *in vitro* induction experiments are telling us that appropriate thymic extract (or analogs that increase cyclic AMP in stem cells) leads to expression of T antigens. The emergence of TL antigens and the lack of immunologic reactivity in the induced cells indicates that the *in vitro* differentiation mimics an intrathymic event that is probably one of the steps by which cells are generated within the thymus to eventually become competent.

On the other hand, in Boyse's and Basch's laboratories mouse yolk sac cells could not be induced to express T antigens. Thus truly prethymic stem cells seem to be devoid of "prothymocytes." One can assume that the prothymocyte is an already committed stem cell and that the commitment may be related to the thymic presence.

MOORE: I would take issue with the suggestion that the yolk sac derived stem cell may have to take up residence elsewhere before acquiring thymic colonizing capacity. That is simply not true in the developing chick embryo, both using chromosome markers and tritiated thymidine autoradiography. The yolk sac cells colonize the developing thymic rudiment within minutes after intravenous infusion into the chick embryo and subsequently undergo proliferation and lymphoid maturation.

I suspect the timing of mammalian fetal thymus development is so close to the time when yolk sac stem cells colonize the liver that it would seem unlikely that the yolk sac stem cell went to the fetal liver, resided there briefly, and then went back to the thymus.

SPRENT: Where does the cell described by Loor and Roelants, i.e., Thy-1 positive cells in spleens of nude mice, fit into Stutman's scheme?

CHAIRMAN STUTMAN: These workers have studied a cell most easily detected in the nude mouse, expressing small amounts (detectable only by sophisticated immunofluorescence) of Thy-1 antigen, which accumulates in the absence of thymic function. This cell was designated as a prethymic cell committed to T differentiation. It is accumulating because of the absence of thymus-induced differentiation.*

METCALF: In this scheme, is Stutman implying that the postthymic precursor has a greater proliferative capacity than the subsequent T cell upon stimulation?

CHAIRMAN STUTMAN: The only thing we know is that it is a rapidly dividing population.

METCALF: Most assume that when stimulated, T cell populations proliferate and produce large numbers of progeny in the periphery. Does Stutman have any reason to discriminate between these two populations as to proliferative capacity?

CHAIRMAN STUTMAN: To get expansion of precursor cells you need the thymic humoral influence. With respect to the competent T cells, this can be accomplished easily via antigen. So in that sense, the precursor is antigen-insensitive. Such effect as we did obtain with antigen could all be accounted for by contamination with competent T cells.

METCALF: What about the responsiveness to PHA?

CHAIRMAN STUTMAN: The precursor population displays high background and poor response to mitogens.

METCALF: Claesson, in my laboratory, has been looking at the properties of the cells in human peripheral blood that generate T lymphocyte colonies *in vitro,* and thereby are expressing a considerable capacity for proliferation. The stimulus used is PHA. But the properties of the T-colony-forming cells are, so far as it is possible to match them in the human, almost exactly the same as those of your T

Afterthought by Stutman: The reagent used to detect the weakly Thy.1+ cells in nude mice by Roelants and Loor, (*Nature* **251**:229, 1974; *Eur. J. Immunol.* **5**:127, 1975; **6**:75, 1976) was mainly the IgG fraction of rabbit antimouse brain (Theta-Br), which although having clear anti-T cell activity, also reacts with hemopoietic stem cells, as was shown by Golub (*J. Exp. Med.* **136**:369, 1972). Thus, it may be postulated that hemopoietic stem cells with low amounts of Theta-Br or other antigens, shared with brain, and not cells of the T lineage, are those detected in the nude mouse.

cells, in that they are slowly sedimenting with a sedimentation velocity of about 3.5 mm/hr. They are non cycling cells. They form rosettes with sheep red cells, as the equivalent of Thy-1. Thus, they would belong to your third category. Yet, by analogy with other colony-forming systems, one would have expected them to be earlier in the differentiation sequence. But it does not seem so.

CHAIRMAN STUTMAN: I would not eliminate the possibility that one actually can drive this precursor cell with other stimuli. Another important difference between the precursor and the competent T cell is that the former is retained on nylon columns.

CLINE: In reference to Metcalf's findings, there must be a subset of T cells that are proliferating in the lymphoid colonies, because if one looked at the entire population there are perhaps 1 in 100 cells that actually proliferate. Does Metcalf agree?

METCALF: In the system that Claesson uses, which involves the addition of sheep red cells, one cell in ten proliferates.

CLINE: Does Metcalf mean one cell of ten with T cell characteristics, or one cell in ten altogether?

METCALF: I refer to one cell in ten mononuclear cells, unfractionated.

VAN BEKKUM: Blankwater has done thymus transplantation experiments in noninbred nude mice (two or three thymuses per recipient). The animals deteriorated from GVH disease. Irradiated thymus grafts effected a satisfactory immune restoration and prolonged survival. So, I think that if Stutman were able to remove competent T cells, he would obtain different results.

CHAIRMAN STUTMAN: 12- or 13-day-old embryonic thymus provided good restoration in the thymectomized F_1 hybrid model without GVH.

CUDKOWICZ: Is the cell described by Loor and Roelants the only Thy-1 positive cell of nude mice, or does one find others after antigen stimulation?

CHAIRMAN STUTMAN: After infection there is an increase of such cells. Agents that increase cyclic AMP will also induce expression of T cell markers; however, one never generates competent cells in this way. The nude mice remain incompetent with or without Thy-1 positive cells.

BORANIC: Some have claimed that thymus also interacts with hemopoietic stem cells to increase colony formation in recipient spleens. Do you account for such a T cell in your scheme?

CHAIRMAN STUTMAN: I am rather skeptical about experiments suggesting that hemopoietic stem cells from thymectomized animals or from nudes are less efficient than the normal counterparts. I could not confirm these results. Infections and autoimmunity in thymectomized animals yielded spurious results.

BORANIC: I would only add that thymus–stem cell interaction seems to be a strain-related phenomenon. I don't know whether viral infections or genetics are the relevant variables.

TRENTIN: I would like to clarify this issue. Much of the data in the literature showing beneficial effects of thymus cells on hemopoietic colony formation are a manifestation of genetic resistance to bone marrow transplantation. One can get this effect only if one uses a bone marrow donor and recipient strain combination in which there is genetic resistance to the bone marrow transplant. Then the thymus has to be from the bone marrow donor. It does not work if it is from the recipient strain. It is known that one can override resistance simply by using a very large dose of bone marrow cells. Or, one can use a small dose of bone marrow, plus a large dose of some other cell type that has no CFUs, but has comparable Hh antigenicity, like thymus cells.

BORANIC: But this is true only in nonsyngeneic combinations, for instance, parent into F_1 hybrids, as Goodman's experiments have shown. Thymus influence on colony formation is, however, also present in syngeneic situations, where the overriding of resistance, or whatever it is, could not contribute to the results.

TRENTIN: But the effect in syngeneic mice is of a different order of magnitude. If one eliminates the data in resistant combinations, one is left with very small effects of thymocytes on hemopoiesis.

O'REILLY: Is there any evidence to suggest that the permanently resident population of the thymus exerts a trophic influence on the thymic epithelium, facilitating its elaboration of differentiative factors? I am asking that inasmuch as repeated fetal thymus transplants into patients with combined immunodeficiency and lacking normal stem cell populations result in persistence of very low thymic hormone levels. Engraftment of a suitable stem cell population and its development is the only means for increasing these levels.

GOLUB: I am addressing the issue that in the thymus there are two sets of cells, one cortisone-sensitive and nonfunctional, and one cortisone-resistant and functional. The functional population is not the one that goes into the periphery, rather it is this cortisone-sensitive population that gets out. Does this merely represent technical artifacts, i.e., the fact that the thymus is implanted under the kidney capsule or in the peritoneum?

CHAIRMAN STUTMAN: I agree that grafting thymuses and similar procedures are nonphysiological. The precursor in the periphery isolated from newborn spleens is from normal and not transplanted animals. Thus, the precursor had been exported from a thymus *in situ*. Moreover, the postthymic precursor in the periphery can be destroyed by treatment with cortisone.

DICKE: I would ask Stutman to elaborate on the nature of the prethymic cell. Is it the stem cell, or is it really a committed cell that might go into the thymus?

CHAIRMAN STUTMAN: I think that the cell induced *in vitro* to express T markers may be a committed stem cell. Enriched preparations (the AB fraction of a discontinuous BSA gradient), further depleted by means of antisera and complement, lost the capacity to repopulate the thymus of irradiated recipients. This is a critical experiment indicating that the cell that has the ability to migrate to thymus is one step away from the conventional colony-forming unit (CFU-S).

DICKE: One could use the anti-stem cell serum of Golub to verify this possibility.

WARNER: I would like to clarify what is or is *not* known in regard to our previous subject of Hh expression. It seems that one of the major concerns of this conference is to determine what types of antigens can result in rejection of hemopoietic grafts.

    Is it clear that all we know is that the stem cell expresses some component of the cell surface, which we equate with an antigen. We have no evidence of its molecular nature. Furthermore, we do not know exactly when its expression is lost on maturation.

    If Hh components are not on red cells, what do we know about the rest of the lymphoid cell series in terms of possible Hh expression on the T cell subpopulations? I am wondering if some of the data might not already be in the literature. For example, in T/B cell collaboration studies using irradiated hybrids, I wonder whether there might have been any combinations where, for example, C57BL T cells were inoculated into irradiated F_1 hybrids. Is this area really quite unknown? For example, might Hh represent a differentiation antigen on the stem cells?

SPRENT: In contrast to marrow cells, C57BL T cells proliferate well in irradiated (CBA × C57BL)F$_1$ mice.

CUDKOWICZ: Claman has shown that T helper cells do express Hh by transferring parental helper cells into F$_1$ hybrids and noticing their failure. He did this experiment not to search for Hh antigens, but to obtain collaboration in an F$_1$. In addition, Trentin showed that parental cells with GVH potential behaved as if they did express Hh antigens. In particular, he noticed that the impairment of growth, and consequently of the ability to produce GVH, was best demonstrable when the host reached 21 days of age or became older. This duplicates the late maturation of resistance to stem cells. Systematic investigation of resistance to GVH cells was carried out in my laboratory, confirming that GVH cells do express Hh specificities.

I would like to consider the question of whether the T cells that were discussed are in anyway involved in anti-Hh responses. Now, this is surely not the case *in vivo* since we don't see any requirement for T cells in marrow graft rejection. Indeed they are stronger in the *absence* of T cells. However, in an *in vitro* model where the end point is lysis (CML) rather than cytostasis, the effectors of F$_1$ and antiparent responses are Thy-1 positive cells. In trying to relate properties of the postthymic precursor with those of the prekiller cells in the F$_1$ antiparent *in vitro* system, it appears that the two cell types differ. Stutman finds that the precursor is nylon adherent but the prekiller is nonadherent. The precursor is insensitive to ALS but the prekiller is sensitive. Stutman's precursor is cortisone sensitive but the prekiller is cortisone resistant.

CRITICAL ISSUES IN CLINICAL BONE MARROW TRANSPLANTATION

Discussion Introducer:

Rainer Storb

CHAIRMAN STORB: I propose to explore the critical issues in clinical bone marrow transplantation as we presently see them on the patient ward, and ascertain how we can approach these issues in large animal models.

Clinical teams all over the world are now committed to bone marrow transplantation for the treatment of patients with three basic diseases—severe combined immunodeficiency, severe aplastic anemia, and acute leukemia. In almost all instances, siblings are used as donors who are matched with the patient at the MHC. In Seattle we have limited ourselves strictly to matched siblings because of our experience in dogs, where grafting results were dismal with mismatched littermates as donors. In that situation, almost all animals died with GVH disease or sequelae. In contrast, recipients of histocompatible littermates have excellent survival.

The first of the three diseases treated with bone marrow transplantation is severe combined immunodeficiency, a rather rare disease. Only a few clinical teams have been concentrating on these transplants. The experience of the transplant team in Seattle has been with the two other disease categories, severe aplastic anemia with approximately 90 transplants, and acute leukemia with approximately 180 transplants from either allogeneic or syngeneic donors.

Over the past six years during which these transplants have been carried out we have been confronted with the critical problems that prevent success in all cases. And what are these problems? Some are common to patients with aplastic anemia and with acute leukemia. These are (1) the GVH disease (GVHD), which occurs in 60–70% of the cases despite matching at the MHC, and which sets the stage for another complication, (2) profound immunodeficiency and fatal infection. A most prominent (and presumably infectious) complication is interstitial pneumonitis.

Apart from these two problems, another is predominantly encountered in aplastic anemia patients and occurs only infrequently in patients with leukemia. This is the phenomenon of marrow graft rejection. I do not think that it is due to Hh incompatibility, as it was discussed earlier. I rather think—based on our animal data—that it is due to transfusion-induced sensitization against minor histocompatibility antigen systems. This immunity is simply not overcome by our conditioning regimens—most frequently cyclophosphamide in high doses. In aplastic anemia patients, rejection occurs in 30% of the cases and is associated with high mortality. The problem unique for leukemic patients is the recurrence of the original disease in about 30% of the cases.

With this cursory introduction, the four major clinical problem areas are identified: marrow rejection mainly seen in the aplastic anemia patient; neoplastic recurrence in leukemia patients; GVHD; and accompanying fatal infections in both aplastic anemia and leukemic patients, presumably related to the patients' poor immunologic performance.

A number of research groups have been concerned with the problem of marrow rejection. Van Bekkum's team has done experiments in monkeys and mice. Mathe's group and Barnes and Loutit have done experiments in mice. We have carried out experiments in the dog using histocompatible littermates. These studies convinced us that marrow graft rejection is most likely the result of transfusion-induced immunity of recipient against donor.

When a dog is given 1,000 R total body irradiation followed by a graft from a litter mate donor matched at the MHC, sustained engraftment is the rule and graft rejection the rare exception. However, if we expose the prospective recipient either to a single transfusion from its intended matched donor 10–20 days before the transplant, or to several transfusions from unrelated donors, marrow graft rejection occurs in a high proportion of cases. In these dogs, we first see good engraftment, as documented by recovery of the leukocyte and platelet counts and genetic markers. Suddenly, however, the counts begin to decline and the marrow becomes aplastic. Dogs then die of infectious complications or bleeding.

These and many other studies support the concept that marrow graft rejection is the result of transfusion-induced sensitization to one or more minor histocompatibility systems that is not overcome by total body irradiation alone. We can overcome sensitization by utilizing a combination of procarbazine and antithymocyte serum in addition to total body irradiation, a regimen elaborated in collaboration with Floersheim.

In man, the concept of transfusion-induced sensitization is much more difficult to prove because most aplastic anemia patients have had multiple transfusions. In our initial survey of 73 transplants carried out before October 1975, there were only three patients who had not received transfusions. All three accepted the grafts and survived. The other 70 patients all had had multiple transfusions so as to preclude meaningful investigation of the transfusion effects.

We carried out a retrospective multivariant analysis in these 73 patients, searching for prognostic factors that might predict graft rejection or sustained engraftment. We entered 24 factors into the analysis, among them the duration and etiology of aplastic anemia, the number of transfusions, the sex and age of recipient and donor, the number of grafted marrow cells, and the conditioning regimen. We also entered the results of *in vitro* tests of cell-mediated immunity of the recipient against the donor. We have two such tests. One is a relative response index in MLC, which simply sets the proliferative response of the patient to his marrow donor in relation to the maximum response of the patient to unrelated individuals. In MLCs among 162 healthy HLA identical siblings we found the relative response index to be 0.1 ± 0.8 (S.D.)% of the response to unrelated subjects.

When the MLC response of marrow graft recipients was analyzed, we found that there were a number of patients who had a rather high relative response index to cells from their HLA identical marrow donor. For the most part these turned out to be patients who later rejected their marrow graft. In fact, a subsequent prospective study indicated that the results of the relative response index in MLC predicted acceptance or rejection of the graft in 85% of the cases. Specifically, using a discriminant analysis, we found that a relative response index of higher than 1.6% predicted rejection, while one lower than 1.6% predicted engraftment. The relative response index was also entered into the multifactorial analysis.

In addition, results of another test of cell-mediated immunity of patient against donor cells, the direct and antibody-dependent cellular cytotoxicity assay (^{51}Cr release), predicted the fate of the graft. Results were not entered in the multivariant analysis since only 26 patients had been studied.

First we examined the relationship of each of the 24 factors with marrow graft rejection. We found that nine factors correlated with rejection, too many to be credible. We then entered these nine factors in a binary logistic regression analysis to separate the factors that were really predictive from those that were spurious. Two factors showed significant association with graft rejection. One was the relative response index, which was significant at the $p < 0.01$ level, and the other was the grafted marrow cell number, which was significant at the $p < 0.05$ level. All the other factors that had shown an association with graft rejection in the simple analysis no longer were significantly correlated: patient age, number of blood units, transplant year, androgen treatment, prednisone treatment, ABO match, age difference, sex match, and duration of aplasia.

As for the two significant parameters, i.e., the negative (low) response index, and less than 3×10^8 marrow cells/kg body weight, three of nine patients rejected; with higher numbers of marrow cells none of 16 patients rejected. With a positive relative response index, and less than 3×10^8 marrow cells/kg, nine of ten patients rejected; while with higher marrow cell numbers only three of six patients rejected.

The findings suggested more powerful immunosuppressive conditioning regimens for those patients who are sensitized according to the results of *in vitro* tests. This would take the form of using the regimen of procarbazine, ATG, and total body irradiation found to be effective in the dog. Finally, it would be advisable to graft the greatest possibile amount of donor marrow, perhaps supplemented by stem cells derived from the peripheral blood.

The nature of the antigenic system detected by the *in vitro* tests involved in rejection is unknown. Whether it involves Hh genes is not clear. I think that family studies are necessary to ascertain whether segregation is independent of HLA, sex, ABO, etc.

We had the opportunity to carry out a similar logistic regression analysis, called haphazard regression analysis, in those patients with aplastic anemia who did not reject their marrow grafts. We first examined 24 possible prognostic factors, and we found nine or ten that seemed to have correlation to GVH disease and death. When entered in the logistic regression only two factors with signifi-

cant association emerged: sex mismatch between donor and recipient and refractoriness to random donor platelets at the time of grafting predicted GVH disease
and death. Sex matched recipients had a 92% survival compared to only 36% of
the sex-mismatched situation. Female to female and male to male grafts yielded
similarly good survival, while female to male and male to female grafts yielded a
similarly poor survival. Refractoriness to random donor platelets adversely influenced survival of the sex-mismatched recipients. These data suggest that X- and
Y-associated transplantation antigen systems are significant determinants of the
outcome of marrow grafting between HLA-identical siblings. The mechanism by
which refractoriness to random donor platelets influences survival is currently
unclear.

CLINE: Has Storb been referring to the incidence of GVH disease or to survival?

CHAIRMAN STORB: Up to this point I have been referring to survival. However, a separate regression analysis showed that sex mismatch had a significant
association with GVH ($p < 0.01$) whereas sex match was associated with the
absence of GVH disease. I should emphasize that our results are to be interpreted
with caution, in view of the small number of patients.

   The important unanswered question is how to prevent or treat GVH disease.
We are currently using methotrexate to prevent and antithymocyte globulin to
treat GVH disease, both with only moderate success. I think that innovation and
breakthroughs in this area have still to be made.

   I want now to report survival data of 100 transplanted leukemia patients
with acute myelogenous or lymphoblastic leukemia. All had had the maximum
chemotherapy before transplantation and all had been conditioned with a combination of cyclophosphamide and total body irradiation prior to receiving marrow
from an HLA identical sibling and immunosuppressive therapy for 100 days. Not
unexpectedly for such end stage patients, the mortality was high. The survival
curves show roughly three slopes. The first, steep slope during the first 100 days
is related to death from GVH disease and associated infections. The second,
gentler slope during the first two years reflects death from leukemic recurrence.
The third, relatively flat slope extends from the second to now more than six
years. This essentially horizontal slope at the 18% level represents survival in
unmaintained remission, i.e., these patients required no further treatment.

   How can one raise this horizontal line; i.e., how can one avoid the GVH
problem and the associated fatal infections and prevent the recurrence of
leukemia?

   We, and the UCLA group as well, have tried to reduce leukemic recurrence
by treating the patient with additional chemotherapy before the conditioning with
cyclophosphamide and total body irradiation. Our experience was not encourag-

ing since there was an increase of toxicity without significant decrease of leukemic recurrence. The patients should be transplanted earlier in the course of the disease, at a time when the number of leukemic cells is sufficiently small to attempt eradication by the conditioning regimen.

Patients with acute leukemia given allogeneic grafts have a 50% incidence of interstitial pneumonia, which is highly fatal. The incidence in patients with aplastic anemia is 32%, and 50% of these die. However, the incidence of interstitial pneumonia in patients with acute leukemia given syngeneic grafts is low, on the order of 8%, despite a pregrafting treatment identical to that of the allogeneic recipients. Immunological recovery postgrafting was quicker in syngeneic than in allogeneic recipients. It was generally complete within the first year in syngeneic, while in allogeneic recipients it may take several years. We consider that the immunodeficiency is most likely the major contributor to the frequently fatal interstitial pneumonias often associated with the presence of cytomegalovirus in the lung.

I have sought to outline the dominant clinical problems, as I see them in the hope that they could serve as a focus for the discussion of the presensitization issue, the GVH disease, the immune deficiency issue, and perhaps even the issue of leukemic recurrence.

BACH: Would Storb tell us a little more about the relative response index as a test of incompatibility, of the 1.6 cut-off, and specifically, what about the reproduceability of the test? Were he to find values greater than 1.6, would it be so also in the opposite direction, i.e., the donor responding to the recipient?

CHAIRMAN STORB: In the opposite direction of the donor responding to the recipient we rarely have seen a relative response index above 1.6. I would remind you that in Seattle, Mickelson has shown that cells from patients with aplastic anemia do not stimulate as well as cells from normal individuals.

DUPONT: The relative response index of Storb is not the same as the relative response. The formula is different, isn't that correct?

VAN BEKKUM: Is Storb using the third-party disparity test?

CHAIRMAN STORB: No. We compare the response in MLC of patient cells to sibling donor cells with the response to unrelated cells, and then express it as a ratio—the relative response index.

DICKE: I am aware of a possible complication in the test, namely, the large variations in the controls. Cells of the aplastic patient yield from 54 to, say, 900 cpm. Does this influence the reliability of the test?

CHAIRMAN STORB: I cannot answer that question.

CLINE: It may be worth mentioning that when Gale analyzed UCLA data, he did not obtain the same correlation. Therefore, we could not predict which patients were going to reject the donor marrow and which would accept it.

CHAIRMAN STORB: The fact remains that we could predict graft rejection with 85% certainty. We believed that this was sufficient reason to change the conditioning regimen in patients who were considered sensitized.

CLINE: Of course; my intent was to point out that the technical way these things are done is critical in generating such an index. One cannot necessarily extrapolate from institution to institution with respect to an absolute value.

PARKMAN: We have been doing a prospective direct chromium release study for the last two and one-half years on 25 patients, 16 aplastics and 9 leukemics. None of the leukemics have been positive in the assay, while 11 of the 16 patients with aplastic anemia have been positive. A positive assay is one with more than 4% specific chromium release. When the recipient peripheral blood lymphocytes are positive, the bone marrow cells are also positive. There is, however, a small number of recipients in whom peripheral blood lymphocytes are negative, but the bone marrow cells are positive. We feel that a positive chromium release with either peripheral blood lymphocytes and/or bone marrow cells in a person with aplastic anemia indicates presensitization. We have now transplanted 11 aplastics and one leukemic who had six white cell transfusions from her donor. Immunosuppression consisted of the procarbazine-cytoxan and intravenous antithymocyte serum protocol. Among those 12 people at increased risk of graft rejection, there have been only two actual rejections. One of these patients experienced recovery of his own marrow function.

I think the only two differences between our immunosuppressive regimen and the one from Seattle is the use of intravenous ATS, and not having given buffy coat. Whether either of these factors accounts for the differences is not known. We feel that the direct ^{51}Cr release assay detects this high-risk group, and that the favorable results we have had are due to the multiagent immunosuppression.

We have not observed rejections wherever the direct ^{51}Cr release assay gave negative results.

BACH: Storb said that he did not have as much data on cytotoxicity as on MLC. Is it possible that the very low-level proliferative responses to HLA-identical cells might be elicited by cytotoxic cells responding to a cytotoxic target antigen, rather than to an LD-like proliferative inducing antigen, in the terms of how we usually think of MLC? This is an important distinction, and since CTL (cytotoxic lymphocytes) do divide, one would wonder whether you are dealing here with the proliferation of CTLs to the non-HLA–CTL target, which we know exists after *in vivo* sensitization.

CHAIRMAN STORB: I guess that could be so.

BACH: I wonder whether it is worth studying the kinetics of CML to establish whether one is dealing with a secondary response.

CHAIRMAN STORB: Yes, Bach's point is well taken. We have tested 26 patients and ten of these were positive. That means that in ten cases the patient's cells, or the patient's serum in the ADCC, released ^{51}Cr from the donor's cells without sentization *in vitro*. Of these ten patients, eight rejected their graft.

Negative results in the ^{51}Cr release test did not ensure sustained engraftment.

BACH: Storb may be detecting a cytotoxic target antigen, in which case he should be able to markedly boost a secondary-type CML response, by adding any allogeneic LD stimulus.

GALE: Regarding Bach's point on the kinetics of the MLC, we have looked at it in a slightly different setting, i.e., in patients who rejected their grafts and then had their own hemopoiesis restored. In this situation we sought to determine whether they had in fact acquired an MLC reactivity via the *in vivo* sensitization. We have not been able to show the acquisition of MLC reactivity in six recipients of MLC matched-sibling transplants after rejection of their grafts.

I find it especially interesting that Storb was unable to establish a correlation between the clinical parameters of acquired in vivo sensitization, i.e., numbers of blood transfusions or duration of aplasia, with rejection. The positive correlation with the relative response index brings up the question of whether the transfusions really sensitize or whether the test detects genetic disparities at loci that are not on the MHC chromosome.

CHAIRMAN STORB: As I said before, we had three patients who did not have any blood transfusions, a number too small for a meaningful analysis. However, in patients receiving a greater number of pretransplant blood transfusions there was a higher incidence of rejections.

More recently, we have transplanted a total of seven patients who had never had pretransplant transfusions. So far, all of them have sustained their grafts.

This finding supports our hypothesis that transfusion-induced sensitization is a major factor in graft rejection.*

Accordingly, we seek to accumulate 20–30 patients without preceding transfusions. If the incidence of rejection is as high in these patients as it is in pretransfused patients, I shall then begin to be concerned about other factors affecting the fate of a graft, such as Hh determined resistance.

DUPONT: Storb's relative response index measures the patient's responsiveness toward the donor. Now, he feels that the test reflects presensitization against some histoincompatibilities, which is raised as a consequence of transfusion therapy. But I think it is also possible that there could be considerations other than genetic for this phenomenon. For example, a subgroup of aplastic anemia patients with a special type of aplasia have in their circulating blood, lymphocytes that differ from the normal. This situation could result in increased MLC responsiveness. Moreover, Storb's patients could have had a loss of suppressor cells, or radioresistant or chemotherapy-resistant cells. The point is that his observation does not need to involve a genetic mechanism or to reflect presensitization, but it could represent a different etiology for these aplasias.

CHAIRMAN STORB: The hypothesis that transfusion-induced sensitization is a major factor in marrow graft rejection derives from solid evidence in dogs. These studies in dogs were done in a prospective fashion. Similar data exist in monkeys and mice. Nevertheless, I would not disagree that other factors such as a defective microenvironment and autoimmune disease could play a role. Against this possibility speaks the fact that we have not encountered marrow graft rejection among the nontransfused patients. In addition, all four identical twin recipients grafted in Seattle without conditioning have shown sustained engraftment.

DUPONT: But several case reports demonstrate that some type of autoimmune mechanism could operate in aplastic anemia patients.

CHAIRMAN STORB: I agree.

PARKMAN: First, is it fair to say that Storb considers the relative response

*Editors' comment. Although the importance of presensitization as an impediment to effective hemopoietic repopulation is recognized, there has been no deliberate investigation of its effects in the murine model. It is known, however, that resistance can be dramatically enhanced in the mouse by specific transfusion of donor-type spleen cells, but whether the mechanism involves familiar immune phenomena (T cell mediated allograft reactions, cytotoxic antibody formation) or systems such as Hh genes and natural killer cells is quite unknown. The readiness with which resistance can be enhanced in the dog and the mouse, the magnitude of the effect, and the likelihood that it would compromise engraftment, warrant its serious investigation.

index as a measure of an intrinsic genetic difference? Is it "natural" or induced?

Second, has Storb determined whether transfused dogs have increased relative response indexes? This would discriminate between a natural and induced response to a genetic difference.

CHAIRMAN STORB: Well, the dog is a bit more difficult to deal with in regard to MLCs and we do not have good data regarding the predictive value of the relative response index in this species.

CUDKOWICZ: One of the significant correlations in Storb's aplastic anemia patients with multiple transfusions was the number of bone marrow cells transplanted. This means that he got engraftment despite presensitization. In the mouse, such presensitization would result in rejection so strong that it could not be overcome by simply increasing the number of transplanted cells. We have explored this situation repeatedly in many strain combinations. If by simply increasing the number of cells one overcomes resistance, this would be an indication that the incompatibility is of Hh type. On the other hand, if resistance cannot be broken in this way, the incompatibility would be of the more familiar H type.

Thus, in a way, it seems almost as if there is a contradiction. Storb's favored hypothesis is that whatever he is measuring in these patients, it is the product of presensitization. Yet the most obvious expectation that results from presensitization fails to materialize.

CHAIRMAN STORB: I do not know how to apply Cudkowicz's comment to the human situation. I can only present our data and seek to develop a hypothesis that is based on studies in dogs.

VAN BEKKUM: Did Cudkowicz sensitize across or within H-2 differences?

CUDKOWICZ: Both, with essentially similar results.

VAN BEKKUM: Is he sure that a sufficient number of cells could not overcome sensitization in H-2 identical combinations?

CUDKOWICZ: If the presensitization was multiple, then even H-2 identical pairs develop immunity such that the host, after irradiation, will still reject up to 100 million marrow cells. Those are the limits of the experiment.

DAUSSET: I would like to contribute the results on aplastic anemia patients of Gluckman, who is working in our institute. Up to the present she has transplanted 18 patients with HLA identical sibling marrow. She had ten rejections, eight takes, two with severe and two with mild GVH disease. Five patients have survived for more than one year, and all of the eight patients with takes were alive at three months after grafting.

Eleven of 17 patients developed antileukocyte antibodies and those were designated high responders. All of these individuals had received transfusions. It is difficult to know the precise number of transfusions, but in the present instance, all of the patients, high and low responders, had received at least 50 transfusions. It is of interest that about 50% of such patients do not develop HLA antibodies even after a great number of transfusions. Table 16 illustrates the correlation between the presence of such antibody (not necessarily directed against the graft) and graft rejection. It is evident that in the majority of these patients antibodies remain in spite of the conditioning for the graft. In this event rejection occurs. In contrast, in four patients in which antibody had disappeared after the conditioning, engraftment took place.

Table 17 deals with a third category of patients, those without antibodies from the start. Here there were four takes and two rejections. Thus, based on this overall experience, we believe that there is a very strong correlation between the presence and persistence of anti-HLA antibody in the serum of recipients and marrow graft rejection. The presence of anti-HLA and other antibody should therefore be considered primarily as an indicator of immune responder status, since host and donor were always HLA identical.

VAN BEKKUM: Doesn't Storb think that the priming with buffy coat should be discontinued whenever the recipient has signs of being sensitized? It is not always possible to inhibit with radiation a secondary response, but it is relatively easy to inhibit the primary response up to two days after the sensitization. It may be that one is, in fact, reinforcing with the buffy coat regimen whatever resistance the sensitized recipients posesses.

CHAIRMAN STORB: We have in fact discontinued the buffy coat regimen for patients in whom we have recognized sensitization. Patients who are sensitized are either randomized into receiving procarbazine, ATG, and total body irradiation (effective in the dog), or given cyclophosphamide and total body irradiation as used for conditioning leukemia patients. Nonsensitized patients are randomized into receiving cyclophosphamide with or without buffy coat.

DICKE: Two patients in Houston who received extensive granulocyte transfusions from family members rejected marrow transplants. Conditioning was with an alkylating-like agent and total body irradiation.

SANFORD: Despite the overall pessimism about bone marrow transplantation in leukemia, Storb has shown us data on 100 acute lymphatic leukemia patients in whom chemotherapy had failed and who subsequently received marrow trans-

TABLE 16

Correlation between Capacity to Develop High Antileukocyte Antibody Titers and Rejection of Marrow Grafts

Presence of HLA antibodies at intervals (days) preceding and subsequent to marrow transplantation

Aplastic anemia patients	-10	-5	0	5	10	15	20	25	30	35	40	60	100	Engraftment	GVH	Survival (days)
LOY	++++	++++	++++	++++	++++	++++	++++	++++						rejection day 10	—	25
TAR	++++	++++	++++	++++	++++	++++	++++	++++	++++	++++	++++	++++		rejection day 25	—	70
MAG	++++	++++	++++	++++	++++	++++	++++	++++	++++	++++	++++	++++		rejection day 15	—	80
CAS	++++	++++	++++	++++	++++	++++	++++	++++	++++	++++	++++	++++		rejection day 17	—	86
GRI	++++	++++	++++	++	+	+++++	+	++++	++++	+++++	+++++			rejection day 7	—	45
DELM	++	++	++	++	+	+	+	+	+	+	+	+		rejection day 90	+day 9	>118
DELAF	+++	+++	++	++	++	++	++	++	++					rejection day 20	—	>39
POE	++++	+++	++	—	—	—	—	—	—	—	—	—	—	take	—	>474
DOU	++++	++++	++++	—	—	+	++	—	—	—	—	—	—	take	+day 58	>394
GUI	++	++	(+)	—	—	—	—	—	—	—	—	—	—	take	—	>464
MEU	++++	+++	+++	+	—	—	—	—	—	—				take	+day 9	36

59

TABLE 17

Correlation between Lack of Development of Antileukocyte Antibodies and Subsequent Bone Marrow Engraftment

Aplastic anemia patients	Absence of HLA antibodies at intervals (days) preceding and subsequent to marrow transplantation													Engraft-ment	GVH	Survival (days)
	−10	−5	0	5	10	15	20	25	30	40	50	80	100			
SUY	—	—	—	—	—	—	—	—	—	—	—	—	—	+	+day 120	>851
CAR	—	—	—	—	—	—	—	—	—	—	—	—	—	+	+day 17 chronic	448
CAU	—	—	—	—	—	—	—	—	—	—	—	—	—	+	+day 50	>205
MES	—	+	—	—	—	—	—	—	—	—	—	—	—	+	—	>70
NOU	—	—	—	—	—	—	—	—	—	—	—	—	—	rejection day 60	—	150
COL	—	—	—	—	—	—	—	—	—	—	—	—	—	rejection day 25	+++ day 60	70

plants. I am rather impressed that 20 or more of these patients are still alive after two years or more.

CHAIRMAN STORB: The present figures are 18 patients with the longest being five years.

SANFORD: I do not think that is so discouraging; does Storb agree?

CHAIRMAN STORB: Yes, I do.

CLINE: Back to the issue of failure of engraftment vs. graft rejection. We have been considering these as one entity; however, they really seem to sort out as two distinct clinical syndromes. The great majority of the patients accept grafts and do very well for perhaps two weeks or so, and then they lose the grafts. There is a subset of patients, smaller in number, who never really engraft. This latter situation may reflect quite a different mechanism.

One of our recent experiences was with individuals who were presumed to be identical twins. Marrow from one twin was given to the aplastic twin and failed to produce engraftment. From the experience, I wonder if in this discussion we have not been lumping together two situations, one in which there is graft rejection, perhaps on an immunological basis, and a second, quite distinct phenomenon in which there are other possibilities, e.g., the environment may not be conducive.

CHAIRMAN STORB: I agree with Cline. The problem is to recognize these patient categories before transplantation by appropriate *in vitro* tests.

CUDKOWICZ: Shouldn't we have further information on the chromium release tests that were used by Storb and Parkman. Is it a natural killer cell type that is assayed, an inducible cytotoxic cell, or an antibody of the prospective recipient?

PARKMAN: PHA-stimulated lymphocytes of the donor and of control individuals are used as targets and fresh donor and recipient peripheral blood leukocytes as well as ficoll-separated bone marrow cells are used as effectors. The assay is done with and without 1% heat-inactivated recipient serum. Therefore, one is testing both for antibody-dependent and antibody-independent cell-mediated immunity. One usually does not get good antibody-dependent lysis using either the bone marrow or the peripheral blood leukocytes of aplastics since they seem to be missing the necessary effector cells.

We have previously done family studies and shown that the CML antigen may be genetically determined (that is to say, cells of one parent will be lysed

TABLE 18
MLC between Donor and Recipient in Five Successful Bone Marrow Transplants with Donors
Other Than HLA-Identical Siblings

Donor	HLA incompatibility	MLC Donor × recipient			References
		Control (cpm)	MLR (cpm)	SR[a]	
Sibling	Bw37	16	17	1.0	Gatti et al., 1968
Maternal Uncle	B7,B12	321	117	0.4	Dupont et al., 1973
Unrelated	A2	611	1364	2.2	L'Esperance et al., 1975
Father	None	52	95	1.8	Barrett et al., 1975
Father	None	168	75	0.5	Polmor et al., 1976

[a] $SR = \dfrac{MLC\ (cpm)}{control\ (cpm)}$.

while those of the other parent will not) and that the target antigens are not linked to either HLA, MLC, the known red cell blood groups, or the sex chromosomes.

Attempts to increase the reactivity of this system by co-culturing recipient and donor cells did not succeed.

DUPONT: There are now described five patients with severe combined immune deficiency who are long-term survivors following bone marrow transplantation. Donors were relatively histocompatible but not HLA identical siblings. The actual imcompatibilities are shown in Table 18. Two of the patients were given paternal bone marrow that was phenotypically but not genotypically HLA identical.

All pairs were weakly reactive in MLC with stimulation ratios from 2.2 to 0.5 (Table 18). The patterns of immunologic reconstitution are outlined in Table 19. In three of the patients the bone marrow seems to be the specific target of GVH reaction as inferred from the development of aplasia. In most of the recipients of MHC-incompatible marrow, immunologic reconstitution was extremely slow. Finally, there was a split between the T and the B cell reconstitution though all of the patients were fully reconstituted in the end. I think this could be a reflection of some type of genetic resistance to engraftment in a clinical situation.

PARKMAN: It is not clear to me that the rate of immune reconstitution in Dupont's patients is different from that in children we have transplanted with

TABLE 19
Immunological Reconstitution and GVH Disease in Five Bone Marrow Transplants
with Donors Other Than HLA-Identical Siblings

D.C.	Fast immunological reconstitution followed by bone marrow aplasia and moderate to severe GVH disease; subsequent complete immunological and hematological reconstitution
KRN	Slow immunological reconstitution; very delayed for the B-lymphoid system; mild to moderate GVH
MR	Slow immunological reconstitution; secondary bone marrow aplasia followed by complete immunological and hematological reconstitution; moderate to severe GVH, which subsided; chronic GVH in skin
WH	Fast T-cell reconstitution but delayed B-cell reconstruction; severe GVH in skin and liver, which subsided with subsequent complete immunological reconstitution
C1. Oh.	Fast immunological reconstitution; mild to moderate GVH; late onset granulocytopenia

compatible sibling marrow; that is, the delay in B cell reconstitution and onset of maturation are not necessarily related to MHC incompatibility.

O'REILLY: I would like to return to Cline's proposition that there may well be a variety of factors that contribute to rejection. Dupont referred to patients who do not have a functional lymphoid system and yet demonstrate either partial or very slow engraftment in a situation where it would not be expected that they have any significant measure of resistance, apart from classical lymphoid mechanisms.

We have recently succeeded in immune reconstitution of a patient with severe combined immunodeficiency using marrow from an unrelated MLC-matched donor. The critical feature was that during the first four transplants, this patient had partial engraftment of donor cells, but never evidence of sustained PHA responsiveness or sustained production of immunoglobulins. In this immunologically inert patient, cytoxan and a very large dose of marrow was necessary to produce a T cell engraftment. Prior to this fifth transplant, we could demonstrate a phagocytic, adherent, recipient-derived cell population capable of suppressing both differentiation of plasma cells and production of immunoglobulin by allogeneic normal marrow cells. B cell reconstitution was achieved after a seventh transplant and conditioning with a high dose of cytoxan. Following this graft, suppressors were no longer demonstrable and immunoglobulin and antibody production ensued. The suppressor cell here was host-derived and apparently nonlymphoid. Its action may have been local, since at the time we could see few if any donor cells or immune responses in the circulation, whereas the lymph nodes were highly cellular, and 90% of the cells were donor-derived and functional.

I want to offer an example of what we observed in two successful fetal liver transplants in patients with severe combined immune deficiency. All of the patients' T cells were fetal in origin, whereas all of the patients' B cells were of recipient origin. In these patients we were also able to demonstrate populations of host-derived adherent cells capable of inhibiting differentiation of B cells. Thus, there may be cell populations, even in recipients with abnormal lymphoid systems, capable of markedly inhibiting engraftment. This mechanism may be especially applicable to the situation of grafts from MLC-matched unrelated marrow donors or clearly allogeneic fetal donors. This also may apply to HLA-identical sibling donors.

METCALF: I would make a plea to those working with marrow transplants to use modern technology whenever possible. Reference is constantly made to "engraftment" and the criteria used were the appearance of mature cells in the circulating blood. This is a very indirect estimate of engraftment and cell proliferation. Colony-forming cell assay will directly estimate progenitor cells capable of proliferation.
    Peripheral blood levels of cells, particularly those of granulocytes and lymphocytes, are influenced by many interacting processes, some of which are unrelated to engraftment or cell proliferation. Clearly, patients are not analyzed as fully as could be done. This is our collective fault and we must now use our separate skills and techniques more effectively in team studies on these valuable patients.

CHAIRMAN STORB: I appreciate Metcalf's comments. Since these are important points, would he want to make a constructive proposal?

METCALF: I would put the general proposition that if one wishes to ask the question "Has the marrow transfusion *taken?*" what one really is asking is whether there is a population of cells of a particular class that is proliferating. Further, what cloning methods are available for measuring the various subpopulations of human hemopoietic cells? There are at least four available right now. There is no reason why any one of the transplant patients should not have erythroid cloning, granulocytic cloning, eosinophil cloning, and T cell cloning performed routinely. Is it going to tell one anything else that peripheral cell counts cannot? Yes, in the sense that one is measuring *directly* the proliferating population.

CHAIRMAN STORB: Some of these things are being done. They cannot all be alluded to in a crowded program such as this.

MOORE: For the record, I think that CFU-C assays have proved of value, at least in the Sloan-Kettering transplantation program. Certainly, if one sees evidence of recovery of CFU-C growth in aplastic or leukemic patients within one to two weeks after transplantation with a well-defined overshoot in CFU-C numbers, and then stabilization back to normal levels, it is fair to say that these patients are engrafted. In other cases, despite cytogenetic evidence of engraftment within the first week, and even hematological evidence of engraftment, the absence of this pattern of CFU-C regeneration in the posttransplant period seems to be related to the eventual failure of the graft.

In the context of marrow transplantation in the leukemic patient, the CFU-C assay can identify the recurrence of the original leukemic clone, days or sometimes weeks before this becomes evident by change in hematologic status or reversion to the original host cytogenetic status.

CLINE: I would mildly disagree with Metcalf and with Moore. Unfortunately, the measurements they propose do not have as much value as one would like. If one can see cells in the marrow, then one can eventually culture them. If, however, there are no cells detectable, as in the patient with aplasia, then there is nothing to culture. The limitation, I think, is in how we express CFU-C and CFU-E. It is as the number of colony-formers per unit number of nucleated cells. What one really needs is a measure of the total number of CFU-C or CFU-E in the hemopoietic system. This information is easy enough to obtain in the mouse, but unfortunately not in man. Sampling is particularly difficult in aplastic patients as they regenerate their marrow only after bone marrow transplantation. Crude as they are, marrow morphology and peripheral cell counts (reticulocytes and granulocytes) happen to be, at the moment, just as good as measuring colonies of random and multiple marrow aspirates.

METCALF: All of what Cline says is fine, if he thinks he knows the etiology and the pathogenesis of aplastic anemia. None of us in this conference would claim to know this, so in a sense we are still investigating. My message is that with new technology it is possible to ask more discriminating questions than looking at a bone marrow smear and counting cells. It may give us a clue to the nature of this disease, or then too, it may not. It may tell us that some of our patients with apparent failed grafts have, in fact, had aplastic anemia reinduced.

We have to make use of whatever parameters we can to assess the abnormalities in the hemopoietic populations. Some abnormalities are not related only to numbers of colony-forming cells, but to their nature. Thus, I do not agree that morphology is still as good as anything else. I know what Cline is getting at, and I agree in one sense, of course. It gives you a numbers estimate, and a numbers estimate agrees with the colony estimate. The advantage of the other technology is that in the long run it will give more information.

BENNETT: According to Storb, the Hh system may not be important in rejection of aplastic anemia and acute leukemia patients. Does O'Reilly have evidence that some of the children with SCID may actually reject marrow grafts, as they do not receive such intensive immunosuppressive therapy? Could such rejections be due to Hh incompatibility?

O'REILLY: We have observed partial or complete failure to engraft despite the use of well over the 10^7 cell/kg usually adequate for lymphoid engraftment in SCID patients. Thus, in one of the patients previously discussed who received unrelated HLA-D compatible marrow, even 1.2×10^8 cells/kg produced a partial graft of T cells only. Full engraftment was finally achieved after lethal doses of cytoxan. Since no lymphoid function is demonstrable in such an immunodeficient host, we feel this represents resistance mediated by nonlymphoid cells.

I do not know whether this is resistance analogous to that described for the Hh system in mice. If one applies certain restrictions to the definition of Hh incompatibility, such as how homozygous expression of Hh genes occurs in donor cells, it would be unlikely. Buf if one is talking about a more general phenomenon of cell-mediated resistance to engraftment, then I think that there are analogies. The adherent host-derived phagocytic cell with suppressor activity for differentiation and/or proliferation of other cell types may be the link between the two phenomena.

We have observed the suppressor cells in three cases of combined immunodeficiency. We are wondering whether this actually contributes to the pathogenesis of the disease, or whether it is a phenomenon secondary to transplantation. However, in two cases, the existence of suppressor cells preceded transplantation.

TRENTIN: Sixteen years ago, Fernbach and I reported a well-documented case of a child with longstanding aplastic anemia who would not sustain marrow from an identical twin given on two occasions. We pointed out at the time that there might be factors other than stem cells and erythropoietin important to hemopoiesis, including organ stromal factors that make the marrow and spleen "home" for hemopoiesis.

Since then there has accumulated a large body of evidence indicating that there are hemopoietic organ microenvironmental and humoral factors that are as important as stem cells for hemopoietic differentiation. Cline has provided us with still another case of an aplastic anemia patient who did not sustain marrow from an identical twin. Thus, it would seem that the mouse does give us valid messages regarding man, but at times we tend not to listen too well. We will continue to find that major immunobiologic situations worked out in the mouse are relevant to man, including "genetic resistance" to bone marrow transplantation.

CHAIRMAN STORB: In some aplastic anemia patients the microenvironmental defect could be a consequence of autoimmune disease. I believe, however, that such patients are the minority. In most cases, aplastic anemia is probably the result of a stem cell defect.

ELKINS: I am addressing the issue of interstitial pneumonia, which often follows bone marrow transplantation. At the experimental level one can make a case that many kinds of virus infections are activated by GVH disease. Interstitial pneumonia virus should be viewed in this framework and not as a separate problem.

CHAIRMAN STORB: Chronic myelogenous leukemia patients grafted with their own stored (frozen) marrow also experience interstitial pneumonia with an incidence similar to that seen in allogeneic recipients. Hematologic and immunologic recovery was generally very slow in these patients, a strong argument for the views that immunodeficiency is really the major factor for the development of interstitial pneumonia. As GVH disease potentiates immune deficits, there is, of course, an association between severe GVH disease and interstitial pneumonia.

Oldstone's recent evidence of activation of latent CMV (cytomegalovirus) infection by GVH disease and similar data from our recent studies of lymphoid cell infection by *Herpes simplex* would indicate that in an allogeneic interaction the lymphocytes become susceptible to infection by a variety of DNA viruses, including CMV, and we ourselves have shown that T and B cells are also susceptible to *Herpes simplex*.

Thus, susceptibility of patients to these viruses may be a manifestation, not so much of immunedeficiency as classically defined, but rather a manifestation of acquired susceptibility of GVH reactive lymphocytes to viral infection.

WARNER: In considering the types of target cells used, one has to recognize that differential expression of surface markers occurs on different cell populations. From the cytotoxity studies described, it seems that T cells have been the principal target type used. Consequently, reactivity against T cells is being detected, whereas the actual grafting is with stem cells that express other types of differentiation antigens. Thus, I would question Storb whether the prescreening is biased by the use of target cells that are not, in fact, the type of cells being grafted.

CHAIRMAN STORB: I think Warner's point is well taken. Warren in our laboratory has begun looking into this.

FESTENSTEIN: That one can get viral activation following alloimmune interaction, immune suppression, irradiation, etc., is well known. Many explanations have been offered. We have new findings that should put quite a different view on the urgent topic of GVH in marrow transplant patients. We have observed the appearance of additional (inappropriate) H-2-like specificities of foreign haplotypes on prospective target cells taken from mice with vaccinia virus infection. These and other H-2-like determinants can then act as targets for cytostasis and cytotoxicity. Were such a mechanism to operate in marrow transplant patients, it could contribute to the GVH disease. Our findings on virus-induced histocompatibility changes will be reported in detail later in the conference.

CHAIRMAN STORB: We have two kinds of syngeneic transplant patients: those who receive autologous frozen marrow, and those who receive fresh marrow from the identical twin. The former are poorly and slowly reconstituted and the latter are reconstituted promptly and well. Incidence of interstitial pneumonia parallels their immune situation.

O'REILLY: The possibility remains that in the autologous marrow graft there may be lymphocytes sensitized to and reactive against the patient's own leukemia or other viral infected cells, whereas in the twin graft situation that would not be the case, since the twin would not have been presensitized and his cells reconstitute promptly.

GALE: I want to address the question of leukemic recurrence. Relapse rates should be analyzed in an actuarial fashion. While the uncorrected overall relapse rate is about 30%, the actuarially determined relapse rate is probably greater than 50% and may be as high as 60–70%. Therefore, leukemic recurrence is a major cause of treatment failure.

   One remedy Storb has alluded to is the use of more intensive conditioning chemotherapy. A second one is to transplant patients earlier. These procedures are not mutually exclusive. Our experience, which differs from that of the Seattle group, suggests that there may be some advantage of supplementing cyclophosphamide and total body irradiation with additional chemotherapy. Since such a regimen is more toxic, intensive supportive therapy including granulocyte transfusions and provision of air flow environment is indicated.

CHAIRMAN STORB: GVH disease is a phenomenon that occurs in 60–70% of the HLA-identical recipients and is associated with a high incidence of mortality. I have already suggested that X and Y chromosome associated transplantation antigens may be involved. However, our means of preventing or treating this disease are limited. Are there any ideas or suggestions in this regard?

BORANIC: Presently, aplastic anemia and leukemia patients to be transplanted are treated in the same manner. The regimens for post-transplantation immunosuppression should perhaps be different in these two diseases.

In aplastic anemia patients, we should strive for a stable graft with as little immunosuppression as possible, whereas in leukemia patients, we should try to exploit the immunosuppressive effects of the drugs with their antileukemic effects and combine this with antileukemic action of grafted immunocompetent cells. An optimal *time* schedule for posttransplant chemotherapy in leukemia patients should be tailored to the dynamics of proliferation of grafted cells.

VAN BEKKUM: We have found no evidence in dogs for the importance of "sex match" in relation to GVH disease.

CHAIRMAN STORB: The number of DLA-identical littermate recipients treated in an identical fashion has not been sufficient for analysis.

FESTENSTEIN: Our experience with kidney transplants shows the opposite sex pattern. In other words, male to female transplants do better than female to female.

CHAIRMAN STORB: We were aware of mouse data showing that the Y associated antigen plays a role in organ graft rejection and even in GVH disease.

WARNER: In response to the query of other approaches to eliminate GVH disease, I want to discuss differentiation markers on lymphocyte subpopulations.
   In the mouse, the cell that induces GVH disease bears a cell surface phenotype identified by Ly markers as an Ly-1,2,3 positive cell. If the human GVH reactive cell is also a distinct T cell subpopulation, it may well bear specific differentiation markers. Accordingly, if appropriate reagents were available, they could be used in conjunction with cell separation methods to remove such cell types or their precursors from the marrow inoculation.

VAN BEKKUM: I want to emphasize that in the mouse there is no evidence whatsoever that removal of the cells that produce GVH reactions influences the occurrence of the delayed type of GVH disease that is associated with weak incompatibilities, as we expect to deal with in the matched sibling situation.

LANDY: For the record, would Storb summarize for us the overall experience to date on the opposite approach of coping with the realities of GVH disease, that is, by germ-free or by life-island techniques?

CHAIRMAN STORB: In Seattle we have been investigating over the last two years the value of laminar-flow rooms in a randomized study with regard to two questions: (1) Is the incidence of infection reduced and survival improved? (2) Is the incidence of GVH disease decreased? Over the years, it had been shown by a number of investigators, Van Bekkum included, that the germ-free environment prevented fatal secondary disease in mice receiving allogeneic bone marrow.

The study in Seattle is still in progress, but thus far the study has not given a strong indication that "protected environment" drastically reduces the incidence of GVH disease.

With regard to infections, there can be no question that the incidence of bacterial sepsis is far less in patients in a protected environment than those outside.

DICKE: In Storb's setup the time between decontamination and marrow transplantation is very short. On the other hand, groups that have prolonged the period of decontamination of patients and large experimental animals have had on the whole better results.

GALE: It should be clear that the leukemic reoccurence being discussed is due to leukemic cells that escaped chemoradiotherapy. This is not *induction* of leukemia in donor cells. Available data do not indicate a beneficial antileukemic effect of GVH disease. However, this is not necessarily excluded, since patients with severe GVH disease die and are therefore not at risk.

CHAIRMAN STORB: Gale is quite right. Early death from GVH disease complicates any such evaluation. In this context, I would like to identify an ongoing randomized immunotherapy study in twin transplantation. Immunotherapy includes weekly injections of the host's own leukemic cells that had been stored in liquid nitrogen and then inactivated by irradiation with 10,000 rads. Patients are also treated twice weekly with injections of fresh, viable donor lymphocytes in the expectation that these lymphocytes will become sensitized to putative leukemia-associated antigens and exert an antileukemic effect.

O'REILLY: Storb showed that patients refractory to infusion of exogenous platelets had a higher incidence of severe GVH disease. Does he feel that the associated mortality is merely due to the thrombocytopenia, or to host-derived components of the GVH syndrome?

CHAIRMAN STORB: My answer is a speculative one. Refractoriness to random donor platelets could be the expression in man of "strong" general responsiveness as determined by Ir genes within the MHC. Since marrow donor and recipient are identical at the MHC, strong immune responsiveness in the recipient might also be present in the donor. In the case of a sex mismatch, strong immune responsiveness would be directed against X- and Y-chromosome associated transplantation antigens, resulting in a high incidence of GVH disease and death. It should be remembered that "refractoriness" need not always reflect immunological responsiveness but also could be the result of platelet consumption.

PARKMAN: We have noticed platelet refractoriness in patients with acute GVH disease. If one uses ^{51}Cr-labeled platelets from the donor, it is possible to show shortening of platelet survival. A part of GVH disease is nonspecific activation of the RES and, in severe cases of acute GVH disease, a shortening of red cell survival is also seen. Platelet refractoriness would then not be primary, but only a secondary consequence of GVH disease.

BORANIC: I would like to emphasize that any antileukemic effect of GVH reactions is associated with the acute (immediate) form of GVH, where there is proliferation of the grafted immunocompetent cells, whereas the chronic (delayed) form of GVH, associated with infections, pneumonia, and other complications, has a weak (or none at all) antileukemic effect in experimental animals. Thus, if one is to make use of the antileukemic effect of GVH reactions, it has to be limited to the proliferative phase in the early posttransplantation period, when GVH is amenable to chemotherapy.

WERNET: A number of the presentations referred to "MHC matched donors" where, in fact, there is no such match in unrelated host–donor pairs. At best there is a match for the A, B, C, and D loci. The definition and manipulation of genetic and immunologic effects of the MHC remain critical for the use of nonsibling donors. Here we may have an opportunity for adoptive immunotherapy particularly in the leukemia situation. If we consider the series of Ia markers in man, both the complexity and the potential for adoptive immunotherapy are evident. Matching for specific linkage disequilibria in and around the HLA region would eliminate mismatching effects from undetected recombination. This should also be valid for Hh-type matchings.

BACH: I would like to comment on the problem of parent–child combinations, where there is phenotypic identity for HLA-A,-B, and -D. In such cases of phenotypic identity we can never be sure whether the pair is also genotypically identical.

GRAFT-VERSUS-HOST DISEASE
AS A CONSEQUENCE OF BONE MARROW GRAFTING

Discussion Introducer:

William L. Elkins

CHAIRMAN ELKINS: Graft-versus-host reactivity and disease state are a very complicated subject for both biologic and semantic reasons. In introducing this subject, I shall be giving my way of thinking about it.

We would all agree that the basic process here is an immune response of donor cells to foreign alloantigens of the host. As defined here, the GVHR (GVH reaction) involves antigen recognition by B and T cells, the formation of humoral effectors (lymphokines and antibodies) and cellular effectors cytotoxic for host cells. As is well known, the T cell component of this response seems to be of paramount importance for initiation. Once unleashed in the host, this immune response has very complex effects, some of which become clinically apparent as GVHD (GVH disease).

Some of the effects of the GVHR are outlined here:

GVHR: immune response to host alloantigens by donor T and B cells.
GVHD: the effects of the GVHR upon the host:
    (1) death of host cells due to activity of cytotoxic lymphocytes and macrophages,
    (2) activation of host RES,
    (3) activation of host B cells, including those which make autoantibody (allogeneic effect),
    (4) control of autocytotoxic cells is diminished,
    (5) immunodeficiency,
    (6) virus activation,
    (7) lesions develop in skin, GI tract, and liver,
    (8) neoplasia.

Certain cells in the host are presumably killed by specifically cytotoxic T cells (CTL) that are generated in the GVHR. We also believe that macrophages are activated by lymphokines released from T cells mediating the GVHR. These macrophages may contribute to the destruction of host "target cells." In unirradiated recipients, host B cells are also stimulated by the T cells mediating the GVHR, and included in this polyclonal response are cells that make autoantibody.

We are now becoming aware of a killer cell that may be unleashed in GVHD in irradiated hosts. This autocytotoxic cell appears to differ in specificity from the CTL that would be generated in the GVHR. I refer here to the recent data of Parkman suggesting that such autocytotoxic cells should be considered as candidates to be added to the list of effector cells important in GVHD.

GVHR produce an immunodeficiency in the host, which may reflect to some extent the activities of the suppressor T cell component in the GVHR, but which undoubtedly comes about by other mechanisms as well.

Under some circumstances viruses are activated during GVHD in mice. The viruses may have a role in tissue injury either by a direct cytopathic effect or by eliciting a graft vs. "altered self" cytotoxic immune response. As suggested by Festenstein, viruses might induce the expression of additional "inappropriate" MHC antigens in the host and so trigger new sets of donor T cells into a GVHR. Some viruses may also induce the development of autoreactive lymphocytes and some may contribute to immunodeficiency in GVHD.

As a consequence of the GVHR, the usual lesions of the skin, GI tract, liver, and to some extent other organs, develop during GVHD. It is generally assumed that these lesions are caused by alloaggressive cells generated in the GVHR, and I suspect that to some extent this is true, but this certainly is not proven. In view of the complexity of GVHD, we should remember that there are other mechanisms that might account for these lesions. It is noteworthy that GVHR can lead to neoplasia in mice under certain circumstances. To my knowledge, this has not been described as a consequence of GVHR in irradiated recipients of allogeneic marrow.

An important point I want to make is that although the GVHR is a necessary trigger for the development of GVHD, this progression is not inevitable. Since we are here concerned with bone marrow transplantation, it is GVHD to which we direct our attention. I want, therefore, to consider the variables that regulate the development of GVHD.

The first is, of course, the intensity of the primary event, the GVHR. If all other factors are kept constant, the intensity of GVHD will be controlled by the immunogenetic disparity between the donor and host, the number of T cells injected, and the immune status of the donor. If the donor has been rendered specifically tolerant of host alloantigens by injection with host type bone marrow at birth, his T cells will be specifically unresponsive when tested in a GVH assay against such hosts. Moreover, preimmunization of an adult donor increases the capacity of his lymphocytes to induce GVHD.

A second important variable is the conditioning regimen used prior to inoculation of donor cells. As Trentin and others showed years ago, one can inoculate an adult F_1 hybrid mouse with parental lymphoid cells and not see any clinical sign of GVHD, whereas in a sublethally irradiated host the same inoculation causes lethal GVHD. Resistance of the F_1 host to the induction of GVHD by parental cells seems to develop in the third week after birth and as mentioned earlier is an indication that the Hh system may be involved.

We have recently studied parent into F_1 combinations in which different regions of the H-2 complex are the source of the antigenic disparity that could elicit a GVHR. We noticed that genetic disparities that appeared ineffective when the F_1 hosts were conditioned by 400 R total body irradiation, elicited lethal GVHD when Cy (cyclophosphamide, 150 mg/kg) was included in the conditioning regimen. As shown in Table 20, AQR spleen cells failed to induce GVH mortality in (B10.A × AQR)F_1 hosts conditioned by 400 R, but the same cells killed hosts conditioned with Cy plus irradiation. In this combination, genetic

TABLE 20

Relative Importance of Conditioning and Genetic Disparity
on the Induction of GVHD in Parent-to-F_1 Hybrid Combinations

		60-Day mortality in hosts conditioned by	
	Disparity	400 R^a	Cy + 400 R^b
AQR →→ (B10.A × AQR)F_1	H-2K^k	0/7	4/6
Controls^c		1/6	0/5
AQR →→ (6R × AQR)F_1	H-2I^k	1/5	6/6
Controls		1/4	1/6
AQR →→ (B10.A × 6R)F_1	H-2K^k,	4/4	5/5
Controls	H-2I^k	0/3	0/3

^{a}400R TBI from ^{137}Cs source 2 hr before injection of 20 × 10^6 spleen cells i.v.

^{b}Cy, 150 mg/kg day 1; 400 R TBI day 0, cells day 0.

^{c}Drug/radiation controls are uninjected litter and pen mates of experimental mice.

disparity was limited to the H-2K region. Similarly, in the case of disparity in the H-2I region AQR spleen cells induced mortality only in the Cy conditioned (B10.T(6R) × AQR)F_1 hosts. On the other hand, (B10.A × B10.T(6R)F_1 hosts, in which disparity to the injected cells occurred in both K and I regions, conditioning by 400 R sufficed. These results cannot be accounted for in terms of abrogation of genetic resistance of the F_1 to the donor cells by Cy in the first two combinations. For if the resistance was due to Hh genes in the K and I regions, respectively, this should then have been also evident in the third combination. Additional evidence comes from the work of Harrison, who achieved lymphoid repopulation of genetically anemic (CBA × C57BL)F_1·W^vW^x mice by injection of 10 million CBA spleen cells (*Transplantion* **22**:47, 1976).

Despite extensive colonization of the lymphoid system of F_1 hybrids by donor type lymphocytes, there was no sign of acute or chronic GVHD unless the hosts had been previously irradiated. This conditioning fostered the development of acute lethal GVHD in all the hosts.

Now, what are the possible explanations for these conditioning effects? The possibilities are multiple and not mutually exclusive.

First, there is the matter of Hh or genetic resistance to donor lymphocytes. Such resistance can be abrogated by appropriate conditioning regimens, including Cy. While resistance of this type requires more intensive conditioning in some parent-to-F_1 combinations, it does not account for the results given in Table 20, nor does it account for the Harrison experiments. In the latter, it is clear that stem cells from the donor do in fact colonize the spleen, lymph nodes, and thymus without causing GVHD in the nonconditioned host.

Second, perhaps the capacity of the host to mount an antiidiotype response that could control the GVHR is impaired by conditioning procedures.

A third possibility is that the more extensive the destruction of hemopoietic cells of the host, the fewer cells remain capable of tolerizing donor T cells. It has long been known from the studies of Silvers and others that the induction and maintenance of transplantation tolerance depends upon the continuance of hemopoietic chimerism.

A fourth possible mechanism of conditioning is simply that two insults are more pathogenic than one. If we think of the GVHR as providing one insult to the host and the conditioning a second, then the effects on the host may be additive or synergistic.

Just imagine that on a given day the GVH-reactive killer cells have the capacity to destroy 20% of the intestinal epithelium of the host. In the unirradiated situation, the epithelium may be readily regenerated; hence the GVHR is reasonably tolerated. If, however, the host has been previously subjected to total body irradiation, this regenerative capacity is going to be impeded.

In addition to the severity of GVHR and the conditioning regimen, there is another variable, the microbial flora, that determines the severity of GVHD. It is well known that mouse radiation chimeras can be induced across H-2 barriers without development of GVHD, provided these animals are raised and maintained in a germ-free state. It seems likely that the proliferative phase of GVHR occurs in the irradiated germ-free recipient, but that the GVH syndrome does not materialize. There are reasons for believing that bacterial endotoxin is required for the full expression of the GVH syndrome.*

Thus, the GVHR itself seems to be the primary mechanism responsible for GVHD, but it can be well tolerated by the host unless other factors (which we term conditioning) and microbial flora of the intestinal tract intervene. In the clinical situation, of course, all three factors may be operative and it is hard to determine which is dominant in any given case. There are three areas in which the relationship of small animal studies to their clinical counterpart need clarification.

There is the precise role of the activated T cell that mediates GVHR. How long do these cells persist as functional entities in a foreign host and how are they distributed? Do they home to the liver, GI, and skin to cause the lesions that we see there? Certainly there would be little reason to treat patients with immunosuppressive agents designed to control the GVHR if the relevant cells had already set the stage for GVHD, virus activation, etc., and had disappeared. We

---

Editors' footnote: Attention is directed to the extensive discussion of this topic in the *Editors' comment* on pp. 265–266.

need to delineate in patients, as they develop lesions, whether these are in fact being caused by alloaggressive cytotoxic T lymphocytes, or whether some other mechanisms are intervening.

There is also the idea, prevalent among clinicians, that stem cells in the allogeneic recipient retain the capacity to generate GVH-reactive cells over a prolonged period and that these constitute the effectors of chronic GVHD. This notion seems to conflict with the assumption that relatively immature immunocytes are more readily tolerized by antigen. If the assumption is correct, it would be unlikely that chronic GVHD could be mediated in marrow chimeras by the progeny of stem cells differentiating in the host. A practical as well as basic issue is the nature of the alloantigenic stimulation in the case of MHC matched-sibling donor–host pair that confronts the clinician.

Most research still is done in the model with H-2 incompatibility, while not enough attention has been given to disparities at other loci. In man, the latter disparities seem to be particularly troublesome. Storb has indicated that H-Y and H-X (sex associated alloantigens) may be implicated.

This outline is now best extended by Parkman, whose findings provide new approaches to understanding the pathogenesis of the GVHD.

PARKMAN: The acute GVHD is produced by lymphocytes that are the progeny of the donor peripheral lymphocytes infused at the time of the transplant. Chronic GVHD has been assumed to be produced by T lymphocytes that are derived from the newly engrafted lymphoid system. Clinically acute GVHD may be modified by methotrexate and other immunosuppressive agents, the same agents that failed to control chronic GVHD. Five of our long-term survivors of allogeneic bone marrow transplants suffered from chronic GVHD and were refractory to conventional therapy. From studies of these patients we have established that the effector cells in human GVHD are neither mature T nor B lymphocytes, that their cytotoxicity is directed toward "antigens" found in donor as well as recipient cells, and that they are a naturally occurring subpopulation of autocytotoxic cells in most normal individuals. These autocytotoxic cells are normally suppressed by a "regulator" subpopulation that is inadequate for such control in some transplant recipients with acute or chronic GVHD. The regulator cells are most probably of thymus origin. The involuted thymic state of bone marrow transplant recipients may contribute to the pathogenesis of GVHD by decreasing the number of regulator T cells.

The test system we used was a microtiter cytotoxicity assay, employing ^{14}C-amino acid labeled fibroblasts as targets. Cultures of fibroblasts in logarithmic growth were labeled, trypsinized, plated in microtiter wells, and allowed to attach overnight. The medium was replaced with test lymphocyte suspensions and incubated overnight; the plates were then washed and fixed. The residual radioactivity was then a function of the number of cells that remained.

TABLE 21
Cytotoxic Specificity of Lymphocytes from Patients with
Acute GVHD

Lymphocyte source	Residual radioactivity in target fibroblasts (% of control)		
	Recipient 1	Recipient 2	Control
Recipient 1	75.2 ± 9.2	93.5 ± 8.2	84.9 ± 5.8
Donor 1	101.7 ± 3.2	103.0 ± 10.6	96.8 ± 2.7
Recipient 2	69.5 ± 3.4	39.6 ± 4.6	59.1 ± 1.9

In this system, the normal range of residual radioactivity was 80–120% of the medium control. The standard deviation of control wells was about 10% and, therefore, a residual radioactivity of less than 80% (two standard deviations less than controls) represents specific cytotoxicity.

Table 21 shows results typical of those obtained on patients with acute GVHD diagnosed clinically and by skin biopsies. Fibroblast lines were derived from patients before transplantation. They were used within 6–12 tissue culture passages and then discarded. This restriction enabled us to control their lysability and to avoid any effects of long-term culture. Lymphocytes were obtained from recipients undergoing acute GVHD, generally three to four weeks after transplantation. Of course, these recipient lymphocytes are of donor origin after engraftment. Donor lymphocytes were also tested, and donor fibroblasts were used as controls for a different host–donor pair.

There is cytotoxicity on recipient fibroblasts by cells of recipient 1, whereas lymphocytes from the donor were not cytotoxic for any of the target cells. Cells from a second patient (recipient 2) were cytotoxic for all three target lines, but the maximum cytotoxicity was against recipient fibroblasts. We were possibly detecting antigenic differences between donor and recipient, but the donor lymphoid cells acquired reactivity to these antigenic differences only after transplantation. Recipient cell cytotoxicity was specific being directed maximally against recipient (i.e., host) rather than unrelated cells. The lymphocytes of all our patients were 100% of donor origin.

GALE: Did Parkman have a control that doesn't have acute GVHD?

PARKMAN: Recipients with no clinocal GVHD or grade 1 have been negative, whereas patients who by the Seattle criteria had grade 2 or greater skin GVHD have been positive in this assay. Thus far we have encountered only one patient in whom there was not a positive correlation between lymphocytes cytotoxic for recipient fibroblasts and a positive skin biopsy.

WARNER: Would Parkman indicate precisely what constitutes a significant difference from controls in this assay.

PARKMAN: It is a question of how one defines positivity. We have chosen to define a normal range rather than determine the significance of each pair of values.

WARNER: Another variation in cytotoxicity test could be the susceptibility of individual fibroblast lines to release chromium.

PARKMAN: I agree. That is why the finding in Table 21 that control fibro-blasts are lysed by patient 2 is important. It shows that the lack of lysis by patient 1 and donor 1 is not a function of the target fibroblasts being unlysable.

I would now like to proceed to more general aspects of the method. The cytotoxic cells from patients with acute GVHD do not form E rosettes, do form EAC3 rosettes, and do not adhere to either cotton or nylon. Rabbit antithymocyte serum, effective in the clinical treatment of GVHD, inhibits cytotoxic lympho-cytes at a dilution of 1/1000 without complement. It should not be inferred from such inhibition that the effector cell is a T cell, but only that this reagent has a large amount of antispecies antibody. The GVH effector cell is neither a mature T nor B lymphocyte. Separation of these cells on a discontinuous bovine serum albumin gradient yields the effector cells in the middle fractions.

Most patients with severe chronic GVHD displayed cytotoxicity by unfrac-tionated lymphocytes against recipient target fibroblasts. The middle layer of the gradient (fraction 2), which represents 70–80% of the total, contained cells that not only were cytotoxic for recipient, but also for donor fibroblasts (Table 22). Donor cells separated on the same discontinuous gradient also yielded a fraction that was lytic for both recipient and donor fibroblasts.

GOLUB: What are Parkman's findings when he tests normal people?

PARKMAN: Well, the donor *is* a normal person. Patients with chronic GVHD contained a subpopulation of lymphocytes that was cytotoxic for the recipient and the donor fibroblasts. Therefore, the target antigen was not a recipient antigen absent from the donor. Cytotoxic lymphocytes are also present in normal individuals.

WARNER: Parkman's data imply that there is a suppression phenomenon in-asmuch as he has separated two cell types (the effectors of cytotoxicity and their

TABLE 22

In vitro Cytotoxicity for Fibroblasts of Donor and
Recipient Blood Lymphocytes[a]

	Residual radioactivity of target fibroblasts (%)	
Lymphocytes	Recipient	Donor
Recipient		
Unfractionated	99.1 ± 7.6	98.7 ± 4.3
Fraction 1	100.6 ± 10.2	95.8 ± 8.5
Fraction 2	75.9 ± 10.6	71.4 ± 4.0
Fraction 3	83.0 ± 4.0	81.3 ± 5.4
Donor		
Unfractionated	96.0 ± 6.3	106.7 ± 6.4
Fraction 1	95.7 ± 5.4	88.5 ± 2.4
Fraction 2	54.8 ± 7.2	38.2 ± 7.6
Fraction 3	71.6 ± 8.9	66.2 ± 3.9

[a]Recipients undergoing mild chronic GVHD.

suppressors). Might he not have instead only concentrated the effector cells in the particular fraction?

PARKMAN: All assays were done at 100:1 effector:target cell ratio. Fraction 2 represents 70–80% of the cells in the gradient. If the number of unfractionated cells used in the assay is doubled no cytotoxicity is detected. Therefore, the fractionation does not simply result in concentration of effectors. We believe that we are removing a suppressor cell regulating the cytotoxicity in the native population.

GOLUB: I don't understand why the cells in fraction 2 of this donor are reacting with himself.

PARKMAN: One would have to consider that fraction 2 cells are "autocytotoxic."

GOLUB: Or else, it could be that Parkman's assay is not measuring what he believes it is measuring.

PARKMAN: The other alternatives are whether we are detecting a fetal calf serum antigen, whether there is antihistocompatibility antibody in the serum, and whether the fractionation procedures activate nonspecifically the fraction 2 cells.

The fraction 2 cells of an individual can be cytotoxic for his own fibroblasts, as well as cytotoxic for allogeneic fibroblasts. Allogeneic lines can be found that are not lysed at a frequency of about one in four. Therefore, the cytotoxicity of fraction 2 cells does not reflect nonspecific activation nor does it represent an immune reaction to acquired antigens.

GOLUB: So Parkman's proposition is really that there is an autoreactive population and that there is also some distribution of these antigens in the population. Doesn't this complicate the use of his test for diagnostic purposes?

PARKMAN: No, I don't think so. We are asking the test to tell us whether the *unfractionated* cells from GVHD patients produce lysis as opposed to the *fractionated* cells from normal individuals.

When the unfractionated and fractionated lymphocytes of normal individuals are assayed against autologous fibroblasts, the fraction 2 cells of approximately 50% of normal individuals lyse autologous fibroblasts, whereas their unfractionated cells are inactive (Table 23). Although the cells in Fraction 2 are predominantly T cells, the autocytotoxic cell is not removed by E rosette formation, and by passage through cotton or nylon, but is blocked by aggregated gamma globulin, and is removed by EAC3 rosette formation. It thus appears that the autocytotoxic cell of normal individuals is not a mature T or B lymphocyte. It has surface characteristics in common with the cytotoxic cell of patients with

TABLE 23

In vitro Cytotoxicity for Autologous Fibroblasts of Unfractionated and BSA Gradient Fractionated Normal Peripheral Blood Lymphocytes[a]

Age of donor (yr)	Residual radioactivity ± 1 S.D. (%)			
	Unfractionated	Fraction 1	Fraction 2	Fraction 3
12	99.7 ± 13.4	99.2 ± 2.0	*66.0 ± 7.0*	89.9 ± 9.6
15	106.7 ± 6.4	88.5 ± 2.4	*38.2 ± 7.6*	*66.2 ± 3.9*
15	86.3 ± 16.6	*74.7 ± 2.5*	*50.6 ± 6.0*	101.6 ± 23.5
3	85.5 ± 7.5	105.4 ± 9.4	*75.1 ± 7.7*	93.1 ± 2.4
9	112.9 ± 7.8	113.0 ± 4.0	82.2 ± 9.4	96.9 ± 12.1
45	113.7 ± 18.4	110.3 ± 6.5	114.4 ± 16.2	98.9 ± 9.4
24	93.5 ± 6.6	126.6 ± 9.3	107.2 ± 7.3	111.6 ± 8.6

[a]Lymphocytes were assayed overnight at a 100:1 ratio with 1000 ^{14}C-amino acid prelabeled autologous fibroblasts in microtiter tissue culture plates. The plates were washed three times in HBSS, fixed, and the residual radioactivity determined. 100% equals residual radioactivity in control wells incubated with medium alone. Italic values represent significant cytotoxicity.

acute and chronic GVHD. We advance the proposition that GVHD may involve a relative excess of these autocytotoxic cells.

BACH: Parkman says that on the average one of four allogeneic fibroblast lines will not lyse. Is there any pattern to this finding? Has he examined enough different individuals to establish genetic control?

PARKMAN: There is no correlation between HLA types and fibroblast susceptibility to lysis. Family studies were not done.

GALE: Obviously, fibroblasts are not the target in GVHD. Therefore, Parkman's test is difficult to relate to the pathogenesis of this syndrome.

PARKMAN: We chose fibroblasts because they are one of the few cell types we could establish as lines from recipients of transplants. Admittedly, this choice was partly of necessity.

The issue of correlation between the naturally occurring autocytotoxic cell and the cells that are causing GVHD continues to surface. If conclusions had to be based entirely on human studies, it would be exceedingly difficult to answer. However, we have been able to establish a mouse model. BSA gradient-separated spleen cells from normal C57BL/6 mice yield a lymphocyte subpopulation strikingly similar to the human fraction 2 population. When the BSA-fractionated cells are injected into either neonates or into older animals partially immunosuppressed by sublethal irradiation or cytoxan, a disease ensues that is microscopically and clinically analogous to allogeneic GVHD. Thus, we have an animal model providing cells that are cytotoxic *in vitro* for syngeneic fibroblasts and that are capable of producing what we call "syngeneic GVH" in C57BL mice in the course of three to four weeks.

EIJSVOOGEL: In our Institute, Hall has been studying a similar phenomenon with the Tagasuki–Klein method. In six of seven patients, there were cytotoxic or cytostatic cells at certain periods. However, there seemed to be no correlation between positive reactions and GVHD. It is, however, noteworthy that a number of these patients have been decontaminated, and this might account for the absence of clinical GVH despite *in vitro* cytotoxicity.

WIGZELL: I would add a comment about this kind of naturally occurring cell in man. It has been known for some time from the work of Jondal and Svedwyn that in man such a cell has the C3b receptor. These workers sought specific cytotoxic cells in the blood of infectious mononucleosis patients. It turned out that these patients and normal human subjects have in their blood natural killer cells acting against a variety of human and mouse cell lines. Leukocytes of certain donors were particularly prone to kill some cell lines but not others. To find specificity in these reactions, C3b-positive cells had to be removed, because they were providing noise-making background. Once removed, specific cytolytic T killer cells were demonstrable during the acute phase of infectious mononucleosis. I therefore question whether Parkman has really shown specificity by his test.

PARKMAN: I think that one person's noise is another person's specificity. In Jondal's assay it was interfering, but that does not mean that in another system it would not have biological significance. We believe that in acute GVHD there is a positive correlation between fibroblast lysis and clinical state.

FESTENSTEIN: Parkman alluded to work on an experimental mouse model. Surely, that is where the question of specificity can be resolved. Would he comment on that?

PARKMAN: In the mouse model, we *do* have specificity as the fibroblast lysis is restricted. We have not done studies with recombinants, but the cytotoxicity is restricted to the syngeneic targets.

FESTENSTEIN: In genetic terms, what does Parkman view as the target in the syngeneic animal?

PARKMAN: I would have to assume it is an autoantigen.

VAN BEKKUM: I think these interesting results of Parkman perhaps do have biological support. I would point out that we and others have shown multiple evidence for autoimmune aggression in neonatally thymectomized mice. Many years ago we described so-called isogeneic secondary disease, which occurs only if recipients are conditioned with a dose of irradiation over 1000 rad. This had been attributed to a partial deficiency of the irradiated thymus, but I think that the suppressor cell of autoaggression that Parkman described is surely thymus-derived or influenced.

CHAIRMAN ELKINS: So, we have the possibility that the GVHR may in some way trigger the autocytotoxic cell, which has completely different specificity. This triggering could be direct or it could operate by eliminating the suppressor cell that normally controls it. Moreover, as Van Bekkum points out, this whole sequence could take place in a syngeneic system if one simply did something (excessive irradiation) that impaired the suppressor T cell.

STORB: If Parkman's model is correct, one should expect similar events in the syngeneic or autologous situation. However, in the course of some 45 transplants of this type, none showed signs of GVHD.*

GOLUB: It is in the allogeneic system and in the presence of GVHD that the suppressor cell is gone. The effector cell, if fractionated from normal individuals (which would be analogous to syngeneic recipients) is able, in the isolated fraction, to carry out its lytic function, but in the presence of other cells (unfractionated) it cannot.

CHAIRMAN ELKINS: As to Storb's query, it is undoubtedly unusual to get the GVHD in syngeneic transplants. We are really saying that the final endpoint, the GVH syndrome, is essentially a nonspecific one, and can be brought about by several means, perhaps the most efficient being GVHR.

PARKMAN: The autocytotoxic cell is independent of thymic function in its ontogeny. On the other hand, the regulator or suppressor cell in the mouse model and in man appears to be thymus-derived. Our view is that in the transplant recipient there is a decrease in thymic humoral function secondary to age of the recipient, to conditioning regime, to infection, and to preceding T cell-mediated GVHR. This decreased thymic function may delay the appearance of adequate numbers of the regulator T cells. Because of the reduced numbers of regulator T cells, there is a relative excess of autocytotoxic cells which then contributes to the GVHD.

Thus, a hypothymic state leads to a decrease or a delay in the appearance of adequate numbers of regulator T cells in transplant recipients required to reestablish the normal control of the autocytotoxic cell.

WARNER: It would be of interest to determine if the effector cell obtained from the patient with GVH can be suppressed. One should be able to take these cells and add the appropriate fraction from normal individuals and suppress cytotoxicity.

CHAIRMAN ELKINS: We shall now move on to have Sprent develop for us the idea that stem cells of donor origin can mature to GVH reactivity in the allogeneic recipient.

Editors' comment: It should be noted that there *are* circumstances in which a wasting syndrome can follow transplantation of syngeneic marrow. The critical circumstance, described by Loutit *et al.*, is that the number of marrow cells be inadequate for reconstitution. Remarkably enough, such GVHD can be counteracted by transfer of lymphocytes apparently devoid of pluripotent stem cells.

SPRENT: I want to briefly summarize the experiences of von Boehmer, Nabholz, and myself in exploring the antihost reactivity of T cells recovered from allogeneic radiation bone marrow chimeras. We made two types of chimeras, and I shall be referring mostly to "single" chimeras, which we prepared by injecting large numbers (2×10^7) of bone marrow cells treated with anti-Thy-1 serum into heavily irradiated (900 rads) F_1 mice. All of our work has been with semiallogeneic combinations.

We used a variety of strains such as CBA and C57BL, CBA and DBA/2, and C3H and SJL. The chimeras remained in excellent health after irradiation and we saw very few deaths attributable to GVHD for up to two years.

We tested the ability of spleen cells of the chimeras to stimulate normal responder T cells of donor type. Spleen cells from the chimeras were nonstimulatory in MLC. We tested the reactivity of T cells from the chimeras as responders in MLC, CML, and GVH. The experiments were designed to test the hypothesis that the determinants responsible for stimulating the MLC are restricted to hemopoietic cells. It was reasoned that if the host were lethally irradiated, the hemopoietic cells and their progenitors would be destroyed. If that were the case, the stem cells of donor origin migrating into the thymus and then producing peripheral T cells would not meet host-type hemopoietic cells; their reactivity to these determinants would therefore not be deleted. Thus, the parent-to-F_1 chimeras should eventually contain parental cells capable of responding in MLC to cells from normal mice syngeneic with the host.

This is, in fact, what we found. There was indeed a response to host-type alloantigens in MLC, although this was in the range of only 5–30% of normal. On occasion, we found no antihost reactivity. The reactivity to third-party determinants was either normal or slightly less.

Surprisingly, we found no GVH reactivity as assayed by cell transfer of 3×10^7 spleen cells from the chimeras into sublethally irradiated mice.

As far as CML is concerned, the assumption was that the determinants responsible for stimulating the development of cytotoxic cells would not have been eliminated by irradiation, since these determinants presumably are present on virtually all cells. Therefore, differentiating parental T cells should have met these determinants, and this encounter should have resulted in deletion of reactive cells. As predicted, chimeras contained no cells capable of generating killers against host-type targets. Reactivity against third-party determinants, however, was normal. The serum of the chimeras had blocking activity. Moreover, the culturing of cells from the chimeras with normal cells of donor type provided no evidence that the development of killer cells was suppressed.

We concluded that the MLC–CML dichotomy in reactivity against host-type determinants was consistent with the hypothesis of deletion and of selective expression of MLC and CML determinants. There are two explanations for the antihost reactivity in MLC being considerably less than normal. First, that MLC determinants might not be restricted entirely to hemopoietic cells; second, that irradiation did not completely destroy the host's hemopoietic cells.

We prepared "tetra-parental" bone marrow chimeras (or "double" chimeras, as I prefer to call them) by injecting simultaneously bone marrow cells from both parents. In this situation we found that the nonreactivity against host-type determinants occurred not only for CML but also for MLC. Our explanation was that in this model, MLC determinants of the opposite parental strain were present, ensuring complete deletion of reactive cells to "host-type" MLC determinants.

As for the presence of antihost reactivity in MLC in the single chimeras, the question remains of whether parental differentiating T cells can still produce subacute or chronic GVHR that we did not detect. I should emphasize that we have not investigated this question very thoroughly.

FESTENSTEIN: Sprent's presumption about the elimination of LD-bearing cells assumes that only hemopoietic cells are carrying these determinants. But there is evidence that other cells such as macrophages have these determinants as well.

SPRENT: The functional tests performed at six months postirradiation would argue for complete replacement of host macrophages by donor-type macrophages. On the other hand, the fact that antihost reactivity was less than normal could mean persistence of radioresistant macrophages.

FESTENSTEIN: In our own experiments with tetra-parental chimeras we could also demonstrate dissociation between MLC and GVHR. In our mice the GVHR was reduced to zero, whereas the MLC was essentially normal. We concluded that there were different clones of T cells being activated for MLC and GVHR.

SPRENT: I wonder whether the persistence of MLC reactivity might be explained by low-affinity cells that were not deleted. Such cells would be incapable of producing a GVHR because of the low affinity, while still capable of responding in culture.

WARNER: The critical issue is how to prevent GVHR. These data of Sprent clearly show that if T cells are removed from bone marrow, no GVHR is induced, nor is there any evidence of maturation into GVH effector cells. According to Van Bekkum, one could remove T cells and still get chronic GVHD. What then is the difference between these situations? Is it that in mice minor H loci, for example, can stimulate a response even from immature T cells? Are we therefore perhaps distinguishing between the ability of cells to be tolerized by different types of antigens, e.g., products of major vs. minor H loci?

VAN BEKKUM: Löwenberg purified stem cell fractions of mouse bone marrow and of mouse fetal liver of the same strain, and compared these preparations
on the basis of the absolute number of CFU-S present. The strain combination
was C57BL into CBA. The same type of GVHD occurs after injecting these
cells, i.e., the delayed GVHD starting at 30 and ending at 90 days. However,
there is a difference in the incidence and severity of the GVHD induced by
fetal-liver-derived stem cell vs. bone-marrow-derived stem cell transplants.

WARNER: Can one be sure that there are not T cells still present in the
CFU-enriched fraction of bone marrow? It is surely not a pure CFU population.
One would have to use an anti-Thy-1 serum-treated fraction to ensure that con-
taminating T cells were not inducing the chronic disease.

SPRENT: With regard to Warner's previous question, one can use CBA marrow without anti-Thy-1 treatment because there are very few T cells in this
marrow. But should one add only 2×10^5 lymph node cells, then nearly all of the
mice die from GVH disease.

TRENTIN: If one repopulates the irradiated mouse with allogeneic bone marrow, there is no acute GVHD, whereas allogeneic bone marrow plus spleen
yields acute disease with 100% mortality at 14 days. Unlike human marrow,
there are insufficient T cells in murine marrow to give acute GVHD. During the
second month, as a result of differentiation of T cells from stem cells, GVH
mortality ensues. At 60 days GVHD abates and the mortality curve stops rising
because of spontaneous onset of some kind of an adaptive mechanism (originally
called tolerance) by which donor-derived lymphocytes tested by *in vivo* assays
were no longer reactive against the host. We now know that, by *in vitro* assays,
they *are* still reactive against host cells. There are claims that either suppressor
cells or blocking antibodies are responsible.

CHAIRMAN ELKINS: To relate Trentin's and Sprent's comments, it seems to
me that there are at least two mechanisms for GVH tolerance: (1) an active
suppression of the development of T cells competent to initiate GVHR and (2) a
true tolerization (i.e., clonal deletion) of the T cells maturing toward competence
in the allogeneic environment. The distinction is between the descendents of
antigen-stimulated *mature* T cells and the descendents of immature, incompetent
precursors, rather than between early and late GVHD.

TRENTIN: In my view, the decline of chronic GVHD is not due to clonal
deletion, since donor lymphocytes are still present and by appropriate *in vitro*
tests can be shown to be still reactive against the host. They are either blocked by
antibody or suppressed by suppressor cells.

GALE: I propose that we now turn to the problem of GVHD in patients grafted with marrow from MHC compatible siblings. Opelz and I have investigated whether MLC reactivity is acquired in the course of GVHD. The experiment was to cryopreserve recipient cells before the transplant. When patients developed GVHD, the circulating donor-derived cells were tested in MLC against the frozen pretransplant recipient cells. In more than ten patients, we have not found acquisition of MLC reactivity. These donor-derived cells have a normal MLC reactivity against third-party stimulator cells, and are themselves competent stimulator cells. Thus, *in vivo* sensitization and development of GVHD did not lead to acquisition of antirecipient MLC reactivity.

The MLC system was investigated kinetically but there was no acceleration. We have not excluded the possibility that a clone of reactive cells is expanded to the point of being exhausted. It is also possible that the peripheral blood is not the appropriate site to look for GVH reactive cells if the key reactions are taking place in the skin, GI tract, and liver.

To establish whether circulating donor-derived cells have proliferative potential and whether this correlated with GVHD, Opelz and I examined spontaneous DNA synthesis in lymphocytes from transplant patients at various times. The cells were incubated overnight with ^{3}H-TdR. ^{3}H-TdR incorporation of leukocytes from 20 transplant patients as a group was considerably higher than that of 20 controls.

FESTENSTEIN: Has Gale excluded the possibility of contaminating myeloid cells incorporating ^{3}H-TdR?

GALE: We used peripheral blood mononuclear cells (predominantly lymphocytes and monocytes) without identifiable granulocytes or granulocytic precursors. The incidence of circulating CFU-C is very low in man. Myeloid precursors are therefore an unlikely explanation of these findings.

When these data were analyzed with regard to the presence or absence of GVHD, no correlation was found, even if we tried various cutoff levels of ^{3}H-TdR incorporation.

MACROPHAGE HETEROGENEITY:
ROLE IN HEMOPOIESIS AND CYTOTOXICITY
FOR NORMAL AND NEOPLASTIC TARGETS

Discussion Introducer:

Malcolm A. S. Moore

CHAIRMAN MOORE: Macrophage-like cells have recently been implicated as effectors or accessory cells in a number of natural host defense systems including antitumor, antimicrobial, and anti-Hh responses. Moreover, this kind of cell has also been involved in regulating lymphocyte and stem cell proliferation. We shall therefore be exploring several critical areas of macrophage physiology. The first area relates to the development, regulation of production, and heterogeneity of phagocytic mononuclear cells. The term "phagocytic mononuclear" cell may be preferable to macrophage, since many cell types we are concerned with may be in the macrophage lineage rather than typical macrophages. The second area is the role of macrophages in hemopoietic regulation, specifically their involvement both in lymphopoiesis and in myelopoiesis in a stimulatory sense. The final area would be the cytostatic or cytotoxic function of macrophages, specifically the tumoricidal role of activated macrophages. The question of the role of macrophage function in Hh resistance involves the second as well as the third area.

To begin with, we shall consider the life history of macrophages as we understand it using techniques of *in vitro* culture. The favored hypothesis for the generation of monocytes and macrophages recognizes that their committed progenitor cell is the CFU-C, which derives from the multipotential stem cell. The *in vitro* CFU-C represents a "black box" situation because it is heterogeneous in terms of giving rise to macrophages, monocytes, and neutrophilic granulocytes, or of certain subpopulations of CFU-C being restricted to only neutrophilic, or eosinophilic, or only macrophage differentiation. Later Metcalf will address the issue of heterogeneity in this compartment as well as heterogeneity among colony-stimulating factors (CSF) required for the proliferation and differentiation of this granulocyte–macrophage progenitor compartment.

The biochemistry of CSF is presently under extensive investigation. Here, too, they are heterogeneous in terms of their biochemical characteristics and their functional properties. Although it is somewhat peripheral to this conference, we may discuss this topic in more detail.

Thus, we have a cell, called the CFU-PM (CFU peritoneal macrophage) described by Lin and Stewart two or three years ago. Their work provided an assay for a cell type, originally described in the peritoneal exudate of mice, that forms colonies of macrophages.

The CFU-PM is itself a macrophage or macrophage precursor with adherence properties and is elicited by agents such as thioglycolate or BCG. Approximately 5% of the cells in an activated peritoneal exudate are capable of proliferating to form colonies of some hundreds of macrophages. We have recently observed that the CFU-C in culture generate CFU-PM. We actually have a system here where one CFU-C can give rise in a period of seven days to some 1000 macrophages. Of these 1000 macrophages, a proportion are capable of yet further extensive proliferation to yield an additional 200-fold or so amplification of macrophage production.

Again, the proliferation of CFU-PM is dependent on the presence of CSF. It is noteworthy that a higher concentration is required to initiate proliferation of macrophages than to promote proliferation of the progenitor cell. In this context, CSFs also proved to be mitogenic agents for macrophages. A factor identified by Defendi, which initiates DNA synthesis in macrophages, turns out to be identical to CSF.

The emphasis in this area is progressing from initial concern with the bone marrow stem cell compartment to recognition that CSFs are important in initiating or sustaining macrophage proliferation in diverse sites, e.g., alveolar macrophages, Kupffer cells, and possibly the fixed-tissue macrophages in spleen and bone marrow.

As I shall shortly affirm, the effect of CSF on macrophages also involves activation. The functional state of the cells in terms of their cytostatic or cytotoxic capacity is markedly dependent on the concentration of stimulating factor to which they are exposed.

The intriguing aspect of regulation of monocyte-macrophage production is that one of the major sources of CSF happens to be the monocyte–macrophage population itself. So, we have indications of a positive feedback mechanism by which products of the end-cell are responsible for recruitment from the stem cell compartment as well as for initiating proliferation within the macrophage compartment.

We have done studies incubating human monocytes for varying periods of time, measuring their production of CSF and observed that within the first one to two weeks of incubation, two species of CSF were produced. One was active on both mouse and human bone marrow; the other species (of higher molecular weight) was active only on mouse marrow and was therefore not a human CSF. As the cells transformed in culture from monocytes to macrophages, production of human active CSF ceased, but the cells continued to produce large quantities of a CSF for mouse bone marrow.

This sort of finding gives us an idea of mechanism by which positive feedback drive is self-limiting. It raises the intriguing biological question of why human macrophages devote so much effort to producing a molecule that is apparently active only for the mouse.

This goes back to the matter of CSF as a macrophage-activating agent. While this mouse-active CSF does not stimulate human bone marrow, it does cause human macrophages to proliferate, and also greatly activates them as measured, for example, by their listeriacidal capacity. This may be an area of considerable importance in attaining an understanding of effector functions of macrophages.

Another area is the role of the granulocyte. Granulocyte chalone, for example, is a mythical beast that has been claimed by a number of groups to mediate a negative feedback acting at the level of the committed stem cell. We have shown that a granulocyte-derived factor acts at the level of the macrophage, suppressing its capacity to produce CSF. This is one control mechanism that would serve to limit overproduction of granulocytes and macrophages based on modulation of CSF production. It is possible that this granulocyte suppression of the macrophage function may extend to macrophage properties beyond their CSF production.

Now we come to the area where we deal with the problems of defining the role of macrophages in promoting hemopoietic cell differentiation and inhibiting hemopoiesis. I would like to illustrate the kind of experimental data that indicate the functional properties of macrophages both in stimulation and in inhibition.

Since the macrophage produces CSF, if one simply takes mouse peritoneal exudate cells as a monolayer overlayed with mouse bone marrow in soft agar, the peritoneal cells release CSF as a function of cell concentration, and stimulate colony formation in the target bone marrow. However, as the number of macrophages are increased, colony formation declines and at high macrophage concentrations, in fact, drops to zero. This is the sort of observation made frequently when working with added macrophages, be it to cultures of lymphocytes or to cultures of bone marrow cells. At one ratio of macrophages to target cells enhancement occurs, at another ratio, inhibition. In this system of opposing effects the stimulating activity involves CSF, and the inhibitory activity is believed to be prostaglandin produced by macrophages.

Synthetic prostaglandins of the E series produce a profound inhibition of proliferation of granulocytes, macrophages, and T and B lymphocytes. Indomethacin, a potent inhibitor of prostaglandin synthesis, markedly enhances the capacity of feeder macrophages to stimulate colony formation, presumably by inhibiting the synthesis of prostaglandin. The latter is an antagonist of the stimulatory action of CSF.

We have investigated the role of prostaglandin in natural suppressor cell function. Figure 9 shows the relationship between concentration of human blood mononuclear cells and the stimulation of granulocyte–macrophage colony formation by a target population of normal human bone marrow. As the number of mononuclear cells is increased, there is first enhanced stimulation of granulocytic colony formation, but this declines at higher concentrations of mononuclear cells. When we add indomethacin to the mononuclear cell feeder layer, the number of colonies stimulated in the marrow is a linear function of the number of mononuclear cells in the feeder layer. What we are observing here is the production of CSF by the blood monocytes and, at certain concentrations, its inhibition by the release of prostaglandins.

The factors released by mature granulocytes that inhibit CSF production by macrophages also suppress colony stimulation by indomethacin-treated mononuclear cells. Thus, we have here two inhibitory mechanisms, one acting at the level of CSF production and the other (the prostaglandin mechanism) acting at the level of the target cell.

Nonadherent cells in human peripheral blood do not produce detectable

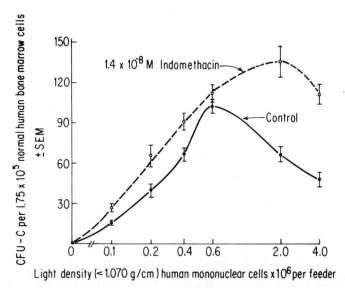

Fig. 9 Human granulocyte colony formation in a two-layer agar culture system with varying numbers of blood mononuclear cells in a feeder layer as a source of CSF. Note the reduction in colony incidence at higher concentration of mononuclear cells on the enhanced stimulation in the presence of the prostaglandin synthesis inhibition by indomethacin.

prostaglandin. Antagonism between release of stimulatory and inhibitory molecules by macrophages extends also to B lymphocytes cloned in agar cultures of mouse spleen cells. When the adherent cells are removed from mouse spleen (Sephadex G10 filtration) or depleted, there is a marked reduction in the number of B lymphocyte colonies developing relative to the native spleen cell population. The addition of macrophages restores to normal the response of the depleted spleen cells. However, as the number of macrophages is increased, a profound suppression of B lymphocyte colony formation is seen, which here too can be overcome by treating the macrophages with indomethacin to eliminate their prostaglandin synthetic capacity.

Turning to the cytostatic or cytotoxic function of macrophages, there are two main issues. One is to define a mechanism that might be tumor cell specific in the sense of antineoplastic rather than generally antiproliferative. Hibbs will tell us more about that particular area, but I shall discuss macrophage-mediated cytostasis because I think this is probably more relevant to the macrophage role in hemopoietic graft resistance *in vivo*.

We used a colony inhibition assay in which leukemic cell lines have been cloned in agar over a basal layer containing thioglycolate-activated mouse peritoneal macrophages. All cell lines tested were sensitive to macrophage inhibition as measured by marked reduction in their cloning capacity. Now, this didn't tell us whether this inhibition was cytostatic or truly cytotoxic. So, we employed the technique of cytofluorometric analysis of tumor target cells using acridine orange to actually monitor directly the DNA and RNA content of the target cell population after incubation with macrophages.

Figure 10 shows that we are indeed dealing with a cytostatic block of tumor cells—in this instance a human and a mouse T cell lymphoma and a mouse myelomonocytic leukemia. The profile of distribution of the leukemic cells in various stages of the cell cycle is shown for control cells in exponential growth (continuous line) and for cells after 48 hr incubation with activated macrophages. After incubation with macrophages, the S phase population was greatly depleted, and cells of one line were blocked in the G_1 phase of the cycle. The EL-4 cells were blocked in the G_2 phase of the cell cycle, and cells of the third line were blocked in G_0.

We therefore have blocks in at least three stages of the cell cycle depending on the type of target cell. These blocks are reversible to varying degree, and I think some of the methodologic problems of demonstrating the specificity of macrophage inhibition of neoplastic cells vs. normal cells can be explained by the degree to which the cells that are placed in a cytostatic block can reverse the cytostasis. Certainly, in some of these leukemic cell lines the cytostatic block is not readily reversible, and it would appear, therefore, that we have an element of specificity whereby the macrophage may particularly suppress leukemic cell proliferation.

I want now to relate what I have said about CSF as an important macrophage-activating principle to the fact that prostaglandin production by this cell may represent the mediation of cytostasis. We have measured via a radioimmunoassay the quantity of prostaglandin produced by peritoneal macrophages, incubated in the absence of CSF. Under these basal conditions, 300 pg of prostaglandin is generated per million macrophages during an incubation period of 40 hr. If we add to the macrophages increasing concentrations of CSF, there is a 10- to 20-fold increase in prostaglandin production, a level sufficient to completely suppress proliferation of lymphoid, granulocytic, and macrophage elements.

With this background, we may now proceed to discuss the three areas I have outlined.

BENNETT: Doesn't prostaglandin inhibit the erythroid elements as well? If I am not mistaken, PGE (prostaglandin E) is known as a stimulator of erythropoiesis.

CHAIRMAN MOORE: PGE markedly increases erythropoietin production and potentiates the action of erythropoietin at the level of the CFU-E, a progenitor of the erythroid series. So we see an opposite effect, the prostaglandins inhibiting granulopoiesis but enhancing erythropoiesis. However, the question remains as

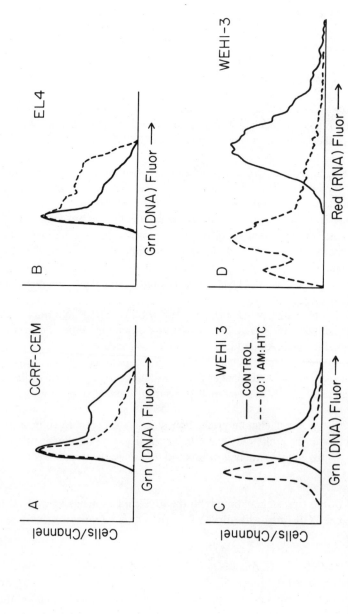

Fig. 10 DNA histograms of leukemic cell lines growing in the presence (- -) or absence (——) of the adherent peritoneal macrophages at a macrophage to tumor cell ratio of 10:1. Analysis performed by flow cytofluorimetry of acridine-orange-stained cells. CCRF-CEM is a human T-cell leukemia line; EL-4, a murine T-cell lymphoma; and WEHI-3, a murine myelomonocytic leukemia cell line. The RNA fluorescence histograms of WEHI-3 cells are shown in D. The histograms have been normalized to the height of the major peak for ease of comparison.

to prostaglandin action at earlier stages of erythroid development, namely, the BFU-E (burst-forming unit), which is more akin to the CFU-C as regards level of differentiation. To my knowledge, there are no data available as to whether prostaglandin enhances or inhibits BFU-E proliferation.

WARNER: Regarding heterogeniety of macrophages and the factors they produce, is it clear whether all the different kinds of macrophages that we recognize are producing PGE? Does PGE production occur only in the terminal stage of macrophage differentiation?

CHAIRMAN MOORE: The production of prostaglandin is one that is modulated, which is to say that at various times in the life history of the macrophage it can either be an active producer or nonproducer. So, we cannot answer the question whether there are subsets of macrophages with totally different functions or whether in a population of macrophages, some cells are activated to produce prostaglandin and others not.

As far as we have been able to establish, all macrophage populations, be they alveolar, peritoneal, or splenic, are capable of producing prostaglandin and the other factors I have described such as CSF and B cell stimulatory activity.

HIBBS: Using the CFU-PM assay, Stewart and I obtained colonies derived from peritoneal cells and found that these colonies, exposed to lymphocyte-mediator-rich supernatants, all develop nonspecific tumoricidal potential. Therefore, there was no evident functional heterogeneity among individual colonies derived from peritoneal macrophages.

CHAIRMAN MOORE: There have been a number of studies on the effect of lymphokines on macrophages. Hibbs has given us an example of one of them. We have looked at numerous sources of lymphokines, mitogen-stimulated lymphocyte products, for example. All of them contain CSF. I have yet to see an experiment in which activation of the macrophages by a lymphokine preparation was not accounted for by its content of CSF.

BACH: How well is CSF defined at present or are there many molecules that can also fulfill this function?

METCALF: If Bach is asking if any old molecule will stimulate CFU-C to proliferate, the answer is no. However, CSF does occur in more than one molecular form. There is moreover, considerable antigenic cross reactivity between those different molecular forms.

If the question is turned around and we ask: Is the action of purified CSF specific? The answer is yes. As Moore said, the historic examples in which a miscellany of procedures has stimulated granulopoiesis and macrophage proliferation, on analysis now all turn out to be situations in which very high levels of CSF production are provoked.

BACH: I do not think that really answers my question. The question, I suppose, would be answered if one had an antiserum to CSF that removed activity from a lymphokine preparation.

METCALF: One can, in fact, completely inactivate CSF with anti-CSF serum. Alternatively, once CSF is removed by fractionation, what remains no longer stimulates proliferation.

ELKINS: Are Moore and Metcalf implying that CSF is responsible for MIF (migration inhibition factor) activity in lymphokine preparations?

CHAIRMAN MOORE: No. We are really talking about crude conditioned media that contain lymphokines such as MIF and will also contain a separate molecule, which is CSF. We should be very careful about the claims we make for this sort of crude soup, because it contains multiple biological activities. What one group would concentrate on as a lymphokine, others would concentrate on as a CSF.

STORB: Does BCG increase not only the number of CFU-PM, but also that of CFU-C?

CHAIRMAN MOORE: Yes, it does indeed. The time course is delayed for CFU-C. I should have indicated that small numbers of CFU-PM are also found in thymus, spleen, and lymph node.

LANDY: Are we prepared to assign major physiological and biochemical functions to CSF activity, or is it essentially trephocytic?

CHAIRMAN MOORE: CSF is an absolute requirement for survival, proliferation, and differentiation *in vitro* of the granulocyte–macrophage series. It is not a simple inducing agent. One cannot briefly expose the progenitor cell to this material and thereby induce differentiation all the way to a mature end cell. The question of a trephocytic role has always been such a hard one to answer, that is, whether an agent is simply required for proliferation and as a consequence of that proliferation, a differentiation sequence results. I do not have an answer to that.

METCALF: To answer that specific question, I think CSF is a specific regulator of granulocyte and macrophage proliferation. I also think it should be regarded essentially as we regard erythropoietin for the red cell series. The situation is a little more complex because the target CFU-C populations are heterogeneous and interrelated in a way we do not quite understand. But erythropoietin and CSF are similar in being neuraminic acid-containing glycoproteins. CSF acts as a proliferative stimulus at the exceedingly low molar concentration of 10^{-11} and has the capacity to quickly induce, like erythropoietin, RNA and protein synthesis in both pre- and postmitotic cells.

WARNER: Given the requirement for these many factors for the complete differentiation and maturation of the hemopoietic cell series, could the conditioning regimes given to recipients of marrow transplants be compromising the sources of these factors?

CHAIRMAN MOORE: Patients with the most severe variants of aplastic anemia, with monocytopenia, are also the patients grossly defective in production of CSF. Such a patient might only be successfully engrafted with a sufficiently large number of donor cells so that hemopoiesis becomes self-starting, thus overcoming the defect in regulator cells that exists.

GALE: Transplant patients are under continuous endotoxin stimulation and receive hundreds of units of blood containing mononuclear cells. Thus, it is unlikely that CSF deficiency is a limiting factor in engraftment.

METCALF: I would like to emphasize two features of the granulocyte-macrophage system that are of particular interest.

The first is the response of the system to microbial products in the course of infection. When endotoxin or endotoxin-containing bacteria are injected into mice, serum and tissue levels of CSF rise very rapidly, reaching a peak within 3–6 hr, and declining over the next 24–48 hr. It is especially noteworthy that in the preimmunized animal exactly the opposite happens on rechallenge. In other words, there is essentially no reactivity, the opposite of what would happen in the immune response.

The CSF response is radioresistant. However, the depressed responsiveness following preimmunization can be broken to a degree by large doses of whole-body irradiation.

The second interesting feature is that in tumor-bearing animals and during GVH reactions, etc., a common pattern of CSF reactivity is seen. The spleen is by far the most reactive organ, followed by the peripheral blood. The bone marrow is a relatively nonreactive organ. Levels of CFU-C rise in the spleen, peaking at about four to seven days, depending on the type of antigen involved, and then decline characteristically. This response will not occur in a preimmunized animal.

In tumor-bearing animals the picture is essentially the same, progenitor cell levels being elevated in the spleen. During rejection of an allogeneic transplantable tumor CFU-C levels rise sharply just prior to and during the actual rejection. This also holds for Moloney-virus-induced sarcoma in C57BL mice, where tumor regression occurs. However, CFU-C are not found in lymph nodes draining the tumor nor in the tumor itself.

The magnitude of these responses to infection and to tumors is quite large. Hundredfold rises both in CSF and spleen CFU-C levels commonly occur. Changes of the same magnitude are seen in mice with GVHD. The response pattern of the CSF–CFU-C axis closely matches many of the features listed by Cudkowicz and characteristic of hemopoietic graft rejection.

There is still another way that proliferation in the granulocyte-macrophage system can be primed. If one stimulates lymphocytes with a mitogen, antigen to which the host has been sensitized, or in MLC, lymphocytes then produce large amounts of CSF. This CSF response includes the type that stimulates neutrophils and macrophages and also the type that stimulates eosinophil and megakaryocyte production. Cell fractionation studies indicate that both T and B lymphocytes are capable of elaborating CSF.

STORB: Can the increased granulopoiesis in GVHR be explained by this excess production of CSF?

METCALF: Yes. However, another possibility is that granulocyte and macrophage precursors may be able themselves to recognize foreignness and respond by proliferation. Now, most are shocked when such a possibility is raised, but I believe that it must be kept in mind. It has been said already that there is heterogeneity in the CFU-C precursor population. I am suggesting that we begin to think about heterogeneity of monocytes and even of granulocytes in the same context as heterogeneity of lymphocytes. McNeill showed in my laboratory that a population of CFU-C from day 10 or day 11 mouse fetal liver, prior to the development of the thymus, was sensitive to antigen. The addition of various antigens to the culture increased colony growth rates and the number of colonies. This is antigen-provoked production of CSF in culture. But which cell in the culture recognized and responded to the antigen? And what sort of antigens will elicit this response by fetal liver cells? The best are bacterial antigens like polymerized flagellin or endotoxin. Now, when an immunologist uses polymerized flagellin, he calls it an antigen. When we do the fetal liver experiment and get proliferation in the granulocyte–macrophage system, this is not viewed as a response to an antigen, but rather a pharmacological effect produced by flagellin.

I still think there is a possibility that cells in the granulocyte–macrophage system, albeit crudely, may be able to recognize some antigens. Whether they do this through their capacity to bind immunoglobulins onto their surface is another matter.

HIBBS: The interest of this conference in macrophage cytotoxicity stems from the findings, albeit indirect, that macrophages—or the macrophage-like cells— are responsible for marrow resistance. In view of the central character of this effector–target relationship, it may be useful briefly to review the state of our present knowledge of the underlying mechanisms by which macrophages kill tumor cells, how macrophages acquire this capability, and the factors that modulate this ability.

Our own involvement in macrophages and host resistance to tumor development stemmed from the observation that mice with chronic infection with the obligate intracellular protozoan parasites *Toxoplasma gondii* and *Besnoitia jellisoni* had increased nonspecific resistance to spontaneous as well as transplanted tumor development (*J. Inf. Dis.* **124:**587, 1971). In mice infected with *B. jellisoni* deaths due to spontaneous leukemia did not begin to occur until ten months after chronic infection was established, by which time practically all control mice had succumbed to leukemia. Chronic protozoal infection also increased resistance to spontaneous mammary carcinoma in C3H mice as well as to several transplanted syngeneic and allogeneic tumors.

This increased tumor resistance seems to be due to the persistent activation of macrophages induced by chronic protozoal infection. Peritoneal macrophages from such mice (as well as mice with *Listeria monocytogenes* and BCG infection) are nonspecifically tumoricidal *in vitro*. It is noteworthy that tumor cells are destroyed by a nonphagocytic mechanism under *in vitro* conditions in which normal target cells are spared and grow to confluency. Intimate contact is required and thus far we have not been able to detect a soluble cytotoxic mediator. Nonadherent peritoneal cells were ineffective, as were macrophages stimulated by treatment of the host with thioglycollate or starch. (*Nature* **235:**48, 1972; *Science* **180:**868, 1973).

The macrophage vacuolar system appears to be involved in tumor cell killing (*Science* **184:**468, 1974). Phase contrast microscopy and lyosomal markers show that lysosomal material is transferred from activated macrophages to the cytoplasm of tumor cells. Such transfer was not seen in normal macrophages. Tumor killing by activated macrophages is inhibited by hydrocortisone, a membrane stabilizer that interferes with the transfer of lysosomal markers to tumorigenic target cells. In addition, the tumoricidal effect of activated macrophages was inhibited by prelabeling their vacuolar system with trypan blue, an inhibitor of lysosomal enzyme action. Activated macrophages transferred the trypan blue lysosomal markers to susceptible target cells but the target cells were not killed. These results suggest to us that the cytotoxic action of activated macrophages can be inhibited either by preventing the transfer of lysosomal contents or by directly inactivating lysosomal enzymes transferred to the tumor cells.

Thus the activated macrophage tumoricidal reaction is nonphagocytic; it requires direct contact with the target cell. Tumor target cells are more susceptible to destruction than are normal target cells, and the mechanism of tumor killing appears to involve the activated macrophage vacuolar system.

A major issue at present is how macrophages acquire nonspecific tumoricidal capacity. Piessens *et al.* recently reported that casein-induced guinea pig macrophages preincubated with MIF-rich supernatants nonspecifically kill tumor cells but not normal fibroblasts or kidney cells (*J. Immuol.* **114:**293, 1975). We used a technique developed by Salvin *et al.* to obtain mouse serum rich in lymphocyte mediator including MIF activity (*Infection and Immunity* **7:**68, 1973); reasoning that mouse serum rich in lymphocyte mediator activity might well provide the signal that induces activation of normal or peptone-stimulated normal mouse macrophages *in vitro*.

Stimulated macrophages preincubated with either 0.1% mediator-rich mouse serum or with 5 ng/ml endotoxin were not tumoricidal. However, the combination of mediator and endotoxin consistently yielded tumoricidal macrophages. This synergistic action of endotoxin and mediator may be relevant to pathogenesis of the GVHR. Could it be that the absence of clinical GVH disease in germ-free animals reflects the absence of this synergistic action of endotoxin and lymphocyte mediator on activated macrophages?

As for the factors other than endotoxin that modulate tumor killing by activated macrophages, we have observed that the serum in the culture medium used has a determining influence on the expression of tumor killing. We find that activated macrophages are only reliably tumoricidal when the medium contains fetal bovine serum. If the culture medium contains serum from adult animals, activated macrophages are not tumoricidal or only variably so. Tumor killing by activated macrophages can therefore be modulated by at least three factors: normal serum components, the amount of lymphocyte mediator in the system, and endotoxin.

Figure 11 illustrates our present understanding of the acquisition and modulation of tumoricidal function of mouse peritoneal macrophages. There is a continuum of functional modification that can result in the expression of tumor killing. Peritoneal macrophages from normal unstimulated mice do not kill tumor cells and do not reliably acquire tumoricidal potential even when exposed to high concentrations of lymphocyte mediators. However, normal unstimulated macrophages that have been cultured *in vitro* for 72 hr, or stimulated macrophages induced by the intraperitoneal injection of 10% peptone can be activated and made tumoricidal by high concentrations (1–3%) of lymphocyte mediator-rich

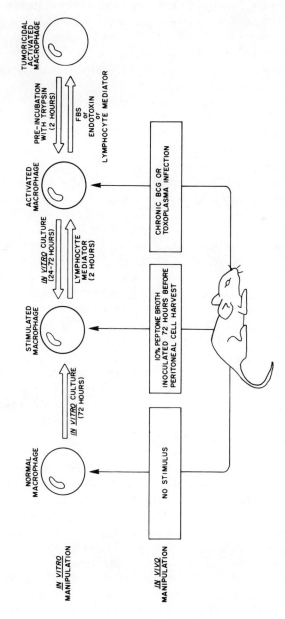

Fig. 11 Schema for the acquisition and modulation of macrophage tumoricidal activity.

105

serum, provided it is present throughout the cytotoxicity assay. However, if stimulated macrophages are preincubated with lymphocyte mediator-rich serum for 2 hr, or small concentrations of lymphocyte mediator-rich serum (0.01–0.1%) are present throughout the assay, then tumor killing depends on the serum and the presence of endotoxin in the tissue culture system. Finally, the attributes of these agents to render activated macrophages tumoricidal can be abrogated by preincubating the activated macrophages with trypsin (50–100 μ/ml).

These findings lead us to conclude that there is bidirectional control of tumor killing by activated macrophages and that the functional differentiation of macrophages is continually being modified by signals from the host environment.

CUDKOWICZ: I mentioned in my introduction at the outset of this conference that the dependence of resistance to marrow grafts on the integrity of macrophages is such that a single administration of an antimacrophage agent is sufficient to abrogate resistance. The conceptual difficulties voiced by Metcalf prevent us, however, from thinking that macrophage-like cells could be the effectors of F_1 antiparent responses *in vivo*. The main difficulty is that one must assume that such a cell is able to recognize foreignness in a rather sophisticated way, since Hh genes are quite polymorphic and the anti-Hh response is always specific. This is not a property ordinarily attributed to macrophages.

Shearer will discuss later an *in vitro* model that we regard a correlate of the *in vivo* rejection of bone marrow grafts in an F_1 antiparent situation. So, I shall not address myself to the evidence that justifies this conclusion, but give, quite briefly, the evidence we have accumulated for an important role of macrophages also *in vitro*. We were actually able to establish that the macrophage-like cell is not the effector of F_1 antiparent cytotoxicity but an accessory though indispensable cell. Experiments with silica were done in collaboration with Shearer and H. Waksal, whereas experiments with carrageenan were done by Yee Pang Yung in my laboratory. The setup is one in which F_1 hybrid responding spleen cells are co-cultured with parental-strain irradiated stimulating cells. After five days, the cultured cells are harvested and assayed in a ^{51}Cr release test on target cells sharing with the stimulators the H-2D/Hh-1 phenotype. Cytotoxic effector cells are generated with specificity for the Hh-1 products of parental type.

When silica particles or carrageenan are added to the cultures, no cytotoxic effector cells are generated, but only if the antimacrophage agents are added at the outset or within the first two to three days of culture (Table 24). At later intervals the agents are no longer effective and the cytotoxic cells themselves are insensitive to these antimacrophage agents. The conclusion is that an early inductive event was disturbed by silica and carrageenan, but not the function of the mature effector cells. The latter turned out to be a lymphocyte positive for the Thy.1 marker.

TABLE 24

Time-Dependent Abrogation of (C57BL/6 × DBA/2)F_1 Antiparental C57BL/6 CML
by Antimacrophage Agent[a]

Antimacrophage agent	Dose (μg/ml)	Specific lysis (%) for cultures given antimacrophage agents on day						
		None	0	1	2	3	4	5
Silica[b]	125	24.8	9.1	−2.7	10.0	21.1	23.8	20.6
ι-Carrageenan[c]	100	53.2	1.8	2.8	12.0	28.4	40.2	61.8

[a]Responder:stimulator cell ratio, 1:1. Cytotoxic effector cells were assayed on H-2[b] lymphoma cells labeled with ^{51}Cr. Effector:target ratio, 40.
[b]Data from Shearer, G. M., Waksal, H., and Cudkowicz, G.
[c]Data from Yung, Y. P., and Cudkowicz, G.

The effect of adding antimacrophage agents to cultures of F_1 cells stimulated by allogeneic instead of parental cells is shown in Table 25. Under the same conditions used for the F_1 cultures stimulated by parental cells, silica particles failed to prevent the generation of cytotoxic cells for allogeneic targets, but carrageenan did. By repeating the experiments under conditions designed for maximum sensitivity (high responder:stimulator ratios; low effector:target ratios) it is possible indeed to consistently prevent the generation of cytotoxic effectors

TABLE 25

Time-Dependent Abrogation of (C57BL/6 × DBA/2)F_1 Antiallogeneic C3H CML
by Iota Carrageenan[a]

Antimacrophage agent	Dose (μg/ml)	Responder: stimulator ratio	Specific lysis (%) for cultures given antimacrophage agent on day					
			None	0	1	2	3	4
Silica[b]	125	1:1	25.0	23.3				
		10:1	33.3	27.0				
		100:1	30.5	25.3				
		1000:1	8.9	9.4				
ι-Carrageenan[c]	100	1:1	39.6	1.1	5.1	12.1	19.5	38.1

[a]Cytotoxic effector cells were assayed on H-2[k] lymphoma cells labeled with ^{51}Cr. Effector: target cell ratio, 4, in assays of silica treated cultures, and 40 in the others.
[b]Data from Shearer, G. M., Waksal, H., and Cudkowicz, G.
[c]Data from Yung, Y. P., and Cudkowicz, G.

TABLE 26

Incompetence of Macrophage-Depleted (C57BL/6 × DBA/2)F_1
Spleen Cells for Antiparental C57BL/6 CML Despite
Competence for Antiallogeneic C3H CML[a]

Treatment of responding cells	Specific lysis (%) in separate experiments			
F_1 Antiparent CML[b]				
None	48.0	40.2	67.2	59.6
Nylon wool	58.8	54.2	58.7	Not done
Nylon wool and cFe	6.7	2.9	9.5	17.4
F_1 Antiallogeneic CML[c]				
None	54.7	60.8	36.5	43.9
cFe	50.5	48.3	31.4	
Nylon wool and cFe				37.9

[a]Data from Yung, Y.P., and Cudkowicz, G.

[b]Responder:stimulator cell ratio, 1; effector:target (H-2^b
lymphoma) cell ratio, 40.

[c]Responder:stimulator cell ratio, 20; effector:target (H-2^k
lymphoma) cell ratio, 40.

in both the F_1 antiparent and F_1 antiallogeneic CML setups. It is quite clear,
however, that the dependence on macrophages is far greater for the former than
for the latter cell mediated response.

We regard this evidence as circumstantial since it is obtained by adding to
cultures of spleen cells substances that could well have multiple biological effects
on cells other than macrophages. Thus, we resorted to a different type of experiment to avoid this pitfall. We attempted to remove macrophages from F_1 spleen
cells prior to culture using several techniques, such as filtration through nylon
wool or rayon columns, carbonyl iron and magnet (cFe), and adherence to
plastic. The most consistent results are obtained by first filtering the spleen cells
through nylon wool columns and then exposing them to cFe. The results of a few
experiments are given in Table 26. Nylon wool filtration alone does not sufficiently deplete F_1 spleen cells of macrophages so as to render the population
incompetent for F_1 antiparent cytotoxicity, but improves the effectiveness of cFe
subsequently applied. Responding cells so treated lose their potential for F_1
antiparent CML. As with silica, macrophage removal by nylon wool filtration
and cFe was not as effective in preventing the development of F_1 antiallogeneic
CML.

Macrophage-depleted spleen cell suspensions were reconstituted by the addition of spleen cells in which prekiller cells were inactivated by exposure to 1000–2000 rads of gamma rays.

In summary, the present evidence for the involvement of macrophages in anti-Hh responses derives from *in vivo* and *in vitro* experiments. No direct experimental evidence is yet available in support of macrophage–lymphocyte interaction *in vivo*. One would have to assign a recognition function to macrophages, however, to interpret the data otherwise. In contrast, the data from *in vitro* experiments are convincing and conclusive since antimacrophage agents, removal of adherent/phagocytic cells, and reconstitution experiments all point to the accessory role of macrophages interacting with T prekiller cells.

PARKMAN: Has Cudkowicz taken this experiment one step further? That is to do the lymphocyte–macrophage or lymphocyte–erythroid interaction, remove the supernatant and add it to a purified macrophage population.

CUDKOWICZ: No, we didn't. The only other maneuvers along these lines were the appropriate controls. When we tried to complement two cell populations, each treated with a different antimacrophage agent, or with two different antilymphocyte agents, they did not complement each other.

WARNER: Has it not been shown by other workers, however, that activation of CML to allogeneic determinants also required macrophages in the culture? This would therefore be the same in Hh and allogeneic CML stimulation.

CUDKOWICZ: The allogeneic CML indeed has a requirement for macrophages. However, it is not the same requirement as the F_1 antiparent CML. Suffice it to say that the macrophages for the former are present in the spleen of infant mice, whereas the macrophages for the latter are not.

BACH: I would like to return to the comment made by Warner on the requirement for macrophages in the allogeneic system. This may well depend on how thorough a macrophage depletion one achieves. There is little reason to doubt that depleting macrophages lowers an allogeneic CML.

Now Cudkowicz has taken the step that all of us tend to take when we are comparing two systems. He has sought to desensitize the stronger one, the allogeneic system. However, the relevant question remains whether the antigenic stimulus is equally strong. If it is not, the allogeneic situation still provides a stronger stimulus. Removing the macrophages is therefore not as critical in this instance as where one has a weaker stimulus.

CUDKOWICZ: I agree that the nature of the stimulus in an F_1 antiparent and F_1 antiallogeneic setup is going to be different no matter what we do in terms of trying to weaken the stronger. Nevertheless, we felt that the comparison was more valid between apparently similar responses in terms of cytotoxic activity. This was accomplished by weakening both the stimulus (high responder:stimulator ratio) and the effector phase.

BENNETT: There are two points I would make. According to Metcalf and Moore, in the allogeneic system, even if one removed *all* the macrophages that were present initially, if CSF is being produced one might have a macrophage precursor that would become a macrophage a couple of days later. So if macrophages are required, it could be that killing or removing macrophages on day zero would not completely rule out the possibility that macrophages are important in the allogeneic situation.

I came across a report in the RES Journal recently to the effect that in addition to suppressing macrophages, silica also suppresses B cell function in a system of antibody responses to T-independent antigens. It seemed to operate via the generation of a factor in serum. Thus it may not be a macrophage poison, strictly speaking.

BACH: I think that what one really has to do is to view this at the single-cell level of the CTL, or the effector cells that are being generated. No matter what we do to try to desensitize the system (and I do think that desensitization at the generation level is better than simply adjusting the number of effector cells), if we have a potent antigenic stimulus in the allogeneic system and a weaker one, and we ask "Do we need help to allow a prekiller cell to become an effector cell?" then we do not have comparable systems. I think that needs emphasis; we do not want to add complexity to an already enormously complex field.

WARNER: Now we come back to the general theme of an earlier discussion, which is macrophage heterogeneity. It is fairly clear that there are multiple functions of macrophages in these various *in vitro* inductive systems, and that mercaptoethanol can replace only some of these functions. It may therefore be that there is an additional macrophage function required in the activation of the Hh systems that is not replaced by mercaptoethanol, whereas mercaptoethanol is sufficient in replacing the need for macrophages in the allogeneic CML system.

CUDKOWICZ: I think that at this stage a number of possibilities should be kept in mind. Operationally there is no doubt that the dependence on macrophages of the F_1 antiparent and the allogeneic CML are different. This may be only a quantitative difference; at this point we can't be sure. However, it is also possible that there is something more fundamental, as Warner has said. There may well be different subpopulations of macrophages, and some would be more easily depleted than others.

To my knowledge, the only clear-cut instance of a procedure aimed at depleting macrophages that abrogated both F_1 antiparent and antiallogeneic CML responses is the treatment with ^{89}Sr. Admittedly ^{89}Sr does a number of things. Among others, it depletes the M cells, which we may consider precursors of macrophages. It also may promote generation of suppressor cells. One or two months after giving ^{89}Sr to F_1 mice there is no potential for an antiparent response, but there is no potential for an antiallogeneic CML response either (Table 27). If we look at this kinetically—these were experiments done in collaboration with Bennett and Paul Evans—we see that the two responses come down in parallel, but not at the same rate. The antiparent response comes down sooner than the antiallogeneic response.

CHAIRMAN MOORE: My impression is that macrophages are essential to every facet of hemopoietic proliferation and differentiation. I suspect that what we have to consider is the very intimate relationship between differentiating hemopoietic cells and stromal macrophages within the marrow and spleen environment. What we observe in our various *in vitro* systems may be artifactual to a degree, since such matters as cell contact or population density are not strictly addressed in a physiological way.

It may be that the release by macrophages of a variety of factors that we are looking at in these systems may not occur under normal conditions. This might be a very local thing with presentation of these factors on the surface of the cell.

TABLE 27

Failure of (C57BL/6 × DBA/2)F_1 Spleen Cells of ^{89}Sr-Treated Mice to Generate *in vitro* Antiparental C57BL/6 or Antiallogeneic C3H Cytotoxic Effector Cells. Evidence for Suppressor Cells[a]

Donors of responding spleen cells	Time after treatment (wk)	Specific lysis (%[b]	
		F_1 Anti-C57BL/6	F_1 Anti-C3H
Normal	—	50.2	46.8
^{89}Sr treated (200 μC)	12	0.1	0.8
Normal and ^{89}Sr treated[c]	12	4.2	7.6

[a]Data from Cudkowicz, G., Evans, P. D., and Bennett, M.

[b]Responder:stimulator ratio, 1. Cytolytic cells were assayed on ^{51}Cr-labeled lymphoma cells at the effector:target ratio of 80. For F_1 antiparent CML the target cells were H-2^b and for F_1 antiallogeneic CML H-2^k.

[c]Mixture of 3 × 10^6 spleen cells of normal mice (responding by themselves as indicated in first line) and 2 × 10^6 cells of ^{89}Sr-treated mice.

Thus, whether one gets a proliferative response or an inhibition might indeed be a very local affair within the marrow rather than a diffusely distributed situation. That is my opinion on the ramifications of macrophage function.

CUDKOWICZ: I am in general agreement with Moore's analysis. If I were to focus it more directly to the unnatural situation of bone marrow grafts, I would say that our present thinking—and I am reflecting now also Shearer's thinking on this as well—our present thinking is that it is entirely possible but unlikely, that *in vivo*, where our endpoint is cytostasis or modulation of proliferation, the primary role, the effector role, in the anti-Hh responses is that of a macrophage-like cell.

In vitro, where we are dealing with a somewhat artifactual situation, in which the endpoint is lysis of a target cell, an endpoint that may have very little relation to the endpoint *in vivo*, the effector cell is a thymus-derived cell. Still it cannot mature into an effector cell without the interaction with the macrophage-like cell. This macrophage may well be the same cell we are dealing with *in vivo*. However, *in vitro* it is exerting unquestionably a role similar to that of the macrophage in other immune responses, namely, an accessory role.

IN VITRO MODELS OF Hh-MEDIATED RESISTANCE AND MHC INCOMPATIBILITY

Discussion Introducer:

Fritz H. Bach

CHAIRMAN BACH: In this session we shall first deal with the Hh system, typing for the Hh gene products, etc. When those issues have been covered, we shall turn back to the general problem of measuring gene products of the MHC.

SHEARER: A better understanding of the mechanisms responsible for the rejection of parental marrow grafts by F_1 hybrid recipients could be possible were an *in vitro* system available for study of this phenomenon. For example, the immunological basis of the *in vivo* anti-Hh reaction could be verified if an *in vitro* model existed in which immunological specificity could be tested, such as the specificity of cytotoxic effector cells. Two years ago, we developed in my laboratory, in collaboration with Gustavo Cudkowicz, a technique for generating and detecting F_1 antiparental cytotoxic responses *in vitro*. Details of the method have been published (Shearer and Cudkowicz, *Science* **190**:890, 1975). Briefly, F_1 and irradiated parental splenic lymphocytes are co-cultured for five days in supplemented RPMI-1640 at 37°C in a CO_2 incubator. The F_1 cytotoxic effector cells generated are assayed for 4 hr on a series of ^{51}Cr-labeled lymphoid tumor or mitogen-stimulated spleen target cells. The specificity of the F_1 antiparent cytotoxic reaction is illustrated in Table 28. Effector cells were consistently generated when (C57BL/6 × DBA/2)F_1 (BDF$_1$) spleen cells were stimulated with C57BL/6 parental spleen cells. These effectors were specific for H-2^b tumor or mitogen-stimulated spleen target cells and did not appreciably lyse H-2^d, H-2^k, or H-$2^{b/d}$ targets. In general, DBA/2 parental spleen cells did not generate a response of F_1 responding cells, although weak F_1 anti-DBA/2 effectors were detected in some experiments (Shearer *et al.*, *J. Immunol.* **117**:754, 1976). These *in vitro* cytotoxic results are consistent with those reported for the selective rejection of C57BL/6 parental marrow grafts by (C57BL/6 × DBA/2)F_1 hosts, and add a dimension of specificity for target cell killing that could not be assessed by the available *in vivo* techniques.

In order to more extensively compare the *in vitro* generation of BDF$_1$ anti-C57BL/6 parental cytotoxic effectors with the rejection of C57BL/6 parental

TABLE 28

Specificity of *in vitro* F_1 Antiparental Cell-Mediated Cytotoxicity

Responding and effector cells	Stimulating cells	Lysis on target cells of H-2 haplotype[a]			
		H-2^b	H-2^d	H-2^k	H-$2^{b/d}$
(C57BL/6 × DBA/2)F_1	C57BL/6	+	−	−	−
(C57BL/6 × DBA/2)F_1	DBA/2	−	−	−	−

[a](+) indicates from 15 to 45% specific lysis; (−) indicates from −5 to 5% specific lysis, at effector:target cell ratio of 40:1.

TABLE 29

Effect of Different Parameters on the Rejection of C57BL/6 Parental Marrow by (C57BL/6 × DBA/2)F_1 Recipients and on the Induction of F_1 Antiparental and Allogeneic Cell-Mediated Cytotoxic Responses[a]

Parameter investigated	Variable	In vivo F_1 rejection of marrow		In vitro F_1 cytotoxic response		
					Effector cell lysis of targets	
		Parental cells injected	Rejection of parental marrow	Stimulating cells	$H\text{-}2^b$ (Hh-1)	$H\text{-}2^k$ (allogeneic)
Maturation (age of F_1 mice)	20–21 days	C57BL/6	−	C57BL/6	−	
	24–25 days	C57BL/6	+	C57BL/6	+	
	20–21 days			C_3H		++
	24–25 days			C_3H		++
Unresponsiveness (F_1 mice preinjected with spleen cells from:)	C3H or DBA/2	C57BL/6	+	C57BL/6	+	
	C57BL/6	C57BL/6	−	C57BL/6	−	
	C3H or DBA/2			C_3H		++
	C57BL/6			C_3H		++

[a]For in vitro cytotoxicity (+) indicates from 15 to 30% specific lysis; (−) indicates from −5 to 5% specific lysis; (++) indicates from 60 to 90% specific lysis. Effector:target cell ratio, 40:1.

marrow grafts by BDF_1 hosts, a number of unusual parameters, which are known to affect bone marrow graft rejection, were investigated in F_1 antiparent and allogeneic cytotoxic systems. These include late maturation of F_1 antiparent reactivity, the induction of specific unresponsiveness of the F_1 by preinjection of parental cells, and, as discussed earlier, loss of reactivity by treatment with macrophage-inhibiting agents (e.g., silica particles), as well as loss of reactivity by treatment of F_1 mice by rabbit antimouse bone marrow serum. The effect of some of these parameters on the *in vivo* and *in vitro* models of Hh reactions as well as in *in vitro* allogeneic cytotoxic reactions, which have been published in detail elsewhere (Shearer *et al., Transplant. Proc.* **8**:469, 1976) are summarized in Table 29. The ability of irradiated F_1 recipients to reject parental marrow developed between the twentieth and twenty-fourth day of life. Preinjection of F_1 recipients with C57Bl/6 parental spleen cells, but not with DBA/2 parental spleen cells, induced specific unresponsiveness in the F_1 mice. Injection of F_1 recipients with silica abolished resistance to parental marrow cells. The abrogation of resistance *in vivo* by injecting F_1 recipients with rabbit antimouse bone marrow serum was dependent on the amount of antiserum injected. Injection of 0.6 ml of serum significantly reduced resistance to C57BL/6 parental marrow cells, whereas 0.1 ml of serum had no detectable effect. Injection of 0.3 ml of rabbit antimouse bone marrow serum slightly impaired resistance. The effects of these same parameters on the *in vitro* generation of F_1 antiparent and allogeneic cytotoxic responses are shown in the two right columns of Table 29. Responding spleen cells from 20–21-day-old BDF_1 mice were incapable of generating a cytotoxic response against parental C57BL/6 stimulating cells, although lymphocytes from the same donors generated a strong allogeneic CML against C3H stimulating cells. In contrast, responding cells from 24–25-day-old F_1 donors generated effectors against the Hh-1 determinant of $H-2^b$, as well as against C3H alloantigens. Three intraperitoneal injections of BDF_1 responding cell donors with 10^7 C3H or DBA/2 spleen cells at weekly intervals did not reduce the ability of the F_1 cells to respond either to the parental C57BL/6 or to C3H allogeneic stimulating cells. However, similar treatment of F_1 donors with C57BL/6 spleen cells selectively abolished responsiveness to parental C57BL/6, but not to allogeneic C3H stimulating cells. Addition of either silica or rabbit antimouse bone marrow serum to the cultures at the initiation of sensitization selectively abrogated the response to the Hh-1 determinant, but not to the C3H alloantigens.

It is worth discussing briefly the dependence of these *in vivo* and *in vitro* models on the presence of an intact thymus or of theta-positive cells. The ability of irradiated athymic nu/nu mice to reject marrow grafts is greater than that of normal littermates (Cudkowicz, unpublished observations). Likewise, irradiated thymectomized recipients reject hemopoietic grafts as strongly as nonthymectomized controls. (Cudkowicz and Bennett, *J. Exp. Med.* **134**:83, 1971). These observations suggest that marrow graft rejection *in vivo* is not a thymus-dependent process and raises the possibility that the effector mechanism does not involve a theta-positive cell. In contrast, F_1 antiparent cytotoxic responses are effected by theta-positive cells and are also dependent on a theta-positive cell at the time of sensitization, since both the effector and the sensitizing phases of the F_1 antiparent cytotoxic responses are abrogated by antitheta serum and complement (Shearer *et al., Cold Spring Harbor Symposia Quant. Biol.* **41**:511, 1977).

It can be concluded from these studies that the F_1 antiparent cytotoxic response exhibits certain characteristics that make it similar both to marrow graft rejection by an Hh mechanism and to conventional allogeneic cytotoxicity. From the same studies it appears that there are features of F_1 antiparent cytotoxicity that distinguishes it from the *in vivo* Hh and conventional allogeneic reactions. A comparison of the effects of the various parameters thus far considered has been tabulated:

Parameter studied	Marrow rejection *in vivo*	F_1 Antiparent cytotoxicity in *in vitro*	Allogeneic cytotoxicity *in vitro*
Response maturation	Fourth week of life	Fourth week of life	First week of life
Preimmunization	Suppressed	Suppressed	Enhanced
Silica	Suppressed	Suppressed	No effect detected
Antimarrow serum	Suppressed	Suppressed	No effect detected
Response by nu/nu mice	Enhanced	No response	No response
Response generated by	Unknown cell type	Thy-1 + cell	Thy-1 + cell
Response effected by	Unknown cell type	Thy-1 + cell	Thy-1 + cell

Considering our present knowledge of these systems, it would appear that marrow graft rejection in irradiated host mice and the generation of Hh-specific cytotoxic cells are effected by different cellular mechanisms, although certain aspects of the cellular events in both systems are common. For example, it is possible that both allogeneic and Hh cytotoxic reactions are generated and effected by T-lymphocytes, whereas marrow graft rejection is effected by a radioresistant null lymphocyte in cooperation with a phagocytic (e.g., silica-sensitive) cell, which matures after the third week of life. In addition, Hh cytotoxicity *in vitro* could be dependent upon this late-maturing cell, which could serve an accessory function necessary for generating Hh effectors, but which would be irrelevant for allogeneic cytotoxicity. One of the cell populations involved in the generation of F_1 antiparent cytotoxic reactions could be the one relevant for natural resistance to tumors (to be considered in a later session), since the naturally occurring cytotoxic cells for leukemias share several properties with both Hh cytotoxicity and with marrow graft rejection (Keissling *et al., Eur. J. Immunol.* **7**:655, 1977).

CHAIRMAN BACH: Does Shearer have any data on proliferative responses of various kinds in this system?

SHEARER: So far it has not been possible to detect a proliferative response associated with the F_1 antiparent cytotoxic reaction.

The F_1 antiparent cytotoxic system exhibits another unusual feature which could be interpreted as lack of specificity at the level of stimulation. As was discussed earlier, the BDF_1 effector cells generated by sensitization with C57BL/6 parental stimulating cells are specific, since they will lyse only $H-2^b$ homozygous target cells. It is possible, however, to activate BDF_1 effectors with allogeneic C3H stimulating cells, which will lyse $H-2^b$ but not $H-2^d$ parental target cells, in addition to the relevant $H-2^k$ targets. The F_1 effectors that lyse the $H-2^b$ targets appear to be specific for $H-2^b$ at the lytic phase, since inhibition of lysis of the $H-2^b$ targets was not obtained using $H-2^k$ cells as cold target inhibitors. This observation raised the possibility that allogeneic stimulation of F_1 lymphocytes activates anti-Hh clones of effectors as well as the antiallogeneic clones. In order to pursue this further, the generation of BDF_1 anti-C3H effectors that lysed $H-2^b$ target cells was investigated with respect to some of the unusual characteristics associated with F_1 antiparent cytotoxic responses, i.e., late response maturation, induction of unresponsiveness, and sensitivity to silica. It was found that spleen cells from 22-day-old BDF_1 mice did not generate effectors that lysed $H-2^b$ targets when stimulated with either C57BL/6 parental or C3H allogeneic spleen cells. In contrast, responding cells from 24-day-old BDF_1 animals generated good cytotoxic responses detected on $H-2^b$ targets when activated with C57BL/6 parental or C3H allogeneic cells. Spleen cells from $B6C3F_1$ mice made unresponsive for Hh cytotoxicity by preinjection of C57BL/6 spleen cells also did not generate effectors that lysed $H-2^b$ targets when sensitized with DBA/2 allogeneic stimulators (although the spleen cells exhibited normal response detected on the relevant allogeneic $H-2^d$ targets). The period of Hh unresponsiveness induced by C57BL/6 parental spleen cells can be time dependent. In the same group of $B6C3F_1$ mice, it was found that the F_1 anti-C57BL/6 Hh cytotoxic response began to reappear five months after injection of C57BL/6 spleen cells and had returned to normal levels by seven months. The restoration of $B6C3F_1$ anti-DBA/2 response detected on $H-2^b$ (Hh) targets was concomitant with the return of F_1 antiparent Hh cytotoxic potential. Finally, silica administered to F_1 mice or added to the *in vitro* cultures had identical suppressive effects on F_1 anti-C57BL/6 parent and or F_1 antiallogeneic responses detected on $H-2^b$ targets. The striking parallels observed with the activation of F_1 cells either by C57BL/6 parental or allogeneic stimulator cells raises the possibility that Hh clones can be triggered by alloantigens and may be activated by immunization with alloantigens. This system provides the potential for investigating Hh reactions *in vitro* in situations not requiring F_1 and parent cell combinations. Such an approach might be useful for typing Hh determinants in human populations.

CHAIRMAN BACH: It should be noted that the issue is whether this two-cell system is really different from alloimmunity, and that issue is still open.

One would like to know whether the late maturation regarded as distinctive of Hh is not also paralleled by events in an alloimmune system. Shearer showed us that the alloimmune system was fully functional throughout the development, presumably because conditions ensured maximum lysis of targets. Instead, when suboptimal conditions were used so as to render the assay more sensitive, Auerbach and I got the impression that there was a gradual increase in CML reactivity during the first four weeks of life.

SHEARER: We were aware of the work of Auerbach and Bach, and indeed it had occurred to us that their results possibly reflected an Hh mechanism. While not discussed extensively here, it should be emphasized that Hh is not at all restricted to F_1 antiparent situations. It is, in fact, demonstrable in allogeneic and xenogeneic combinations as well.

Our data showed 90% lysis or more because the effector:target ratio was 40:1. By lowering this ratio we rendered the assay much more sensitive. Despite this, the alloimmune system did not manifest the delayed maturation consistently manifested by the Hh system. We know that the alloimmune system is already functional during the first week of life, whereas the Hh system consistently emerges during the fourth week. We therefore are dealing with a major difference.

WARNER: In the system described, can Shearer "tolerize," with third-party cells, and obtain nonreactivity as detected by challenge *in vitro* with either the parental or third party? Does the third-party strain share Hh alleles with the parental strain and are these detectable *in vivo?*

SHEARER: The answer to Warner's first question is that we have been unable to tolerize with third-party cells. This holds for both *in vivo* and *in vitro* situations and constituted one of the first justifications for claiming that the anti-Hh response was antigenic-specific. If one seeks to tolerize with H-2^b parental cells, this is successful, but with the contralateral parent, it does not work. Attempts to tolerize with a third party are also unsuccessful.

So, the system does show a specificity with respect to tolerance induction that is not manifest in activating the clones of Hh-reactive cytotoxic precursors. The reply to Warner's second question is that parental and third-party strains capable of activating antiparent responses do not share an Hh allele. The requirements for this nonspecific activation are still under investigation.

FESTENSTEIN: We have typed EL-4 cells and another $H-2^b$ tumor and found that they have additional "inappropriate" H-2 specificities on them. Could these be involved in anti-Hh responses?

SHEARER: No. $H-2^b$ blasts (PHA, LPS) serve as targets equally well as tumor cells.

SANFORD: If one produces resistant F_1 mice from C57BL and DBA/2 parents carrying the *nu* mutant allele, would the *nu/nu* F_1 still be resistant *in vivo* and develop anti-Hh responses *in vitro?*

SHEARER: Athymic *nu/nu* F_1 mice are indeed resistant *in vivo*. However, spleen cells of such mice do not generate cytotoxic cells *in vitro*. This is the only apparent discrepancy between the *in vivo* and *in vitro* tests, that is, the involvement of T cells in F_1 antiparent *in vitro* cytotoxicity. It is possible that lysis of target cells, as detected by release of ^{51}Cr, is an endpoint requiring T cells, irrespective of the nature of the sensitizing antigen. This endpoint is, however, quite different from resistance *in vivo*, where cytostasis is paramount.

NAKAMURA: I shall be identifying another aspect of F_1 antiparent CML additional to the properties of this system elaborated by Shearer. Specifically, I shall be concerned with the events leading to stimulation of F_1 responder cells. The experiments were done in collaboration with Cudkowicz.
    We first sought to determine whether parental cells taken from different hemopoietic sites would all function as stimulators. $B6D2F_1$ responding cells were cultured for five days with irradiated stimulators, and the effectors were then assayed on ^{51}Cr-labeled L5MF-22 lymphoma targets. The data in Table 30

TABLE 30

Induction of (C57BL/6 × DBA/2)F_1 Antiparental C57BL/6 CML
by Stimulator Cells of Different Lymphoid Organs[a]

Stimulator cells	Specific lysis (%) at responder:stimulator ratio				
	8:1	4:1	2:1	1:1	1:2
Spleen	10.1	17.0	31.3	40.3	37.5
Lymph node	37.9	51.7	50.0	61.7	Not done
Bone marrow	−0.3	−0.5	−0.6	−1.3	−1.5
Thymus	−8.3	−9.0	2.7	3.5	Not done

[a]Responding spleen cells were co-cultured for five days with irradiated (2000 rad of γ-rays) stimulating cells. Cytolytic activity was assayed on ^{51}Cr-labeled $H-2^b$ lymphoma cells at the effector:target ratio of 40.

clearly show that parental spleen and lymph node cells were good stimulators, whereas bone marrow and thymus cells failed to stimulate. This observation was surprising, since we know that all cell populations employed contained Hh-positive cells.

We investigated this matter further by replacing resting lymphoid cells with mitogen-induced blasts (Table 31). Parental LPS blasts from spleen were good stimulators, but not PHA blasts from the same organ (suppression induced by PHA) nor dextran-sulfate blasts from bone marrow. It is to be noted that all these blasts function well as targets for anti-Hh reactions and thus are unmistakably Hh-positive. So we are faced with the fact that cells that are antigenic in the Hh system are not necessarily immunogenic.

A series of additional experiments were done to identify the spleen cell subtypes responsible for stimulation. First, the cells were separated by nylon wool filtration and it was found that the nonadherent fraction was stimulatory, but not the adherent fraction (Table 32). Second, spleen cells exposed to anti-Thy-1 serum and complement lost the capacity to stimulate; third, cortisone-resistant thymocytes were good stimulator cells. It appears then that T lymphocytes are the stimulators or the cell type required for stimulation by some other antigenic cell, the only exception being LPS blasts.

The simplest way of thinking about this stimulation is to postulate that F_1 responding cells are sensitized by Hh antigen presented by parental stimulating cells, presumably in the presence of macrophages. In this case, our data would point to T lymphocytes as the stimulators. The problem with this interpretation is that lympho–myeloid cells other than T lymphocytes are also antigenic, and even immunogenic *in vivo,* yet fail to stimulate *in vitro.*

An alternative interpretation is illustrated by the schema of Fig. 12. It is proposed that parental T cells, though irradiated (2000 rad), recognize alloanti-

TABLE 31

Induction of (C57BL/6 × DBA/2)F_1 Antiparental C57BL/6 CML
by Mitogen-Induced Blasts[a]

Stimulator cells	Specific lysis (%) at responder:stimulator ratio				
	16:1	8:1	4:1	2:1	1:1
LPS/spleen	9.2	10.0	18.9	22.5	18.8
PHA/spleen	2.4	−0.6	−0.6	−1.4	−2.1
DS/bone marrow	−0.3	1.9	0.5	0.4	−0.9

[a]Stimulator cells were cultured for two days with mitogenic doses of LPS or PHA for spleen cells, dextran sulfate for bone marrow cells. Responding F_1 cells were set up for induction of antiparental cytotoxicity as indicated in the footnote of Table 30.

TABLE 32

Requirement of Parental T Cells for the Induction of
(C57BL/6 × DBA/2)F$_1$ Anti-C57BL/6 Cytotoxicity[a]

Stimulator cells	Specific lysis (%) at responder:stimulator ratio		
	4:1	2:1	1:1
Spleen			
Nylon adherent	−1.9	−2.6	4.6
Nylon nonadherent	3.8	15.5	23.5
Nonseparated	9.7	23.0	36.2
Spleen			
Normal mouse serum + C'			27.1
Anti-Thy-1.2 serum + C'			7.0
Thymus			
Cortisone-resistant	15.5	24.4	41.5

[a]See footnote of Table 30 for experimental setup and cytotoxicity assay.

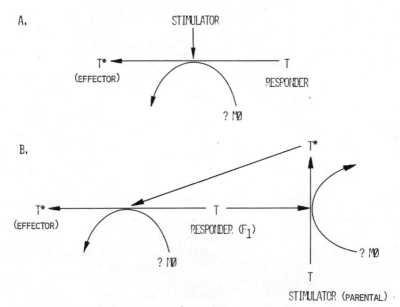

Fig. 12 Schema of events leading to stimulation in conventional allogeneic CML (A) and in F$_1$ antiparent CML (B). In the latter, irradiated parental T cells, activated by alloantigens of F$_1$ cells, release diffusible factors (lymphokines?), which in turn activate F$_1$ cells. Only then will F$_1$ responding cells generate specific anti-Hh effectors of cytolysis in the presence of viable macrophages sensitive to silica particles and carrageenan.

gens of F_1 responding cells and are thereby activated so as to release diffusible lymphokines. Only then will F_1 cells respond to parental Hh antigens presented by the T lymphocytes themselves as well as by other cells of the stimulator population. In other words, there is first "backstimulation" of F_1 responders and then "forward stimulation" against Hh determinants. LPS blasts may substitute for T cells in the backstimulation step; this step may also account for the "nonspecific allostimulation" earlier described by Shearer.

O'REILLY: My query is whether parental cells that have been pretreated with mitomycin C or some other agent that would prevent division and possibly activation, are now no longer a stimulus for the F_1 antiparent cytotoxic reaction.

NAKAMURA: The parental stimulator cells were always irradiated with 2000 rads of γ-rays and thus unable to divide. They were still able, however, to recognize foreignness as would mitomycin-C-treated cells, and this is what matters for their effectiveness. It should be noted, however, that very high doses irradiation, in excess of 5000 rad, did diminish the capacity to stimulate.

CHAIRMAN BACH: Could I add one comment? Both mitomycin-treated and irradiated cells do elaborate the kind of factors that one looks to for help and would therefore fit Nakamura's model. Also, it is noteworthy that very high dose irradiation does inhibit the production of such factors.

Earlier, the question arose why there was recessive expression of Hh, and I suggested as one reason that one could be dealing with a threshold phenomenon. At the time some doubt was left whether the heterozygote could be used as a target.

It seems to me that Nakamura has demonstrated that there are targets, which I presume are specific, that do not sensitize. Doesn't that bring us back to at least supporting the possibility that the reason for recessive expression may have to do with low-level threshold recognition, in terms of immunization requiring something more than simply being a target?

NAKAMURA: If F_1 hybrids were to express small numbers of Hh molecules, it would be difficult to visualize that an *in vivo* and *in vitro* response could be induced against antigens they already possess. As to the target cells that do not sensitize, other explanations may be invoked. For example, the frequency of Hh-positive cells may be suboptimal for anti-Hh stimulation, which is known to be critically dependent on the responder:stimulator ratio.

CUDKOWICZ: I want to comment on Bach's remark that there are some specific target cells that are not stimulating. Of the two cell types mentioned by

Nakamura, PHA blasts are actually suppressing the response. So they may not be stimulating only operationally, as a consequence of the presence of suppressor cells or suppressor factors. Such factors would be irrelevant when these cells are used as targets.

I also want to comment on Warner's query concerning cross reactivity between third-party stimulating cells and specific parental stimulators. It is my feeling that despite the requirement for stimulation, the *in vitro* F_1 anti-Hh response is still a natural response, not one that is induced *de novo*, as is the allogeneic CML. If so, I would regard allostimulation a totally nonspecific stimulus, one that simply provides the final impetus for a prekiller cell, already well advanced in differentiation, to reach the killer cell stage. It may even be possible that allostimulation as such is not essential and that mitogen stimulation would suffice.

WARNER: We now have the input available to directly answer Bach's interpretation. If the difference between parental and F_1 hybrid cells were simply a matter of gene dosage in expression of the molecules bearing this determinant, then in competitive blocking of cytotoxicity, at least twice as many F_1 as parental cells should be required. This is a decisive answer that should be obtainable.

CHAIRMAN BACH: Despite all this input, I feel we are left with two questions. First, can *in vitro* CML be used as a method to type for Hh? Second, to what degree should we regard Hh incompatibility as an *in vivo* phenomenon important for bone marrow engraftment? Are we agreed that CML typing for Hh shows remarkable similarities with the *in vivo* phenomenon, including the determinants with respect to the MHC regions that code for them? Is there further information?

SHEARER: We have obtained more data on mapping within the murine MHC of the *in vitro* F_1 antiparental cytotoxic reaction. As was described earlier, one of the unique features of hybrid resistance-mediated hemopoietic graft rejection was the demonstration by Cudkowicz that the resistant F_1 recipient of the parental graft be heterozygous at the D region of the H-2 complex. It was irrelevant whether the F_1 host was heterozygous or homozygous at the other known MHC regions. Thus, as outlined in Table 33, both (C57BL/10 × B10.A)F_1 and (B10.A × B10.A[2R])F_1 reject C57BL/10 and B10.A(2R) marrow grafts. In contrast, (B10.A[2R] × C57BL/10)F_1 do not reject either B10.A(2R) or C57BL/10 parental bone marrow (Shearer and Cudkowicz, *Science* **190**:890, 1975). A similar mapping pattern was reported in the same study using these F_1 hybrid combinations as responding cell donors and the respective parental strains as stimulator cell donors. However, more recent studies have indicated that B10.A(2R) spleen

TABLE 33

Summary of Hh Mapping Studies Comparing the Rejection of Marrow Grafts *in vivo*
and the Generation and Detection of Cytotoxic Effector Cells *in vitro*

F₁ Hosts of marrow grafts and donors of responding cells in vitro[a]	Strain used as marrow or stimulating cell donor	Rejection of marrow graft in vivo	Cytotoxicity detected on H-2[b] tumor targets[b]
(C57BL/10 × B10.A)F₁ b b b b b b/k k k d d d	C57BL/10 b b b b b b	Yes	Yes
	B10.A k k k d d d	No	No
	B10.A(2R) k k k d d b	Yes	No or weak
(B10.A × B10.A[2R])F₁ k k k d d d/k k k d d b	B10.A k k k d d d	No	No
	B10.A(2R) k k k d d b	Yes	No
(B10.A[2R] × C57BL/10)F₁ k k k d d b/b b b b b b	B10.A(2R) k k k d d b	No	No or weak
	C57BL/10 b b b b b b	No	No

[a] The lowercase letters indicate the haplotypes of origin of the K, I-A, I-B, I-C, S, D, regions of the H-2 complex.

[b] Effector:target cell ratio, 40:1

cells either do not, or only weakly, stimulate (B10.A × B10.A[2R])F₁ or (C57BL/10 × B10.A)F₁ responding cells to generate effector cells that lyse H-2^b tumor target cells. In the same experiments, C57BL/10 parental cells stimulated the (C57BL/10 × B10.A)F₁ responders to generate effectors. Such results indicate that the stimulation of F₁ lymphocytes by nonparental stimulator cells homozygous for the b haplotype at H-2D is not sufficient for optimal generation of cytotoxic effectors detected on parental targets. These observations suggest that the requirements for, or the specificity associated with, the development of an F₁ antiparental cytotoxic response may be more complicated than that involved in the rejection of parental marrow grafts *in vivo*. Such differences in these *in vivo* and *in vitro* Hh models could be attributed to the fact that the effectors of the cytotoxic Hh response and their precursors are Thy-1-positive cells, whereas the cells responsible for marrow graft failure *in vivo* appear to be thymus-independent.

In this context, it may be significant that T-cell-mediated cytotoxic responses directed against antigens other than classical allogeneic MHC-coded products are restricted to MHC-associated self antigens. In murine systems of this type, homology was required at the K or D regions of the H-2 complex either between stimulator and target cells or among responding, stimulating, effector, and target cells in order for efficient lympholysis to occur. In the Hh CML model, one would have expected that any such H-2-associated requirements that might have been anticipated would have been fulfilled for the generation of (C57BL/10 × B10.A)F$_1$ effector by B10.A(2R) stimulators detected on C57BL/10 or C57BL/6 targets, since H-2 homology exists among all the cell types involved at H-2D, in addition to expression of the Hh determinant on both the stimulator and target cells. I would prefer to postpone further discussion of the possible reasons for the failure of B10.A(2R) sensitizing cells to stimulate (C57BL/10 × B10.A)F$_1$ responding cells to generate effectors that lyse H-2^b targets for later consideration of H-2-restricted CML responses. In summary, although these observations are not fully understood at the present time, they do imply that the *in vitro* Hh CML is probably more complex than marrow graft rejection *in vivo,* and raise some problems for the use of the Hh CML model as a method for Hh mapping. It may be that effector mechanisms involving T-lymphocytes with cytotoxic functions exhibit specificity restrictions not required by other types of effector cells, i.e., the cells responsible for Hh-mediated *in vivo* hemopoietic graft rejection. This, in turn, would suggest that *in vivo* hemopoietic graft rejection may not be effected by cytotoxic lymphocytes, which would seem to be the case, since Hh cytotoxic effectors are Thy-1-positive, whereas marrow graft rejection appears to be thymus-independent.

SANFORD: We may be making a serious mistake in insisting on fitting the phenomenon of resistance to marrow grafts into the present immunologic dogma. From what we have heard of the properties of the system, it has become increasingly clear that its many relevant aspects are at odds with its having an immunologic basis in the conventional sense. It would be no less interesting nor less important if it were to turn out that factors pertaining to the graft environment were the ones of paramount importance. In that case, we would of course not be preoccupied with the Hh antigens and instead view the problem in a different perspective.*

Editors' comment: Immunologists have been and continue to be preoccupied with adaptive immunity and its dramatically ultraspecific attributes. It is understandable that *natural* defensive systems of the host, whose function and operation have a quite different basis, would not be so clearly perceived and would be more difficult to work with. Contemporary use of the term immunity has made it synonymous with *acquired* immunity so that it has become somewhat strange even to refer to natural immunity, although the older literature employed this designation and concept. What we are experiencing here is the disclosure of systems (Hh, natural killer cells, resistance to tumors and intracellular pathogens) that could function to assure that the host copes successfully with threats of the environment. It should come as no surprise that the operative mechanisms of these natural systems *would* differ considerably from those of acquired immunity as the former are likely to be phylogenetically far more ancient and therefore still shared with species more primitive than vertebrates.

CHAIRMAN BACH: Now we move on to the problem of defining HLA anti-gens by cellular and serological techniques. We shall be considering the antigens of the A, B, and C loci either as the antigens that are defined serologically or as the antigens that are the targets for cytotoxic T lymphocytes (or serving as markers for these targets). In terms of cellular immunogenetics, then, we shall be dealing with the CML targets as CD (cellular defined) antigens that are as-sociated and perhaps identical with the A, B, and C locus determinants.

For the D locus, we have the MLC reactions, by which the D locus was first defined, and more recently three tests have become available that help define the antigens of the D region: Homozygous typing cells, PLT (primed LD typing), and SLC (sperm lymphocyte culture). The serological approach in relationship to the D region primarily allows measurement of the Ia-like or B cell antigens. To draw the distinction with Hh phenomenology, we should consider two more areas after we have discussed the definition of antigens. First, what are the cellular events that relate to these various antigens? And second, what *in vivo* correlations have been obtained with respect to typing and matching for these different antigens?

Cellular immunogenetics has been the prime approach to HLA-D. The MLC test is still the ultimate cross match for determining whether two people are identical for the LD antigens of the MHC. The homozygous typing cell method was introduced by Bradley and Mempel and their collaborators. They used cells that were presumably homozygous for the LD antigens as stimulating cells so that any responding cell that carried the determinant or determinants present on the homozygous typing cell would not recognize the latter as foreign and there-fore would yield either no response or a much diminished one.

Using a variety of different homozygous typing cells and screening panels, it has been possible to define a series of what I would call the HLA DW clusters or determinant clusters in the population. Table 34 shows data from the 1975

TABLE 34

Frequency of HLA-D Specificities as Defined
by the Sixth International Histocompatibility Workshop

HLA-D Specificity group	Antigen frequency (%)	Gene frequency (%)	Most significant HLA-B association	Delta value
DW 1	19.3	0.102	BW35 (W5)	0.021
DW 2	15.2	0.078	B7	0.031
DW 3	16.4	0.085	B8	0.044
DW 4	15.6	0.082	BW15	0.017
DW 5	14.6	0.075	BW16	0.013
DW 6	10.5	0.054	—	—
"Blank"	—	0.524	—	—

Histocompatibility Workshop, in which there were six different HLA D specificity groups, DW1 to DW6. In addition, two others were less clearly defined and
were referred to as LD 107 and LD 108. The frequency of these antigens varies
between 10 and 20%. Calculating gene frequencies for something as involved as
the HLA-D complex is somewhat misleading.

These various HLA D specificity groups are associated with antigens of the
HLA-B locus as defined serologically, a reflection of linkage disequilibrium.

A second cellular approach to HLA-D which Sondel, Sheehy, and I developed uses a secondary response system. The basis of this technique, shown
schematically in Fig. 13, is to take one haplotype-different family combinations
and set up an MLC that is left for ten days, well beyond the peak proliferative
response. At this time one restimulates the culture with cells of the original
stimulator, thereby obtaining a very rapid response in terms of the incorporation
of radioactive thymidine. It is antigens of the HLA-D region that are primarily, if
not solely, responsible for any strong restimulation of such a primed responding
cell. We refer to this as primed lymphocyte typing—PLT.

The response thus is a measure of HLA-D in that the PLT test is predictive
of a primary MLC. Studies in recombinant families support these conclusions. At
this point, we look for PLT cells that, when tested against a panel of unrelated
individuals, show what we refer to as highly discriminatory responses. On the
top line of Fig. 14 we plot the response of one PLT cell to 50 different unrelated
cells. The majority of cells elicit a relatively small response, i.e., 3000 cpm or
less. There are five cells, however, that restimulate this PLT cell above 5000
cpm. The cell initially used to sensitize the primary MLC leading to this PLT cell
also stimulated in this high range. One can then assign the antigen measured by
this PLT cell to those five highly restimulatory cells.

We have used many different PLT cells of discriminatory type to define
HLA-D region antigens by this method. Figure 15 gives the results of a series of
studies done by several collaborators. Listed across the top of this figure are a
series of 21 different PLT cells, each prepared against an independent HLA
haplotype within family combinations. Listed along the left side of the figure are
48 test cells of unrelated individuals. The solid vertical bars refer to those
instances where a given test cell restimulated a given PLT cell to the same extent
as the cell initially used to sensitize in the PLT preparation (reference cell). Thus
we assign the unknown antigen measured by this PLT cell to the reference cell. It
is evident that these 21 different cells can be grouped in the way that im-
munogeneticists are accustomed to do, into a series of clusters. The first three
PLT cells define one antigen, which we refer to as PL-1, the next two define
PL-2, the next four PL-3, etc. In this way we define seven different antigens.

Of interest is that at least in one case, and I shall relate this to the homozygous typing cells, two PLT cells define an antigen, which, in terms of the individuals carrying it, is completely included within another antigen. There are

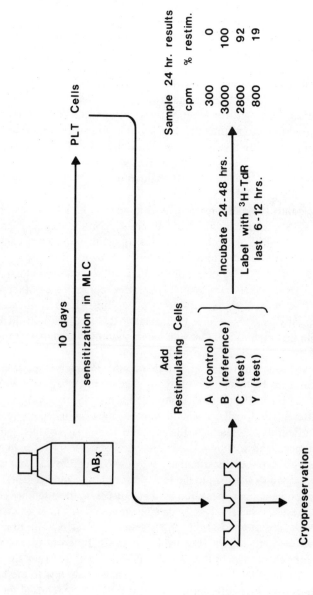

Fig. 13 Schema for primed LD typing.

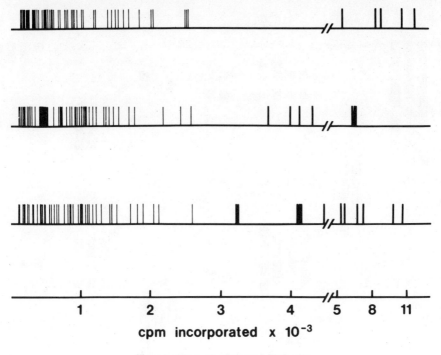

Fig. 14   Three discriminatory PLT cells.

eight individuals who are positive for what we refer to as PL3 defined by four PLT cells; four of those eight individuals are positive for an antigen that we refer to as PL3.1. Thus, we have two individuals in our panel who carry at least three determinants. For instance, individual 43 is PL2, PL3, and PL3.1, and PL4. Individual 11 has PL3, PL3.1, and PL5. The only interpretation of these data is that we are dealing with more than one determinant per HLA haplotype. In addition to these seven PL antigens we have at least six more for which we have only a single PLT cell per antigen.

How do the PLT cells and the PL antigens relate to the homozygous typing cells? The approach that we have taken in collaboration with Yunis, Bradley, Svejgaard, and others has been to restimulate PLT cells with homozygous typing cells. Two of the three PLT cells that define the antigen PL1 were restimulated with a number of different homozygous typing cells. Table 35 gives the results for DW1, DW3, and DW6. The two PLT cells are not restimulated by the homozygous typing cells for DW1, but they are significantly restimulated by homozygous typing cells for DW3, and also very significantly restimulated by the homozygous typing cell for DW6. This speaks for complexity; likewise, the DW6 homozygous typing cell restimulates not only the PLT cells that define

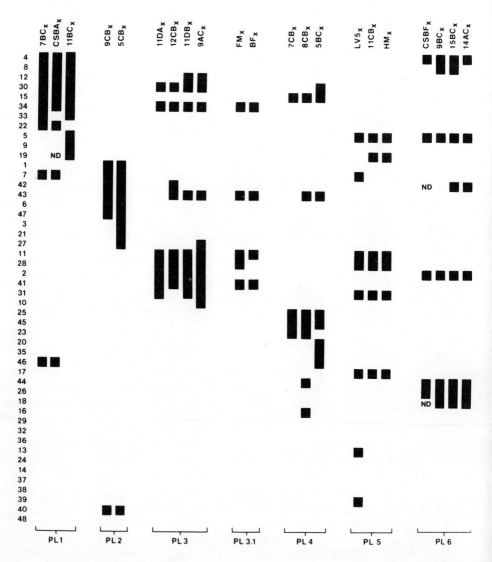

Fig. 15   Results of collaborative studies to define HLA-D region antigens by utilization of PLT 1-6 categories.

PL1, but also PLT cells that define PL3. So we have complexity in both directions. PL1 is associated with both DW3 and DW6 homozygous typing cells, and DW6 is associated with both PL1 and PL3.

My interpretation is that the DW antigens (as defined by homozygous typing cells) are complex in that there is more than one determinant per homozygous

TABLE 35
Restimulation of Primed Lymphocyte Typing Cells
with Homozygous Typing Cells

Restimulating cell	PL1		PL3	
	$7BC_x$	$11BC_x$	$11DB_x$	$9AC_x$
DW1	774	499	951	138
DW3	3509	2181	841	1030
	6431	4833	213	1580
DW6	3232	4331	3299	7948

typing cell; or that the PL antigens are complex or both. I prefer the interpretation that the homozygous typing cells are the more complex, because the phenotype frequencies of these DW clusters are about twice as great as the phenotype frequencies of the associated PL antigens.

Table 36 summarizes these data. By restimulation of PLT cells with homozygous typing cells, and by typing our panel with the PLT cells and homozygous typing cells, we found that PL5 is associated with DW1, PL2 with DW2, PL1 with both DW3 and DW6, and so on. The main point here is complexity in the HLA-D system, which had been suggested by Dupont on the basis of homozygous typing cell testing and by ourselves in the initial PLT studies.

Sassportes, Dausset, and their collaborators have shown an association between the serologically defined Ia-like antigens and PL antigens. In collaboration with Compston and Bachelor, we have done similar studies testing a part of our panel with three different antisera. These sera defined a B cell antigen called 103

TABLE 36
Restimulation of Primed Lymphocyte Typing Cells with Homozygous Typing Cells

	1	2	3	3.1	4	5	6
DW Antigen							
1	—	—	—	—	—	+++	—
2	—	+++	—	—	—	—	—
3	+++	—	—	—	—	—	—
4	—	—	—	N.T.	—	—	—
5	—	—	—	—	—	—	—
6	+++	—	+++	+++	—	—	—
LD 107	N.T.	—	N.T.	N.T.	—	—	N.T.
LD 108	—	—	—	—	+++	—	—

in Bachelor's laboratory and gave very similar patterns of reactivity with the panel.

Some 103 positive individuals are PL6 positive and PL1 negative. Others are PL1 positive and PL6 negative; some are both PL1 and PL6 positive, and there are also double negatives. Nevertheless, there is a highly significant association between the antigens 103 and PL1, and also a significant association between 103 and PL6, both supported by absorption studies.

But I would point out a few notable exceptions. The Ia-like antigens recognized serologically may be different from what is recognized as PL antigens, or else there is really very extensive complexity in this system.

Now we move on to the cellular definition of the target determinants in CML, and briefly consider the evidence suggesting that the SD determinants may not be what a cytotoxic T lymphocyte recognizes.

Edidin and Henney determined whether the SD antigens were the actual target antigens by capping them and then ascertaining that the capped cells, no longer sensitive to antibody-mediated, complement-dependent lysis, could still be killed in CML.

Sondel and I studied unrelated individuals, as others have done, and found that not infrequently cells of sensitized individuals could elicit very strong killing of the specific target, but would also cross-kill target of individuals who shared no SD antigens (Table 37). Khristensen and others also suggest that this is not an

TABLE 37
Cell-Mediated Lympholysis on Targets with no SD Antigens Shared with Stimulator Cells

CTLs	Unit	Number of CTLs $\times 10^4$	10^4 Target cells			
			W	X	Y	Z
	%	25	62.5 ± 2.8	55.9 ± 3.2	38.5 ± 2.7	1.7 ± 3.9
ZW_m	Cyto-toxicity	5	37.6 ± 0.9	29.5 ± 2.3	16.5 ± 3.1	—
	Potency	25	(25)	(10)	(2)	—
	%	25	48.5 ± 4.3	67.6 ± 6.2	29.3 ± 3.5	0.3 ± 3.1
ZX_m	Cyto-toxicity	5	24.7 ± 1.4	46.3 ± 4.3	8.8 ± 2.3	—
	Potency	25	(10)	(25)	(1)	—
	%	25	40.7 ± 3.8	28.6 ± 2.3	68.9 ± 3.4	-1.6 ± 3.2
ZY_m	Cyto-toxicity	5	15.6 ± 2.3	14.0 ± 3.7	50.1 ± 3.3	—
	Potency	25	(6)	(2)	(25)	—
	%	25	0.4 ± 1.7	-3.1 ± 2.3	-1.7 ± 2.5	—
Z--	Cyto-toxicity	5	0.5 ± 1.3	-1.0 ± 1.9	-0.7 ± 2.4	—

infrequent finding; that one can detect sharing of antigens between cells where serologically there is no sharing. This is another line of evidence that the cytotoxic target antigens may not be identical to what is seen serologically.

The cellular reactions that take place against cytotoxic antigens require two T cell subpopulations: a helper T cell, presumably responsive to the LD antigens, and a cytotoxic T cell, primarily responsive to the CD antigens.

Sollinger and I have obtained some evidence that this collaboration between LD-responsive and CD-responsive cells is operative *in vivo* as well.

PARKMAN: Is there an effective way to sensitize MLC identical individuals *in vitro* to CD antigenic differences?

CHAIRMAN BACH: Yes. For example, Shearer pointed out that in the Hh system one doesn't need a proliferative response.

FESTENSTEIN: We found in mice that an I region incompatibility, particularly one not relating to the strong lymphocyte-activating determinants of the I-A region, is required for the amplification process in order to produce effective or good CML reactivity. One can get CML responses without MLC positivity, but it is easier and more effective if one has that incompatibility as well. We have called it ECS (effector cell stimulating) incompatibility because it is genetically separate from the determinants of MLC.

CHAIRMAN BACH: Can Festenstein or others obtain cytotoxic cells against non-MHC target antigens?

FESTENSTEIN: Despite identity at the HLA-D locus, Van Rood and Gaulmy get weak MLC and generate cytotoxic effectors very well.

CHAIRMAN BACH: That is an important issue. Is there really any evidence that without proliferation one can get cytotoxicity in man? In Van Rood and Gaulmy's work there was very weak stimulation.

WERNET: Bach's PLT cells were sent to us in Tubingen and were tested against 30 HLA-ABC D typed unrelated individuals. The clustering of individuals of our panel was very similar to that observed by Bach. Likewise, two D locus specificities defined by MLC typing as identical segregate by PLT typing into two different categories. An interesting question would be whether cells like these would be able to become cytotoxic for each other in a CML test.

DUPONT: We studied the distribution of relative responses obtained in MLC of family members consisting of 77 HLA-identical sibling pairs, 287 one-haplotype-different family members, and 328 two-haplotype-different combinations. We included 59 pairs of unrelated individuals HLA-D identical according to results with two different typing cells of the well-defined specificities DW1, DW2, DW3, and DW4. Our results actually support the idea that one is dealing with a region with multiple genes and/or cross-reacting antigens, and that the D specificities defined by homozygous typing cells are clearly clusters of multiple determinants.

EIJSVOOGEL: One cannot overlook that the data that are accumulating reveal discrepancies between what is demonstrated serologically and what is demonstrated in CML. That is clear. Whether this is due to some cross reactivity that is not detected serologically, we don't yet know, but we should perhaps expect to find different patterns than we are finding now. Otherwise we have to assume that there are other determinants on the same molecule, which are the target specificities of CML or that there is a separate molecule controlled by a distinct locus. But in the latter case, we have to assume a high linkage disequilibrium with the SD genes.

CHAIRMAN BACH: Or, perhaps, it is the same determinant that has to be presented in a somewhat clustered form.

WARNER: Are the data still accepted that in mouse cytotoxicity there is a restriction that only private H-2 specificities can be recognized by cytotoxic T cells? As yet there is no apparent difference in the ability of serological reagents to be capable of reacting with either the private or the public components. Could the cellular competitive-inhibition assay be used to assess the reactivity of the cytotoxic cell? The blocking assay would be a way of looking at the antigenicity of the molecule and not at its immunogenicity.

CHAIRMAN BACH: Competitive blocking of cross reactions by the specific target was obtained by Sondel and myself. Also, one can get killing associated with some public specificities as defined serologically.

FESTENSTEIN: A mouse tumor cell lacking the K private specificity was still a good target for cytotoxicity. Moreover, I region products are also targets in CML.

GALE: I want to pose a question regarding the cellular basis of GVHD. There is a model for generation of secondary CTL (cytotoxic lymphocytes) against MHC antigens without proliferation. If an analogy to non-MHC antigens can be drawn, one could account for graft rejection in presensitized recipients without cellular proliferation. If one examines the situation with GVHD where the donor is not sensitized, it is difficult to understand the mechanism whereby cytotoxic lymphocytes could be generated without a proliferative response. Even if CTL were generated with a proliferative response, one would anticipate a low incidence of CTL without clonal expansion, which would probably not be detectable *in vitro*. Given the constraints of our usual CML assays requiring high effector:target cell ratios, this seems very unlikely. How then does one explain reports of CTL activity in MHC identical transplant recipients with GVHD?

SCHMITT-VERHULST: In those systems in which one doesn't detect proliferation by ^{3}H-thymidine uptake, there is still a requirement for DNA synthesis for the generation of CTL (TNP-autologous and "Hh"). Indeed, if BUdR is added two days after the onset of the culture and one exposes to light one day later, the generation of CTL effector cells is abolished.

WARNER: I would like to return to the issue raised by Eijsvoogel on the molecular basis of the distinction between SD and CML target components. Are these two different molecules on the cell surface, or different determinants on the same molecule?

Perhaps one piece of data already answers this. If the SD determinants are capped, the determinants for killer cells remain available on the target, thus indicating they are on two different molecules. Alternatively, SD capping may have not been absolute and it only takes a few determinants left to act as CML targets.

There are perhaps other methods for solving this problem. Using the approach of cell surface iodination techniques, it is possible to label and isolate the recognition site on a cytotoxic T cell, and then this material could be used as a probe to dissect the nature of the membrane component with which it is reacting. We have already heard that NP-40 solubilized extracts contain molecules that can block the CML.

CHAIRMAN BACH: I think the answer will be obtained soon. Edidin and Henney, in addition to capping the SD antigens, also treated cells with papain for different periods of time to determine when the susceptibility to killing was lost. Cell-mediated and antibody-mediated killing were both lost at the same rate.

GORDON: The H-Y system and Bevans' minor H gene system offer good models for approaching the issue of requirement of a proliferative response for CML. Two facts stand out. First, one cannot get a primary CML response *in vitro* to either H-Y or minor H antigens. Second, according to Cantor, Lyl,2,3 positive cells are required for responses to altered self but not for traditional responses to alloantigens. All of this suggests that these systems start at a point of greater immaturity for CML responses. However, we do not know if there is in fact thymidine uptake in primary cultures for anti H-Y.

ELKINS: It is going to be very complicated to investigate helper effects in CML against minor H antigens. One could use the M locus to cause a proliferative response and perhaps helper function. So, just the idea that proliferating T cells will give a helper effect for killer cells to a minor H antigen is naive.

GORDON: I did not mean to imply that it was merely a matter of inducing proliferation. We need to know more about the specific subsets of T cells involved in these responses, not just general proliferation. I was referring to antigen-specific proliferation required to generate sufficient numbers of educated T cell clones of both amplifier type and cytotoxic effector type.

DAUSSET: It is now clear that the genes coding for B cell specificities are localized around HLA-D. The main question at the present time is to know if PLT and HTC antigens are the same or different from those we detect by serology. We cannot answer this question at the present time. There is good correlation, but it is never complete, and this is the status of the ongoing work. In preparation for the Seventh International Histocompatibility Testing Workshop we are already identifying clusters of sera that define cellular specificities of the B lymphocyte in every region of the world.

Another issue at present is the existence of one or two Ia-like loci. There is some evidence that there are two loci and that each HLA-D specificity is probably the result of interaction of two genes. This may explain the discrepancies and the complexity observed with cellular techniques.

In our laboratory, we tried to approach this problem by immunizing HLA-identical parent–siblings. In one family, the father was immunized with cells of his HLA-identical, MLC-negative daughter yielding an antibody reacting against donor B cells, and not against cells of a second HLA-identical offspring. Thus, we are dealing with a B lymphocyte system that is *not* HLA linked. This system has been found in many other family studies as distinct from HLA. It could be a candidate for some minor locus, perhaps important in bone marrow transplantation.

In another family where the father was immunized against his MLC-positive daughter an anti-B lymphocyte antibody that detects the product of a gene linked to HLA was formed. The specificity defined by this antibody is closely linked to HLA-D as shown by family studies and recombination.

Another approach that we tried in our laboratory is to test systematically all the sera of bone marrow transplant patients. The sera of patients with GVHD react with normal B lymphocytes in seven of eight cases. In all eight cases they also react with lymphoblastoid and leukemic B cell lines. The optimal temperature for these antibodies was 15°C. They react with cells of the donor, recipient, and other members of the family as if they had no specificity.

WARNER: It is relevant to stress some parallel serologic data from studies in the mouse. It is now known that there are at least four, and probably five, distinct I region genetic loci in mice. From an evolutionary point of view, it is very likely that they will also be found in man for the reason that there appears to be differential expression of these I region genes in distinct T cell subpopulations.

DUPONT: We have also identified serum groups defining B lymphocyte alloantigens. There is strong linkage disequilibrium of these determinants with HLA-D, and there is also significant association with the relevant HLA-B antigens.

It is well known that anti-Ia antibodies of the mouse block stimulation in MLC. Also human anti-B lymphocyte antibody blocks the MLC in which two DW4 homozygous typing cells were the stimulators for a panel of six unrelated individuals not carrying any of the known HLA-D specificities. However, the MLC-blocking was not complete, though it was specific, by not blocking MLC with DW1 or DW3 homozygous typing cells. In another series of such experiments we identified B-lymphocyte alloantigens coded for by genes close to the HLA-A locus. These data support the concept that human B-lymphocyte alloantigens are specified by several different genes, and that some are closely linked to the HLA-D chromosomal region, while others are close to the HLA-A locus.

WERNET: By using a human anti-Ia alloantiserum we were able to precipitate from radioidinated NP40-lysed B lymphoblastoid cell membranes two polypeptides that according to markers had a molecular weight of 24,000 to 28,000 daltons. Analogous preparations from Daudi cells yielded only one with molecular weight of 28,000. This peak carries the Ia-like specificity. Peripheral blood B lymphocytes yield two polypeptides. This led us to believe that there are two components to the Ia-like molecule; the larger one is detected by serology and the smaller one seems to be more common. It is possible that the antibody Dausset has observed during GVHD (the one without known specificity) is directed against this common component of Ia.

FESTENSTEIN: Another HLA-D typing technique was developed as a consequence of the finding that sperm stimulate lymphocytes to divide *in vitro*. The question was whether sperm actually express the same kind of antigens on the surface as are recognized by HTC typing, and other methods. Dausset had shown some time ago that HLA antigens were present on sperm in haploid form and this was confirmed by Halim in my laboratory. More recently, we used this principle to separate the sperm into two haploid populations. The method has also been used for genotyping males without having to do family studies.

Sperm are treated with an anti-HLA serum, either an anti-HLA-A or HLA-B locus antibody, and then treated with complement; the sperm are filtered through a nylon column. The dead are retained and the viable sperm coming through are used for HLA-D locus typing. Thus if one eliminates sperm that have a given specificity on one haplotype, the remaining sperm will stimulate lymphocytes from all individuals except those who share the stimulating haplotype.

EIJSVOOGEL: I would like to make a general comment. On exposure to these and similar data comparing B cell antigens with HTC specificities, it is important to realize the following: HTC typing is at present a relatively crude method with technical problems. Dupont just illustrated that individuals that type identical in this manner are very often not really MLC identical.

There are, however, also other aspects that limit the information obtained by the present HTC typing. We too have data indicating that some of the typing cells in international use recognize either broad specificities or even multiple specificities, determined by the same haplotype. This is not so surprising if one is aware of the nature of the reaction underlying HTC typing. As long as the typing cell does not carry any determinant absent from the responder cell, the reaction will be negative, thus characterizing the responder as having one LD haplotype in common with the typing cell. However, this does not exclude the possibility that the responder cell has additional LD determinants controlled by the same haplotype, but absent on the HTC. Our experiments indicate that this indeed occurs. This would explain why individuals that type identical with HTCs may still differ for LD and when tested against each other yield a positive MLC.

So, this implies that for proper recognition of lymphocyte activation, or LD determinants, we should use methods that allow us to further dissect the different specificities. In my opinion, only the PLT assay has this potential, as it develops cells of more and more limited specificity.

The comparison of data obtained in this way with those of B-cell antisera will then be much more informative. Even the fact that Bach still finds discrepancies between his PLT antigens and the Batchelor antiserum is not disconcerting, since it may well be that these PLT cells (though of much more limited specificity than HTCs) still pick up more than one determinant.

WERNET: I agree with Eijsvoogel and this is the reason we also make these comparisons. But as long as the PLT system is not yet defined, we prefer to use complementary methods, particularly the Ia-serology. The real difficulty of evaluating any type of cellular response is the unresolved issue of target antigenic determinants. If they are distinct, then again one is hardly likely to find the full answer by means of immunogenetic typing with one method. An approach based on different and complementary methodologies is still needed.

CHAIRMAN BACH: Before closing this discussion, Elkins should tell us about his studies on correlation between *in vitro* CML and *in vivo* events such as GVHR and GVHD.

ELKINS: We have been looking for a while at the possibility that the factors controlling the generation of CML effector cells, i.e., cytotoxic T lymphocytes (CTL), would also be important in the pathogenesis of GVHD, insofar as they would effect the GVHR. If so, there should be a correlation between the results of the CML and GVH mortality assays as genetic disparity is varied. The problem with this is that one is studying one unknown with another, and the sensitivity of each assay is itself a variable. Unfortunately, genetic disparity is not the sole determinant of the result in either assay.

Despite these difficulties, we looked at combinations wherein there were either partial or complete differences in the H-2 complex. We found a rather good correlation between Bach's CML results and GVH mortality (*Transplant. Proc.* **8:**343, 1976).

In the case of an H-2K or H-2D difference alone, it is quite hard to get GVHD and usually the CML is weak. With complete I region differences, as between AQR and B10.T(6R), there is CML of moderate strength, but lethal GVHD. On the other hand, in the combination B10.A(4R) vs. B10.A(2R), in which there is an I-C region difference causing MLC-like proliferation with very little effector-cell activity, we find no GVH mortality. B10.A(4R) mice also fail to reject B10.A(2R) skin grafts. Thus, GVH mortality is modest in this combination even though a variety of conditioning regimens were employed. It is to be noted that B10.A(4R) T cells are stimulated by I-C differences so as to proliferate in the spleens of irradiated B10.A(2R) mice. So, one could say that there is a GVHR in terms of antigen-induced proliferation, lacking however the effector CTL component. With this experimental setup we are in a position to verify the postulated "helper effect" of an I-C difference.

The AQR chromosome is similar to B10.A(2R) as judged by Ia markers in the I-C subregion. It thus specifies LD antigens that would stimulate B10.A(4R) donor lymphocytes as in B10.A(2R) hosts. AQR also differs from B10.A(4R) at H-2K and H-2D but not in the I-A subregion. Thus, in the combination B10.A(4R) versus [AQR × B10.A(4R)]F$_1$ one might predict a "helper effect" of the I-C region LD antigens facilitating the development of CTL to the CD determinants in the H-2K and H-2D regions. Moreover, this putative helper effect could be eliminated through genetic complementation when [B10.A(2R) × B10.A(4R)]F$_1$ mice are used as the donors. In this case the I-C region difference is lost but the CD differences remain. Accordingly, we have compared the mortality rate of [AQR × B10.A(4R)]F$_1$ hosts injected with B10.A(4R) or [B10.A(2R) × B10.A(4R)F$_1$ lymphocytes in several experiments. We varied the conditioning regimens and the dose and source of donor cells (lymph node, spleen, bone marrow). We found that when conditioning was suboptimal, as with

400 R total body irradiation and relatively small numbers of injected spleen cells, a pronounced helper effect of the I-C stimulus could be demonstrated. This was revealed by more frequent and earlier deaths among the recipients of B10.A(4R) cells compared to those receiving [B10.A(4R) × B10.A(2R)]F_1 cells. However, under more stringent conditions, when conditioning included cyclophosphamide or larger numbers of donor cells were employed, the recipients of the F_1 cells exhibited the same GVH mortality as did those receiving B10.A(4R) cells. Thus, the helper effect becomes irrelevant (superfluous) when the system is optimized for GVHD.

My interpretation is that in the heavily conditioned host the relatively few CTL generated in the absence of LD help are capable of producing lethal GVHD. Amplification of the CTL population by a helper effect would then be superfluous. This reemphasizes the point I made earlier that the intensity of GVHD is a function both of the intensity of the GVHR and the conditioning regimen.

GOLUB: The nature of the "helper effect" postulated by Elkins seems to be unknown as yet. Why then not just assume that conditioning with cyclophosphamide and heavy irradiation substitutes for products of helper cells in some unknown manner? Elkin's experiments were addressed to the basic question of whether or not MLR and GVHR use the same loci. The results suggest to me that for clinical situations the question is irrelevant because the conditioning regimens eliminate the need for "help."

MHC-RESTRICTED CELLULAR IMMUNITY: ALTERED SELF AND MINOR ALLOANTIGENS

Discussion Introducer:

Gene M. Shearer

CHAIRMAN SHEARER: During the past 2½ years a previously unknown functional association between products of the murine MHC and cell-mediated immunity has been recognized. T-cell-mediated cytotoxic reactions were demonstrated against viral-infected (Zinkernagel and Doherty, *Nature* **248:**701, 1974), chemically modified (Shearer, *Eur. J. Immunol.* **4:**527, 1974), and weak-transplantation antigen-associated (Gordon *et al., J. Exp. Med.* **142:**105, 1975; Bevan, *Nature* **256:**419, 1975) syngeneic cells. All of the responses (irrespective of whether they were generated in vivo or in vitro) shared the striking common feature of exhibiting specificity not only for the antigen involved, but also for syngeneic K and D region products of the H-2 complex. More explicitly, the effector cells from viral-infected mice lysed only target cells that were infected with the same or a cross-reacting virus and that expressed the same K and/or D region antigens as the infected source of effector cells. Likewise effectors generated from cultures sensitized with syngeneic chemically modified cells lysed only targets that were modified with the same "hapten," and that shared the K and/or D regions of H-2 with the responding-effector and/or stimulating cells. Similar results were obtained in the weak-transplantation antigen system.

Two basic models have been proposed to account for the H-2 restriction observed in these experiments (Zinkernagel and Doherty, *Nature* **248:**701, 1974; Shearer, *Eur. J. Immunol.* **4:**571, 1974). The "altered self" model proposes that the viral components or chemical agents interact with self H-2 antigens, resulting in significant alterations of the syngeneic antigenic structures, which are then recognized as nonself. This model has been considered to involve a single receptor for recognition of the neoantigen. The second model, known as the "dual receptor" model, proposes that two receptors are involved—one for the "hapten" or viral antigenic determinant, and a second for the recognition of unaltered self structures. The second receptor for self recognition would presumably be important for conferring enough binding energy for an immunological event to occur. A number of experiments have been designed and performed to discriminate between these two alternatives, but none has thus far provided unequivocal proof or disproof of either model, although certain experiments involving fine specificity studies of the TNP-modified self systems tend to favor altered self (Rehn *et al., J. Exp. Med.* **144:**1134, 1976).

The objectives of this discussion will be (a) to review briefly the major features of the H-2-restricted CML, using the *in vitro* generation of cytotoxic effectors to trinitrophenyl (TNP)-modified syngeneic cells; (b) to consider new results of the TNP-self model; (c) to discuss in some detail one of the H-2-associated weak-transplantation antigen systems (the H-Y antigen) for which considerable information is available concerning antibody production and skin graft rejection; (d) to present some recent results from the radiation leukemia virus model, which may be important for this issue; and (e) to consider the possible relevance of the H-2-restricted phenomenon in F_1 antiparental cytotoxicity.

I would like to start the discussion by briefly reviewing the relevant experimental points that have been made during the past three years using the CML model for TNP-modified syngeneic cells. The method employed involves the co-culturing of spleen cells from normal mice with autologous or syngeneic spleen cells that have been modified with trinitrobenzene sulfonic acid (Shearer, *Eur. J. Immunol.* **4:**527, 1974). After five days in culture, the effector cells generated are assayed by the standard four-hour ^{51}Cr-release assay on a series of unmodified or chemically modified target cells expressing different H-2 haplotypes. Our experience concerning the specificity of such effector cells can be summarized as shown in Tables 38–41.

As shown in Table 38, the modifying agent makes a significant contribution to the specificity of the cytotoxic reaction. Cells modified with TNBS do not cross-react with cells modified with N(-3-nitro-4-hydroxy-5-iodophenyl acetyl)-β-alanylglycylglycylazide (N), and vice versa (Rehn *et al., J. Exp. Med.* **143:**127, 1976). In order to define the specificity even further, the TNP group was separated from the cell surface by an alanylglycylglycyl tripeptide spacer (x-TNP). Although responders sensitized with x-TNP-modified syngeneic stimulators generated effectors that lysed x-TNP-modified targets, indicating that x-TNP-modified cells are both antigenic and immunogenic, effectors generated against TNP-modified syngeneic stimulators did not lyse x-TNP modified targets

TABLE 38

Role of the Modifying Agent ("Hapten") in the Specificity of Effector Cells Generated by Sensitization *in vitro* against Modified Syngeneic Spleen Cells[a]

Responding cells	Stimulating cells	Target cells	Lysis
A	A	A	−
A	A-TNP	A	−
A	A	A-TNP	−
A	A-TNP	A-TNP	+ +
A	A-TNP	A-N	−
A	A-N	A-N	+
A	A-N	A-TNP	−
A	A-TNP	A-x-TNP	−
A	A-TNP	A~TSD	−
A	A~TSD	A~TSD	−

[a] A, any inbred mouse strain; -TNP, cells modified with trinitrobenzenesulfonic acid; -N, cells modified with N-(3-nitro-4-hydroxy-5-iodophenyl acetyl)-β-alanylglycylglycylazide; -x-TNP, cells modifieed with TNP separated from the cell surface by a β-alanylglycylglycyl group; ~TSD, cells modified by TNP-stearoyl dextran by noncovalent linkage.

TABLE 39

Role of the Murine Major Histocompatibility Complex in the
Specificity of Effector Cells Generated by Sensitization *in vitro*
against Modified Syngeneic Spleen Cells[a]

Responding cells	Stimulating cells	Target cells	Lysis
A	A-TNP	A-TNP	++
A	A-TNP	B-TNP	−
(A × B)F$_1$	(A × B)F$_1$-TNP	A-TNP	++
(A × B)F$_1$	(A × B)F$_1$-TNP	B-TNP	++
(A × B)F$_1$	A-TNP	A-TNP	++
(A × B)F$_1$	A-TNP	B-TNP	−
(A × B)F$_1$	B-TNP	B-TNP	++
(A × B)F$_1$	B-TNP	A-TNP	−
A	B-TNP	A-TNP	+
A	B	A-TNP	+
A	B	A	−

[a] A and B indicate inbred mouse strains that differ throughout the entire H-2 complex or at H-2K and H-2D.

(Rehn *et al., J. Exp. Med.* **144:**1134, 1976). It is noteworthy that cells modified
with an amphipathic molecule such as TNP-stearoyl-dextran (∼TSD), which
binds to the cell surface by a noncovalent linkage, are neither immunogenic nor
antigenic (Henkart *et al., J. Exp. Med.,* in press). Furthermore, TSD-modified
cells do not serve as targets for effectors generated by sensitization with TNBS-
modified stimulators. Such results suggest that a stable interaction may be required between the interacting agent and the relevant self cellular antigenic
structures. These observations support the altered-self model, since both TNP
groups and self H-2-coded structures were demonstrated on TSD-modified cells.

The importance of the murine major histocompatibility complex (H-2) in
determining the specificity of CML against TNP-modified syngeneic cells is
summarized in Table 39. When lymphocytes from two inbred mouse strains that
do not share K and D region haplotypes and the F$_1$ hybrid are compared for
cross-reactivity, it has been observed that effectors generated by sensitization
with syngeneic modified cells will not lyse (or will lyse much less) target cells
of another inbred strain modified by the same agent, but expressing different K
and D haplotypes (Shearer, *Eur. J. Immunol.* **4:**527, 1974; Shearer *et al., J. Exp.
Med.* **141:**1348, 1975; Forman, *J. Exp. Med.* **142:**403, 1975). Lymphocytes
from F$_1$ mice will lyse modified targets from either parent, when sensitized with
modified F$_1$ stimulator cells. Lymphocytes from F$_1$ mice sensitized against modified parental cells will lyse modified parental target cells only of the haplotype
used for sensitization. Such results indicate that homology between effector and
target cells is not the homology (or at least is not the only homology) that is

relevant for lympholysis, and favors but does not prove the altered-self mode. In this context, it is noteworthy that other experiments have been performed in which parental lymphocytes were made tolerant to alloantigens by engrafting in F_1 hybrid hosts. Such parental cells, while unable to respond to the relevant alloantigens, do generate CML against the allogeneic cells modified with TNP (Pfizenmaier *et al.*, *J. Exp. Med.* **143**:999, 1976; von Boehmer and Haas, *Nature* **261**:141, 1976). These findings also favor altered self, although more complex interpretations are possible.

A more detailed analysis of the involvement of products of the H-2 complex in this system has been made by mapping within H-2 those regions for which homology is important. These results, summarized in Table 40, indicate that either K or K plus I-A represent the regions for which homology is required in the B10.A strain. It is important to point out that homology at regions that include D but not K did not result in appreciable lysis. In contrast, effector cells from the B10.D2 strain lysed TNP-modified targets syngeneic with the cells of the responding phase at I-C, S, and D or at all regions except D, including K. From

TABLE 40

Mapping within the Murine Major Histocompatibility Complex the Specificity of Effector Cells Generated by Sensitization *in vitro* against Modified Syngeneic Spleen Cells[a]

Responding cells	Stimulating cells	Target cells	Lysis	H-2 Homology at
B10.A kkkddd	B10.A-TNP kkkddd	B10.A-TNP kkkddd	+ +	All of H-2
		B10.A(4R)-TNP kkbbbb	+ +	K, I-A
		B10.D2 dddddd	−	I-C, S, D
		A.TL-TNP skkkkd	−	I-A, I-B, D
		C57BL/10-TNP bbbbbb	−	None
B10.D2 dddddd	B10.D2-TNP dddddd	B10.D2-TNP dddddd	+	All of H-2
		B10.A-TNP kkkddd	+	I-C, S, D
		B10.A(2R)-TNP kkkddb	−	I-C, S
		C3H.OH-TNP dddddk	+	K through S
		C57BL/10-TNP bbbbbb	−	None

[a]Lower case letters indicate the haplotypes of origin of the K, I-A, I-B, I-C, S, and D regions of H-2. The more recently described I-J, I-E, and G regions are excluded for simplicity.

these and other studies, it has been concluded that K and D are the regions of H-2 for which homology is important in these CML reactions.

As outlined in Table 41, B10.D2 but not B10.A responding cells generate effectors that lyse modified targets syngeneic with the effector and stimulating cells at H-2D. These results are compatible with there being H-2-linked immune response (Ir) gene control of cytotoxic potential for TNP-modified syngeneic H2D^d. Dominant, H-2 linked, Ir gene control has been demonstrated for the H-2D^d-TNP specificity (Schmitt-Verhulst and Shearer, *J. Exp. Med.* **142**:914, 1975; Schmitt-Verhulst *et al., J. Exp. Med.* **143**:211, 1976). Recent mapping studies for this Ir effect have revealed that the CML response to the H-2D^d-TNP specificity is in fact controlled by at least two distinct H-2-linked genes (Schmitt-Verhulst and Shearer, *J. Exp. Med.* **144**:1701, 1976) as described later.

Thus, the TNP-modified syngeneic CML system provides a unique example of a major histocompatibility-linked control of T-cell-mediated immunity at two distinct but interacting functional levels. One is expressed in the stimulating and target cells, and has to do with the H-2-modified or H-2-restricted antigenic

TABLE 41

Dominant Genetic Expression of Cytotoxicity by (B10.A × B10.D2)F$_1$ Responding Cells to TNP-Modified Products Associated with H-2D^d

Responding cells	Stimulating cells	Target cells^a	Specific lysis^b
B10.A kkkddd	B10.A-TNP kkkddd	B10.A-TNP *kkkddd*	++
		B10.D2-TNP *dddddd*	−
(B10.A × B10.D2)F$_1$ kkkddd dddddd	B10.A-TNP kkkddd	B10.A-TNP *kkkddd*	++
		B10.D2-TNP *dddddd*	+
	B10.D2-TNP dddddd	B10.A-TNP *kkkddd*	+
		B10.D2-TNP *dddddd*	+
B10.D2 dddddd	B10.D2-TNP dddddd	B10.A-TNP *kkkddd*	+
		B10.D2-TNP *dddddd*	+

^{a}Italics indicate target cell H-2 region common to responding and stimulating cells.

^{b}++, >30%; +, 10–20%; −, <5%; effector:target ratio, 20:1

structures. The second H-2 control is expressed in the responding cells and involves immune response potential to these H-2-modified or H-2-restricted antigenic structures. Thus, the generation of an immune response in such a system would depend on at least three levels of control: one concerned with the "modifying" agent and the specificity it contributes (or the first receptor of a dual recognition model); the second, also concerned with the specificity of the antigenic complex, involving H-2-coded products (or the second receptor of the dual recognition model); and the third expressed at the level of the Ir gene(s) control necessary for recognition and response to the antigenic complex formed.

FESTENSTEIN: Does Shearer have serological or other data to show that the H-2K and the H-2D gene products are altered?

CHAIRMAN SHEARER: The answer is that we do not.

UHR: I can mention some work that is pertinent to the question. Foreman, Vitetta, Hart, and Klein have evidence that the H-2 antigens are altered by TNP in the system described by Shearer. They have looked at the capacity of the stimulator or the target cells to act in the TNP-syngeneic system as a function of the extent of derivatization of surface molecules by TNP. They also examined the surface molecules on these cells over a wide dose range of TNP added to the cells to determine which molecules were derivatized. At low doses, non-H-2 molecules were derivatized, and as the concentration of TNP was increased, more non-H-2 molecules were haptenated. However, only at the concentration of TNP where H-2 became derivatized did the cells then begin to function as stimulators or as targets. Therefore, they found a strict correlation between the function of these cells and the capacity of the H-2 molecules on them to be derivatized. The experiment also indicates that the effect of TNP is at the cell surface.

WARNER: In relation to that point, is there any information on the degree of derivatization of the H-2 molecules? What I am getting at is whether the modification of the molecule is so extensive that it might have altered most of the H-2 antigenic determinants. As I understand it, there is no evidence of any loss of H-2 specificities in TNP conjugated cells.

UHR: The H-2 molecule probably does not need to be heavily haptenated. Foreman *et al.* were able to show that one molecule of TNP per H-2 was sufficient for detection by an antibody binding assay. Thus, at the lowest concentrations of TNP, when only a modest derivatization of H-2 had occurred, one already could demonstrate acquired function of the haptenated cells.

DAUSSET: Nonetheless, one can still fix an anti-H-2 on the so-called altered H-2 molecule. Does this mean that the antigenic determinants are not modified? If so, the modifications must involve other parts of the molecule.

UHR: I think the observation Dausset referred to is a recapitulation *in vitro* of very old observations in humans, i.e., a delayed hypersensitive skin reaction can be elicited in the presence of an enormous excess of antibody. Presumably, the eliciting antigen is well covered by antibody. For example, a molecule of diptheria toxoid can probably bind seven or eight antitoxin molecules simultaneously in a normally immunized individual and yet it can elicit a delayed skin reaction. It remains to be explained how the antigenic receptors on T cells can respond to this type of immunogenic complex or, indeed, how such a complex could bind to an MHC product and create a toxoid-specific reaction.

FESTENSTEIN: One would expect that, if there were alteration, the serological reactions with a particular serum would be different, particularly in a quantitative sense. If one had achieved alteration, then one should not expect these things to be the same. But it is not possible to rationalize this properly if one knows that there is an alteration and yet cannot demonstrate by conventional testing a change in antibody binding. This is what I find difficult to understand in this whole system. Those who advance the altered self hypothesis claim that there is a new product, a neoantigen, which is derived from the old antigen and a new chemical grouping.

GOLUB: Doesn't this all get back to the question that Bach raised earlier, whether the CD product is an SD product. In the altered-self situation, we are looking for cell interaction products. It might very well be that reactivity with antibody is not the appropriate parameter.

FESTENSTEIN: It has been implied that the K and the D region products are involved from the mapping that was done by Shearer and others in the viral model.

GOLUB: The inference was not made from the serologic data but from genetic analysis. Shearer knew the haplotype but did not know which product of the MHC region was involved.

CHAIRMAN SHEARER: What we know is that whatever the relevant structure, it is a product of K or D regions, which may or may not be serologically defined.

DUPONT: Is the conventional testing with anti-H-2 reagents sufficiently quantitative that one would expect to pick up such an alteration?

FESTENSTEIN: I think it is.

SANFORD: With so many working on isolating molecules that carry H-2 specificity, isn't information emerging on whether one can detect biochemical differences on supposedly altered H-2 molecules?

UHR: Where the alteration is imposed by TNP, the questions could be asked: What part of the molecule is derivatized with TNP? Which parts carry private and public specificities as defined serologically? Which parts stimulate transplantation reactivity? Does TNP alter these portions? These experiments have not been done. In response to Festenstein's query, I think it *is* possible that one might have portions of the molecule altered by TNP that are distinct from those that normally induce cytotoxic reactivity. Thus, conventional anti-H-2 reactivity could be retained in the face of developing neoantigens. In addition, if the vocabulary for T cell recognition is different from that for antibody formation, we could even have an alteration induced by TNP-derivatization at the same part of the molecule that reacts with antibody and *yet* not lose the reactivity with T cells. One might retain recognition by one dictionary, while inserting a new word to be recognized by the second dictionary.

PARKMAN: Going back to Golub's point, we learned earlier that capping with anti-HLA still allowed the cells to be effective targets for CD antigens. Has anybody capped these cells for H-2 to see if they retain altered self function?

CANTOR: Experiments along that line have indeed been done. I believe it was Zinkernagel *et al.* who showed that one cannot lyse cells conjugated with TNP that do not express H-2. So the absence of H-2 precludes the altered self response.
    I would like to refocus the question in terms of the two models that have been discussed by Shearer, namely, are we dealing with a single antigen recognized by a single receptor, or a bivalent antigen recognized by two receptors. It seems to me that studies of the antigens cannot definitively answer this question. One may demonstrate the antigens as close together as one likes, one can also show considerable H-2 "modification," but one nonetheless may be dealing with two very closely related receptors. The most direct approach involves studying the receptors themselves.

WARNER: Replying to Cantor, don't we already have some information on that issue? It is my recollection that the hapten itself will not block the cytotoxic reaction. This approach might be more rewarding than looking at the inductive stage, where the potential of interaction between many cells is great. Thus, if dual receptors exist, they must also be expressed on the mature cytotoxic cells, and one receptor will be binding the hapten.

CANTOR: We cannot infer that the absence of blocking implies a single receptor for an altered H-2 product. For example, the energy of binding of cells that have two receptors, one binding H-2 and the other TNP, may be considerable. Hence it may be difficult to effectively block this interaction with hapten only.

CHAIRMAN SHEARER: I think we have arrived at the point where we can say that if two receptors are involved, they are not totally independent and must be very close to each other. Attempts to block these receptors in the way that Warner has suggested have not led us to the conclusion that they are separable one from the other.

SCHMITT-VERHULST: The data to be described present evidence for (a) the involvement of genes mapping within the H-2 complex in the control of responsiveness to TNP-self in association with a particular haplotype at the D region of H-2; (b) the differential requirements of H-2 region homology between primary and secondary TNP-modified stimulating cells for the generation of secondary CML and MLR *in vitro*.

The results in Table 41 show that the B10.A strain that has the same d haplotype as B10.D2 at the H-2D region does not express cytotoxicity in association with H-2D^d (as assayed on B10.D2-TNP targets) after sensitization with TNP-syngeneic cells, whereas the B10.D2 does (as measured on B10.A-TNP targets). The (B10.A × B10.D2)F$_1$ responder cells give, however, a H-2D^d-associated CML response when sensitized with either TNP-modified parental cells. These results suggested that there might be genes mapping in K through I-E (where B10.A and B10.D2 differ), which may regulate the ability to respond in CML to TNP modification in association with the H-2D^d haplotype and that these genes would be expressed in a dominant fashion in the F$_1$ mice. Further attempts to map within the H-2 region the genes controlling this response are shown in Table 42. The CML reactivities of the congenic strains A.TH, A.TL, and A.AL, all of which have the d haplotype at the D region but vary in the expression of the haplotypes in K and I regions are compared for both K end-associated and D end-associated TNP-self reactivities. Whereas all three strains produce high lysis of the TNP-modified H-2K-matched target cells, a differential pattern of reactivities is found on TNP-modified H-2^d (H-2D-matched) target cells. The A.TH gives a high response, the A.TL a significant but lower response, whereas the A.AL did not generate a significant response on the D-end matched target cells. Both the responder strains A.TH and A.TL have the s

TABLE 42

In Vitro Cytotoxic Responses to TNP-Modified Autologous Cells in Different Inbred Mouse Strains on the C57BL/10 and A Genetic Backgrounds[a]

Responding spleen cells	Stimulating spleen cells	H-2 Haplotype at:								TNP-Modified target cells[b]	Specific lysis ± S.E. (%)	Range of lysis
		K	A	B	J	E	C	S	D			
B10.A	B10.A-TNP	k	k	k	k	k	d	d	d	$H\text{-}2^d$	2.2 ± 1.1	1–10
										$H\text{-}2^s$	5.2 ± 1.0	2–16
										$H\text{-}2^k$	30.6 ± 1.7	22–46
B10.HTT	B10.HTT-TNP	s	s	s	s	k	k	k	d	$H\text{-}2^d$	38.0 ± 1.4	38–53
										$H\text{-}2^s$	49.9 ± 2.6	50–55
										$H\text{-}2^k$	27.3 ± 2.1	
A.AL	A.AL-TNP	k	k	k	k	k	k	k	d	$H\text{-}2^d$	8.2 ± 1.6	2–8
										$H\text{-}2^s$	3.1 ± 1.9	0–6
										$H\text{-}2^k$	32.5 ± 4.7	23–33
A.TL	A.TL-TNP	s	k	k	k	k	k	k	d	$H\text{-}2^d$	19.9 ± 1.1	20–23
										$H\text{-}2^s$	45.6 ± 0.9	10–46
										$H\text{-}2^k$	11.1 ± 2.5	0–11
A.TH	A.TH-TNP	s	s	s	s	s	s	s	d	$H\text{-}2^d$	33.3 ± 1.4	33–44
										$H\text{-}2^s$	51.8 ± 0.6	16–52
										$H\text{-}2^k$	11.4 ± 1.7	5–11

[a] Effector:target ratio, 40:1.
[b] $H\text{-}2^d$, $H\text{-}2^s$, and $H\text{-}2^k$ target cells were 48-hr PHA-stimulated blast spleen cells from B10.D2, SJL/J or B10.S, and B10.BR donors, respectively.

haplotype at the H-2K region. We verified by cold target inhibition experiments that the CML reactivity detected on the H-2^d targets was not a consequence of cross reactivity between H-$2K^s$ and H-$2D^d$ associated TNP-self reactivities. High responsiveness to H-$2D^d$ associated TNP-self reactivity was also found for the B10 congenic mice expressing the s haplotype at the K end (B10.HTT), whereas nonresponsiveness was associated with the k haplotype at the K end (B10.A).

Table 43 summarizes the mapping within H-2 of the ability to respond to self-TNP in association with the H-$2D^d$ specificity. Responsiveness is found whenever the s haplotype is expressed also in the I-A through I-J regions, as compared to the k haplotype. Therefore, it is suggested that two genes may be involved in the regulation of responsiveness to self-TNP in association with the H-$2D^d$ specificity, one mapping to the left of the crossover between K and I-A (as defined by the A.TL recombinant) and one mapping in the I-A, I-B, or I-J region.

These findings suggest that products of genes mapping within the H-2 region may control the cellular interactions that are required in order to generate cytotoxic effector cells to modified self. Responsiveness involving either a control of the expression of the relevant clones of cells specific for the recognition of TNP modification in association with H-$2D^d$ or a control at the level of a specific cellular interaction with helper or suppressor cells are testable speculations. Further analysis of the cellular interactions involved in the generation of effectors against modified self is required to define the level at which the regulation by these H-2 mapped genes occurs.

The mechanism of the H-2-associated recognition of chemically or virally modified syngeneic cells by cytotoxic effector cells is still debated. It has been

TABLE 43

Mapping within H-2 of Gene(s) Controlling the Level of TNP-Autologous
CML Associated with H-$2D^d$

	H-2 Haplotypes at Subregions:								
Responding and stimulating cells	K	I-A	(I-B	I-J)	(I-E)	I-C	S	D	Specific lysis[a]
A.TH	s	s	s	s	s	s	s |	d	+ +
A.TL	s |	k	k	k	k	k	k̇ |	d	+
A.AL	k	k	k	k	k	k	k |	d	−
B10.HTT	s	s	s	s |	k	k	k	d	+
B10.A	k	k	k	k	k	d	d	d	−

[a] + +, >25%; +, >15%; −, <6% at E/T = 20/1.

suggested that (1) H-2 cell surface products are part of the antigeneic or immunogenic structure resulting from the external modification of the cells (altered self), or (2) that the modifying agent and the self H-2 gene products are recognized by separate receptors of the T-effector cells.

The reactions requiring H-2K and/or H-2D homology that have so far been studied all involved the interaction between cytotoxic effector cells and target cells. It was therefore possible that some cell surface structure coded by the K and/or D region H-2 were functionally involved in the lytic event between effector and target cells (Forman, *J. Exp. Med.* **142**:403, 1975). One approach to define the specificity of lymphocytes stimulated by TNP-modified syngeneic cells, independently from a lytic assay, was to analyze the requirements for restimulation of sensitized cultures into secondary CML and MLR.

The results in Table 44 indicate that lymphocytes sensitized by culturing TNP-syngeneic cells *in vitro* for seven days could be restimulated by stimulator cells presenting the TNP on the same type of cells, but not by TNP-modified cells from a congenic resistant strain of mice differing in the expression of the H-2 haplotype. The inability of the cultures sensitized by TNP-syngeneic cells to

TABLE 44

Triggering of "Memory" Cells into Secondary Cytotoxic Cells Requires H-2
Homology between Primary and Secondary TNP-Modified Stimulator Cells[a]

Responding	Immunogen in primary	Immunogen in secondary	Specific lysis ± S.E. (% on	
			RDM4-TNP H-2^k-TNP	LSTRA-TNP H-2^d-TNP
B10.BR H-2^k	B10.BR-TNP H-2^k TNP	B10.BR H-2^k	0.0 (27.6)	0.0 (1.2)
		B10.BR-TNP H-2^k-TNP	39.3 ± 2.7	5.3 ± 0.6
		B10.D2 H-2^d	−5.5 ± 1.3	0.4 ± 0.6
		B10.D2-TNP H-2^d-TNP	−7.3 ± 1.3	1.1 ± 0.5
B10.BR H-2^k	B10.D2-TNP H-2^d-TNP	B10.BR H-2^k	0.0 (7.9)	0.9 (7.7)
		B10.BR-TNP H-2^k TNP	11.0 ± 1.5	13.4 ± 1.1
		B10.D2 H-2^d	17.3 ± 0.9	88.2 ± 3.5
		B10.D2-TNP H-2^d TNP	6.6 ± 0.9	56.7 ± 1.4

[a]Effector:target ratio, 10:1.

generate a primary allogeneic reaction after restimulation with allogeneic cells is probably due to nonspecific suppressor cells of precursors of primary CML and MLR effectors in unsensitized (Hodes and Hathcock, *J. Immunol.* **116:**167, 1976) or sensitized spleen cell cultures. Such conditions are favorable for the analysis of the H-2 homology requirements for secondary CML and MLR allowing the use of allogeneic stimulator cells in the absence of an allogeneic reaction.

Although the generation of a primary CML reaction against TNP-syngeneic cells is accompanied by only marginal cellular proliferation as measured by thymidine incorporation into the cells, a strong proliferative response could be measured two to three days after secondary stimulation with TNP-modified cells syngeneic to the primary TNP-modified stimulating cells. The results in Table 45 indicate that optimal TNP-dependent restimulation is obtained when the secondary stimulating cells share the whole H-2 (irrespective of the "background") or the K and I-A regions of H-2 [B10.A(4R), results not shown] with the primary TNP-stimulating cells. When only the D region (C3H.OH) or the I region (A.TL) haplotype were shared between primary and secondary TNP-modified stimulating cells, a lower but significant TNP-dependent proliferative response was observed. These results suggest (a) that the specificity of lymphocytes sensitized *in vitro* against TNP-modified syngeneic cells is for TNP and H-2 coded products not only as measured by the lytic interaction between effector and target cells, but also for the restimulation of primary sensitized precursors of CML and MLR responsive cells; and (b) that TNP modification can be recognized in association with I region products by strongly proliferative cells, whereas this recognition did not occur by the cytotoxic effectors.

An approach to distinguish between models involving one receptor for modified self or two receptors (one for the modifying agent and one for unmodified self H-2 products) has been attempted by the selective *in vitro* elimination of clones of cells reactive against an alloantigen by suicide of proliferating cells and by restimulating the cultures with the same alloantigens modified with TNP. The results described in Table 46 indicate that when the clones of B10.BR cells reacting against B10.D2 alloantigens were eliminated after BUdR and light treatment, no cytotoxic effectors could be generated against TNP-modified B10.D2 allogenic cells. It is important to note that CML effectors specific for TNP-syngeneic cells could be stimulated by TNP-modified B10.BR cells in these same cultures. These results indicate that stimulation with B10.D2 alloantigens in the primary culture activates clones that recognize TNP-modified as well as -unmodified B10.D2 stimulators in the secondary cultures. These results do not support the hypothesis that there are separate clones of lymphocytes that are stimulated by modified alloantigens (B10.D2-TNP) that would not be activated by the unmodified B10.D2 alloantigens. At least two interpretations are possible from these results. First, the clones of cells recognizing TNP-modified alloantigens are among the cells that are sensitized by (and probably bear a receptor for)

TABLE 45

Mapping the Regions within the H-2 Complex Responsible for Secondary Mixed-Lymphocyte Reactions against TNP-Modified Stimulating Cells

Primary stimulating cells	Secondary stimulating cells[a]	K	[A	B	J	E	C	S]	D	cpm ± S.E.	Ratio	Δcpm
B10.BR-TNP H-2^k	B10.BR	k	k	k	k	k	k	k	k	2888 ± 279	1.0	0
	B10.BR-TNP	k	k	k	k	k	k	k	k	42,928 ± 1049	14.9	40,040
	C3H/HeJ	k	k	k	k	k	k	k	k	1644 ± 174	0.6	−1243
	C3H/HeJ-TNP	k	k	k	k	k	k	k	k	47,033 ± 2623	16.3	44,145
	C3H.OH	d	d	d	d	d	d	d	k	6366 ± 345	2.2	3478
	C3H.OH-TNP	d	d	d	d	d	d	d	k	26,030 ± 1358	9.0	23,142
	B10.D2	d	d	d	d	d	d	d	d	12,187 ± 222	4.2	9299
	B10.D2-TNP	d	d	d	d	d	d	d	d	9923 ± 419	3.4	7035
	A.TL	s	k	k	k	k	k	k	d	5705 ± 504	2.0	2817
	.TL-TNP	s	k	k	k	k	k	k	d	26,880 ± 1332	9.3	23,993
	A.TH	s	s	s	s	s	s	s	d	3320 ± 188	1.2	432
	A.TH-TNP	s	s	s	s	s	s	s	d	4164 ± 327	1.4	1276

Header spanning columns K through D: H-2 haplotype at[b]

[a] Responding lymphocytes from B10.BR donors were restimulated seven days after the initiation of the primary cultures.
[b] H-2 subregions common to primary and secondary stimulating cells are underlined.

TABLE 46

Inability to Generate Anti-B10.D2-TNP Effector Cells from B10.BR Spleen Cells Selectively Depleted of B10.D2 Reactive Cells

Responder	Treatment[a]	Primary immunogen	Secondary immunogen	Specific lysis (% on Target Cells[b])				
				B10.BR (H-2^k)		P815 (H-2^d)		EL-4(H-2^b)
				—	TNP	—	TNP	—
B10.BR	BUdR + light	B10.D2	B10.BR	[19.6] 0.0	[19.6] 0.0	[10.8] 0.0	[8.8] 0.0	[12.8] 0.0
			B10.BR-TNP	0.7 ± 1.5	36.2 ± 1.5	3.5 ± 1.1	3.9 ± 0.9	4.2 ± 1.6
			B10.D2	6.5 ± 1.7	7.8 ± 1.6	7.7 ± 1.0	9.8 ± 1.1	5.8 ± 1.8
			B10.D2-TNP	1.6 ± 1.2	10.8 ± 1.4	4.5 ± 0.7	7.3 ± 0.9	5.4 ± 1.6
			B10	8.5 ± 1.1	20.0 ± 2.0	5.3 ± 0.8	8.2 ± 0.9	69.7 ± 2.0
B10.BR	no	B10.BR	no	[17.0] 0.0	[26.1] 0.0	[9.1] 0.0	[7.3] 0.0	[12.4] 0.0
		B10.BR-TNP	no	3.4 ± 0.8	62.8 ± 2.4	1.8 ± 1.0	6.9 ± 0.7	5.9 ± 0.4
		B10.D2	no	15.8 ± 0.5	25.6 ± 2.0	61.2 ± 1.1	64.8 ± 1.0	35.4 ± 1.7
		B10.D2-TNP	no	10.9 ± 0.8	23.8 ± 1.5	64.9 ± 4.2	73.3 ± 0.9	36.3 ± 1.8
		B10	no	14.8 ± 0.5	28.8 ± 2.8	16.8 ± 1.1	21.9 ± 1.1	84.5 ± 2.0

[a] BUdR 1 μg/ml final was added to the treated cultures 48 hr after the incubation of the cultures. The cultured cells were exposed to light 24 hr later and harvested, washed, and resuspended in fresh medium with stimulator cells two days later. Cytotoxic activity was measured five days after the incubation of the secondary culture.

[b] Specific lysis (%) is obtained by subtracting percentage of lysis (shown in brackets) measured for unstimulated cultures from the total percentage of lysis. Effector:target ratio, 20:1.

the alloantigen (favoring a dual-receptor model). Second, the possibility can be raised that a particular class of cells is required for the recognition of altered self and that such cells are not generated in primary *in vitro* CML against TNP-modified alloantigens. However, data obtained by *in vivo* depletion of alloreactive cells (negative selection) suggest that such cells may exist *in vivo,* as will be described by Sprent.

BACH: In the combination where Schmitt-Verhulst sensitized with B10.BR and restimulated with A.TL, she got about a ninefold proliferative response. Is it correct that in that particular case she does not generate cytotoxicity against TNP modified targets?

SCHMITT-VERHULST: Well, I am studying that more carefully because the cytotoxicity was measured either on tumor targets or on PHA blasts. Now I want to extend the work to include LPS blasts so as to make sure that there is no I region involved.

SPRENT: I think Schmitt-Verhulst's data are extremely interesting. On the point of whether or not one can get killing to TNP across an allogeneic barrier, mention should be made of the experiments of three groups, von Boehmer and Hass, and Pfizenmaier and Wagner for the TNP system, and Zinkernagel for the virus system. These workers used T cells tolerized to H-2 determinants in the environment of tetraparental bone marrow chimeras. With this system they were able to obtain specific killing for TNP across an allogeneic barrier. The problem with the chimeric system, however, is that one can always argue that T cell differentiation in the chimeric environment is abnormal. For example, the tolerized T cells might express abnormal cell-interaction determinants.

In some preliminary work with Kirsten Fischer-Lindahl we used an approach that differs from both the chimeric experiments and that of Schmitt-Verhulst. We used the method originally described by Ford and Atkins, where T cells from strain A are transferred in large numbers into irradiated (A × B)F$_1$ hybrid animals and then recovered from thoracic duct lymph one day later. At this time the cells in the lymph are almost entirely of donor origin and by all parameters tested these cells are completely unresponsive to the host-type alloantigens. For abbreviation we refer to these cells as having been "negatively selected" against the alloantigens of the host. The question we were now able to ask was: Would these A strain T cells, unresponsive to B strain H-2 determinants, be able to be stimulated by and lyse B strain TNP modified cells?

The system we used was to transfer CBA T cells intravenously into irradiated (CBA × C57BL)F$_1$ mice. The problem that we ran into was one alluded to by Shearer earlier, that of cross-reactive killing. When F$_1$ T cells were stimulated with CBA-TNP, they killed CBA-TNP targets but not C57BL-TNP targets. However, in the reverse situation, i.e., stimulation with C57BL-TNP, there was high cross-reactive lysis against CBA-TNP targets (Table 47).

With respect to the CBA T cells negatively selected againat C57BL H-2 determinants (CBA-C57BL), these cells when stimulated with C57BL-TNP gave no lysis against C57BL targets but lysed C57BL-TNP targets quite well. Regretfully, they also lysed CBA-TNP targets.

So these experiments are a little difficult to interpret. Although I think they are in favor of the view that one can generate cytotoxic cells against modified allogeneic targets, i.e., that they support the one-receptor hypothesis. Until we can repeat the experiments in the reverse direction (i.e., using C57BL cells negatively selected to CBA, where presumably we would not run into the cross-reactive problem), too much emphasis should not be placed on these data.

The problem with doing it the other way around is that for some reason the filtration system does not work well in that direction, i.e., we recover too few cells from the lymph to work with. But I could mention that Wilson at the University of Pennsylvania has begun these sorts of experiments in rats. So far he has done one experiment that does seem to support the general findings that I have shown, but without the troublesome cross-reactive killing we encountered.

TABLE 47

Cytotoxic Activity Generated in Negatively Selected Mouse Lymphocyte Populations against TNP-Modified Allogeneic Target Cells

Responder Population	Stimulator Population	Specific ^{51}Cr release (%) from target cells			
		CBA	CBA-TNP	C57BL	C57BL-TNP
CBA-C57BL TDL	CBA-TNP	2.0	45.9	−3.6	−0.4
	C57BL-TNP	−0.5	21.3	2.5	25.9
	F_1-TNP	−2.2	50.9	−5.3	15.1
CBA normal LN	CBA-TNP	5.0	60.0	3.4	5.5
	C57BL-TNP	3.8	17.2	39.9	36.3
	F_1-TNP	4.1	44.5	36.1	26.0
F_1 normal LN	CBA-TNP	5.7	42.9	0.5	6.2
	C57BL-TNP	5.0	26.8	4.8	45.2
	F_1-TNP	5.8	45.6	0.1	21.0
Maximum release/ spont. release (cpm)[a]		1669/494	2308/614	1574/514	3339/991

[a] 10^4 Targets; killers:targets ratio, 5:1.

FESTENSTEIN: Has Sprent done these experiments with any other strain, because of this quite extensive cross reactivity. His may have been an unfortunate choice from that point of view.

SPRENT: I would dearly like to be able to say I had tried other strain combinations. It just so happens that CBA cells filter extremely well through irradiated (CBA × C57BL)F$_1$ hybrids and for this reason we've concentrated on using this combination.

GORDON: With regard to the H-Y system, Simpson and I recently reported that we can prime B10 female mice, which are good responders to H-Y, with allogeneic male cells, particularly CBA or BALB/c, and then challenge in secondary culture with syngeneic male cells and get H-2-restricted secondary cytotoxic response against H-Y.

So, where the primary sensitization is *in vivo,* the system is not necessarily restricted by the H-2 haplotype of the sensitizing cells. Bevan and also Mitchison have sought to explain this by emphasizing that in the presence of an allograft reaction, the H-Y antigen may be picked up by host macrophages; the phenomenon could thus really be priming against self.

However, we tried to reproduce this kind of experiment in F$_1$ animals such as (B10 × CBA)F$_1$ females primed with BALB/c male cells, and then challenged *in vitro* with either one of the two parental cells or with those of the F$_1$ male. However, we got no response in the several different combinations we have tried. We are at a loss to reconcile this with a macrophage explanation for allogeneic priming.

WARNER: Is it necessary to invoke the H-2 determinant as being involved in the allosensitization system of Sprent? Is there any evidence in favor of another cell surface structure being modified by TNP, or that H-2-TNP is being recognized? I guess the approach would be to determine whether anti-H-2 sera would block at the target cell level.

SPRENT: We have not investigated it.

CANTOR: We have looked at the T cell subpopulations participating in the response to modified autologous cells in comparison with the response to allogeneic cells. The response to H-2 allogeneic cells involves both precursor and effector cells expressing the Ly2,3 phenotype. The response to TNP-modified autologous cells has a slightly different cellular basis. The effector cells express the Ly2,3 phenotype. However, if one examines the generation of this response, it is clear that one cannot generate these effector cells simply with Ly2,3 precursors, nor can one generate a significant response by a combination of helper cells (Ly1 cells) and Ly2,3 precursors. So this suggested to us that a third subclass of T cells, the population that expresses all of the known Ly antigens may be essential.

The question then concerns the function of the Ly1,2,3 cell in this response. Is it helping the response in the sense that it is amplifying the generation of Ly2,3 cells to become Ly2,3 effectors or is it actually the precursor itself in the response to modified self? The evidence suggests that it is the precursor cell.

We can obtain Ly2,3 cells from B6 donors, which express the Ly1.2 phenotype, and we can obtain the Ly1,2,3 population from the B6 congenic mouse, which is identical to the B6 except it has the Ly1.1 phenotype. Thus we can determine whether the effector cell generated has derived from the Ly2,3 cells or from the Ly1,2,3 cells in the mixture. The conclusion is that the effector cells are generated from Ly1,2,3 precursors.

We have not studied whether the generation of these killer cells from Ly1,2,3 precursors is autonomous. For example, this may require a helper effect from Ly1 cells. Our results suggest that there is a difference in the allogeneic and altered-self responses insofar as the precursor of the altered-self killer is relatively immature, perhaps a newly formed thymus-dependent cell.

We suggest an explanation for this result based upon the assumption that the idiotype that recognizes allogeneic H-2 and the idiotype that recognizes conventional antigens, as studied by Binz and Wigzell and by Eichmann and colleagues, seem to be coded for by genes in the same cluster (linked to heavy-chain allotype genes) and seem to have the same physicochemical properties. So consider the possibility that there is a single receptor that is similar to the types of receptors coded for B cells, and that this T cell receptor recognizes both conventional antigens and histocompatibility antigens. In addition, T cells express a second receptor, which can recognize (modified) self H-2 products. As the T cell matures in the thymus, it could be selected for cells that do not have idiotype material for self, but do have idiotypic material for allogeneic H-2 molecules, and these same idiotypes would also have a range of specificity for conventional antigens.

The cells that express the Ly1,2,3 phenotype could be monitoring cells in the organism for cell surface changes, for example, due to viral modifications. T cells that recognize antigens in the context of their own H-2 might be stimulated to differentiate further to become Ly2,3 cells. So in a sense, the Ly2,3 cells are memory cells and large numbers might accumulate during the course of this monitoring process after birth. Because the idiotypes that recognize the antigens or viruses present on autologous cells also cross-react with allogeneic H-2, one would expect the formation of large numbers of alloreactive memory cells, reflected in a vigorous alloreactivity.

BACH: Could Cantor list for us the other lines of evidence for the response to hapten-modified self being mediated by less mature cells.

CANTOR: I think the TNP system might be slightly anomalous as an example of a response to modified self. In almost every other response of this type one has to prime *in vivo* and then challenge *in vitro* to obtain cytotoxicity. For example, this occurs in the H-Y system and in several of the viral systems. Perhaps a more relevant response in the TNP system would be elicited if one were to modify stimulating cells with suboptimal amounts of TNP. If one does not use large amounts of TNP, one cannot get a primary response in culture. In addition, one does not see a strong mixed lymphocyte response even using the heavily conjugated stimulator cells, as one sees, for example in an allogeneic interaction.

WARNER: Would Cantor also predict that Ly1,2,3 cells are the precursors of the cells mediating delayed-type hypersensitivity responses to altered-self antigens?

CANTOR: Yes. In this case the relevant molecules might well be the products of the central MHC region, rather than those of the peripheral regions. Using SRBC, we find cells of the Ly1 sublcass that mediate a primary response. It is possible, however, that SRBC have antigens that are ubiquitous in the environment, and we may be dealing with a partially primed mouse cell population. We say this because in several other systems, it looks as though the Ly1,2,3 cell is required for the generation of Ly1 cells that function in delayed-type hypersensitivity phenomena.

CHAIRMAN SHEARER: We should now move away from the TNP model for considering altered self, and proceed instead to more classical transplantation systems, particularly one that has been studied by Gordon and Simpson, dealing with generation of cytotoxic responses to the H-Y antigens. Skin graft rejections in this system were known for some time and recently a cytotoxic *in vitro* assay was developed that demonstrates H-2 restriction and possibly Ir gene control.

GORDON: Zinkernagel recently published data in which he has shown that in delayed-type responses to certain viruses, K or D region compatibility is required rather than I region compatibility. On the other hand, there are instances, such as delayed-type responses to fowl gamma globulin, where I region determinants seem to be involved. To some extent, then, the requirement for compatibility with central or peripheral MHC regions is dependent on the particular non-MHC antigen in question.

Several times during the conference, concern has been expressed about the potential for cell-mediated and humoral-mediated responses to minor histocompatibility antigens in the context of an MHC-matched donor and recipient. Ir genes should be considered in this context because even though an antigenic difference may exist between two individuals, this does not necessarily mean that there will be an immune response. For example, the H-Y antigen is detectable in CBA male mice, but CBA females do not reject male grafts. Immune response genes may be important in determining the potential for GVH reactions or graft rejection also in a clinical context.

The H-Y antigen is a gene product of the Y chromosome and is expressed on the surface of the male cells of almost all mouse strains. It is also ubiquitous in mouse tissues. It effects the skin graft reaction that, although not as strong as the conventional anti-H-2 reaction, is nonetheless marked in those strains that do mount a response. The rejection usually occurs two to three weeks after grafting male skin onto a female mouse of the appropriate strain. Previous *in vivo* data have implicated the H-2 complex in controlling responsiveness to H-Y.

Three patterns of responsiveness have been observed: strong responsiveness mainly in strains carrying the H-2^b haplotype; intermediate responsiveness, by which significant numbers of animals do reject their grafts more slowly; no responsiveness at all.

We have developed an *in vitro* method for studying T-cell-dependent cytotoxic responses to H-Y in mice. Females must be primed *in vivo,* either by skin grafting or by the injection of male spleen cells intraperitoneally. As few as one million male cells will successfully prime responder females. Then, from two weeks to many months later, spleen cells can be placed in mixed lymphocyte culture with an equal number of irradiated male spleen cells, usually syngeneic. After five days, responder cells are assayed against a panel of chromium-labeled Con-A blast target cells.

Using this system, we first found that B10 females that had been primed *in vivo* and challenged in MLC with B10 male cells would lyse B10 male target cells, but not female cells. We also observed that the response was restricted by the H-2 complex. In fact, one required the H-2^b specificity in the D region of the MHC. We also found that all of the strains that carried the H-2^b haplotype, regardless of their genetic background, showed the same high level of responsiveness and the same requirement for H-2D^b on target cells.

We investigated a number of other strains, so-called nonresponders, which only rarely reject male to female skin grafts. These included CBA, BALB/c, A.SW, and B10.A. In none of these strains were we able to demonstrate the presence of cytotoxic T cells, suggesting that at least in part the failure of these mice to reject their skin grafts might be due to an inability to generate cytotoxic effector cells to H-Y.

We then looked at the congenic and/or recombinant strains. We found that in no case, regardless of the H-2 haplotype, the nature of the recombination, or the non H-2 genetic background (whether congenic with B10 or not) could we find cytotoxic T cells for H-Y. Several of these strains have the appropriate H-2^b target specificity. Thus, B10.A(4R), HTG, and D2.GD all have H-2^b in the D region, but they do not mount discernible cytotoxic responses to H-Y. This suggested to us that the situation was more complex than a mere single H-2 requirement in the D region and that there might be genes involved in regulating immune responsiveness to the male antigen in other regions of the MHC.

We have examined the pattern of responsiveness to H-Y by various F$_1$ females sensitized to parental male as has been done in other H-2 restricted systems. The results are shown in Table 48. First of all, F$_1$ females produced by pairings of nonresponder and responder strains are responders, suggesting dominant inheritance of responder capacity. We found if we sensitized a (CBA × B10)F$_1$ female to the CBA male parent, we got a response restricted to H-2D^k. Male target cells of the other parental haplotype (B10) or of other unrelated haplotypes are not lysed. If we sensitize to B10 parental male cells then we see the same responses seen with a B10 responder, that is, a response restricted to H-2D^b targets.

Next we examined (BALB/c × B10)F$_1$ females. BALB/c is a nonresponder strain. Again, the F$_1$ responds to either parental strain and kills only the cells that match the parental haplotype used to sensitize. If we sensitize to BALB/c we find that we have an H-2K^d restricted kill. When we sensitize to B10 we again have an H-2D^b restricted response.

Thus, we are able to get a response against the H-2^d male haplotype, but the restriction required is different from that seen in the previous examples, since it involves the H-2K region.

TABLE 48
T-Cell-Mediated Cytotoxic Responses to H-Y Antigen by F$_1$ Mice[a]

Strain tested	Antigen	Cytotoxic T-cell response
(Nonresponder × Responder)F$_1$♀		
(CBA × C57BL/10)F$_1$♀	CBA♂	H-2D^k restricted
	C57BL/10♂	H-2D^b restricted
(BALB/c × C57BL/10)F$_1$♀	BALB/c♂	H-2K^d restricted
	C57BL/10♂	H-2D^b restricted
(A × C57BL/10)F$_1$♀	A♂	H-2K^k restricted
	C57BL/10♂	H-2D^b restricted
Nonresponder × Nonresponder)F$_1$♀		
(CBA × BALB/c)F$_1$♀	CBA♂	H-2K^k or H-2D^k restricted
	BALB/c♂	No response

[a]Spleen cells from F$_1$ female mice, primed *in vivo* and challenged in mixed lymphocyte culture with the parental male cells shown, were assayed in triplicate for three hours against a panel of ^{51}Cr-labeled con A blast spleen target cells.

Having found that the restriction for the H-2^k allele is at the D end and that for the H-2^d allele at the K end, we tested (A × B10)F$_1$ inasmuch as A has H-2^k at the K end and H-2^d at the D end. We found that we could get killing of A male targets by (A × B10)F$_1$ females sensitized to A male. This response was restricted to H-2K^k target cells. There was no killing of the H-2^d allele at the D end. Once again, if sensitized to the B10 parental male, the F$_1$ female cells showed killing restricted to H-2D^b as in all of the previous examples.

There is at least one interpretation of altered self that seems to have ruled our experiments: the Y antigen is only capable of modifying or of being recognized in close association with a particular H-2 gene region product. Thus, the modified H-2D^k and H-2K^k gene products are both recognizable by an appropriate effector T-cell. In this sense, the specificity of the response is not limited by the nature of the interaction of H-Y and H-2 on the stimulating or target cell, but by the specificity of the responding T cell receptor.

CBA and BALB/c mice fail to reject male skin grafts, and we have never been able to detect cytotoxic T cells *in vitro* from either of these strains. However, F$_1$ females produced by pairing these two strains respond to one of the two parental haplotypes, the CBA. Apparently, sensitization to CBA male cells produces cytotoxic T effectors for target cells presenting H-2^k at either the K or the D end.

So, two nonresponders give a responder. However, this animal responds only to one of the two parental haplotypes. Sensitization to BALB/c produced no response. The response to H-2K^k and H-2D^k may involve two clones.

Given the previous evidence, both *in vivo* and *in vitro,* implicating the H-2 complex in regulating responsiveness to H-Y, we think it reasonable to suggest that this probably represents complementation involving the H-2 regions of these strains and may be an example, like in the TNP system, of Ir gene control of a cell-mediated response against a naturally occurring minor histocompatibility antigen. Accordingly, the variations in restriction when one changes the nature of the responder (different F$_1$ females) could be the effect of Ir genes altering the specificity of the T cell receptor for self-MHC.

CHAIRMAN SHEARER: Would Gordon summarize briefly the experience thus far, comparing the *in vivo* and *in vitro* models, as pertaining to the H-Y antigen.

GORDON: One may be challenging *in vitro* a restricted and selected population of effector cells, not representative of the total population causing allograft rejection.

FESTENSTEIN: Gordon hypothesized that the Y antigen was modifying H-2 and, on the other hand, that H-2 linked Ir gene may influence cell-to-cell interactions. It is really necessary to refer to MHC modification in the H-Y system, as opposed to the TNP system, which might in fact be operating in this way?

GORDON: Altered self is not a necessary explanation of results in the H-Y system. If anything, I was arguing against one particular type of altered-self model. It is clear, however, that the Y antigen is recognizable for a given MHC allele in the context of either the K or D region, depending on who the responder is.

So the idea that the limitation is imposed by Y-induced alteration of an MHC gene product in a particular region does not seem to be warranted. Other altered-self models, however, are possible, since these data do not discriminate between altered self and dual recognition.

CHAIRMAN SHEARER: It may be appropriate now to consider a distinctive tumor model involving radiation leukemia virus-transformed cells with which Meruelo has been working.

MERUELO: Lilly described the genetic control by H-2 of susceptibility to leukemia viruses, and this work was corroborated by the association with H-2 of susceptibility to other viruses including Gross, Tennant, and Friend. In other words, control over leukemogenesis would involve Ir genes associated with H-2 such that a vigorous cytotoxic response against tumor cells would occur in some strains and not in others. More recent work by Chesebro et al. has demonstrated that recovery from Friend leukemias is controlled by a gene at the D end of the complex. Since no Ir genes are yet mapped within this part of the MHC, it is possible that H-2 controls resistance to leukemia by more than just an Ir gene mechanism.

We shall consider this notion in the context of the altered-self model. I shall briefly summarize some data that localize a resistance gene in the D end of H-2 and then try to ascertain at what stage of the disease the mechanism operates and a possible mechanism. This work was done in collaboration with Lieberman (Kaplan's laboratory) as well as with McDevitt.

We injected radiation leukemia virus intrathymically in animals three to six weeks of age. The percentage of survival as a function of time elapsed after the injection of the virus was recorded in a series of H-2 congenic strains (Fig. 16).

Strains B10.G, B10.S, and 2R are highly susceptible to the disease, whereas strains 6R, 7R, and B10.A are very resiatant. The H-2 map at the top of Fig. 16 shows that the resistant strains differ from the susceptible strains only by the D and TL regions of the H-2 complex. Hence, there is an H-2-Tla effect manifested as delayed onset of the disease, as well as overall survival.

To more precisely map the effect in either the D or TL regions we are now comparing susceptibility or resistance to RadLV (radiation leukemia virus) in TL

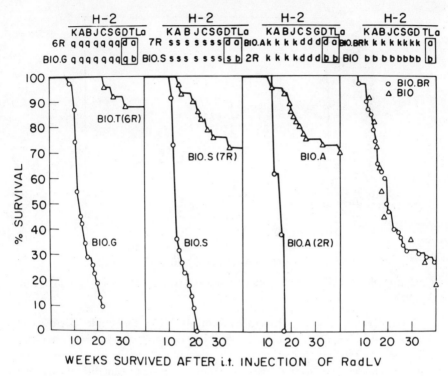

Fig. 16 Correlation between host resistance to intrathymic challenge with RadLV and H-2D genotype.

congenic mice. We have already compared strains B10.BR and B10. B10.BR is Tla[a], which could be associated with resistance, and B10 is Tla[b], which could be associated with susceptibility. In fact, there are no differences in susceptibility (Fig. 16). Additional data indicate that B10 is eventually more resistant than B10.BR, which again strongly suggests that the TL region is not involved. So, these data tentatively map the resistance gene in the D region of H-2.

We have examined a large number of additional recombinant strains and found no exception to the D-region associated resistance. In unrelated strains of mice, segregation analysis places genetic influences on susceptibility on chromosomes other than that of the MHC.

Lilly had shown that, in the case of Friend virus, the H-2 effect was not on virus penetration or replication. The animals from resistant strains could be infected and would develop splenomegaly. The subsequent recovery from the disease, however, was affected by H-2. So, analogous studies were done with RadLV and the results are shown in Fig. 17. The thymus is the predominant site of action of this virus and only in the very late stages of the disease will metas-

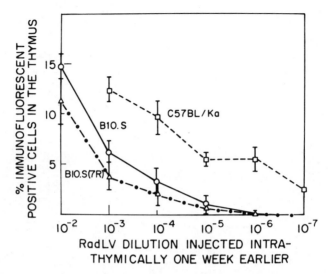

Fig. 17 Lack of correlation between resistance to RadLV and the number of virus-infected thymocytes.

tasis to other organs occur. The virus was injected into susceptible and resistant mice as well as in C57BL/Ka animals, the strain in which the virus is maintained. One week later the number of immunofluorescent cells in the thymus was measured with a specific reagent for RadLV. There is no significant difference in the amount of infected cells in susceptible and resistant strains. On the other hand, the number of virus-positive thymus cells in C57BL/Ka mice is greater, reflecting the adaptation of the virus. Thus, the initial infection step is not affected by H-2. To establish whether H-2 controls later events, various F_1 and syngeneic mice were challenged with tumors from susceptible animals.

F_1 mice from resistant and susceptible parents (e.g., B10.S × 7R) were resistant whereas F_1s from two susceptible strains (e.g., B10.S × B10.G) were as susceptible as the strain of origin of the tumor (Fig. 18).

These experiments, which were done before the genetic analysis of F_1 crosses with respect to susceptibility to virus infection had been carried out, predicted that resistance to leukemia would be dominant. That is exactly what was found.

Whether immunological mechanisms are involved in this resistance is uncertain, but it is known that humoral and cell-mediated responses during the course of the disease appear to be identical in resistant and susceptible strains. Analogously, Chesebro found no correlation between antibody responses and survival in studies with Friend-virus-infected mice.

The question in my mind, then, is: Do genes within the H-2 complex, and primarily the D region, affect susceptibility to RadLV by a predominantly im-

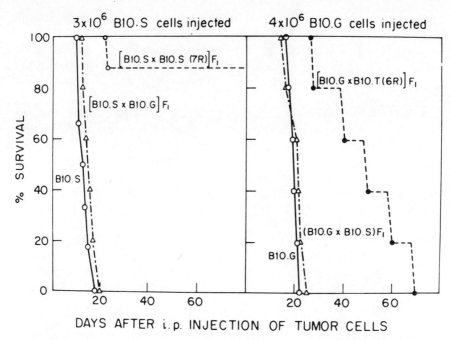

Fig. 18 Inheritance of resistance to RadLV lymphomas in F_1 hybrids. B10.S and B10.G were susceptible parents, whereas 7R was the resistant parent.

munological mechanism of the Ir type or do such genes affect other parameters, such as the expression of H-2 or other antigens, or their modification, or their association with virus in the membrane?

CHAIRMAN SHEARER: Does Meruelo think that an alternative explanation for the F_1 experiments could be hybrid resistance, which is also genetically controlled by the D region?

MERUELO: So far we don't know of any Ir genes associated with the D region, but an Hh-associated phenomenon could be involved. There are two difficulties with this explanation: first, the disease occurs primarily in the thymus and Hh genetic control may not operate in the thymus; second, studies by Lilly demonstrated that as a result of virus infection differences develop between susceptible and resistant hosts in the cell surface expression of H-2 determinants. To me this suggests that one is dealing with an H-2 effect as such, rather than with some Hh type mechanism.

CHAIRMAN SHEARER: Although it is correct that the anti-Hh reaction, as it applies to bone marrow graft rejection, is most strongly manifested in the spleen, this does not rule out the possibility of Hh-like mechanisms for suppression of leukemogenesis operative in other organs such as the thymus. I think that a verification could be obtained by "tolerizing" resistant F_1 mice in the standard Hh way with parental spleen cells to determine whether such animals then become susceptible to the virus infection and tumor cells.

CUDKOWICZ: I would point out that Meruelo has used F_1 strains that are known to be resistant to parental leukemias because of Hh-1 heterozygosity. We and also Warner have set up similar crosses involving SJL instead of B10.S (both H-2^s), and we found, as Meruelo did, that these particular hybrids are susceptible or resistant to parental cells depending on the H-2D alleles involved (see Tables 4, 7–9, 61–63). Thus, Meruelo did indeed encounter hybrid resistance, at least in crosses involving H-2^s and H-2^b.

MERUELO: I agree with Shearer's comments, and I also think that Cudkowicz's comments are most relevant. It will be very important to determine whether one is dealing with an H-2D- or Hh-associated phenomenon. Both are distinct possibilities.

TRENTIN: As Heran-Ghera described, in the irradiated C57BL mouse destined to develop leukemia months later there were almost immediately preleukemic cells held in check for some time by a residual host resistance mechanism. What she described had many of the characteristics of genetic resistance to bone marrow transplants, which several of us will relate later to NK (natural killer) cell lysis of lymphoma targets *in vitro*. We also have evidence that *in vivo* this same mechanism operates specifically against AKR lymphoma. So, there is a good probability that what was recognized for many years as hybrid resistance to parental bone marrow transplants is, in nature, the mechanism by which the C57BL mouse is extremely resistant to leukemia.

    Now, Meruelo found no evidence that resistance in his system was immunological, but his studies do not exclude this natural resistance, this null-cell-mediated genetic resistance to bone marrow transplants, which is apparently analogous to NK cell lysis of lymphoma cells *in vitro*.

NK CELL SYSTEMS AS EFFECTORS OF RESISTANCE TO NORMAL AND MALIGNANT HEMOPOIETIC CELLS

Discussion Introducer:

Hans Wigzell

CHAIRMAN WIGZELL: We shall be concerned with NK (natural killer) cells in mice and rats and how such cells relate to marrow and leukemia resistance. The test system used to detect these cells is a chromium release assay, i.e., a *short-term* cytolytic reaction occuring *in vitro*. We have been using mouse Moloney lymphomas as the targets in this particular system, whereas Herberman and others have utilized other kinds of lymphomas.

Our own system, developed by Kiessling, involves the incubation of lymphoid cells from normal mice with NK-sensitive targets. The initiation of lysis is as fast as that evoked by immune T cells. If the population of NK cells has been sufficiently purified, the initiation of lysis is extremely rapid, indicating that there is some kind of induction of a cytolytic capacity via *in vitro* contact with the target cells.

Contact is essential for this kind of lysis. None of the NK systems so far assayed has yielded any evidence of soluble factors being involved. Actually time-lapse cinematography discloses that NK cells attack tumor targets in a manner analogous to immune T lymphocytes. Any maneuver that separates effector from the target cells prevents lysis. NK reactions are not blocked by immune complexes. Kärre showed that if NK cells are treated with trypsin, capacity to lyse is abolished. However, this attribute will regenerate *in vitro,* despite the fact that NK cells survive rather poorly under *in vitro* conditions.

Thus, it should be emphasized that the NK cell functions as though its lytic ability is mediated via receptors it produces itself. There are conflicting reports on the specificity of this reaction, that is, the kinds of target cells that are sensitive. Our experience is that T cell lymphomas are the best targets, but there are, nonetheless, certain T-cell lymphomas that we have found to be resistant to NK lysis. For the most part, we consider Moloney lymphomas of the mouse to be suitable targets for NK cytolysis.

Herberman and his group claim that target structures somehow involve C-type viruses or C-type regulated products, that tumors positive for C-type virus or such cell lines are more prone to be NK sensitive. There are, however, exceptions to this generalization; some culture lines with endogenous C-type viruses are nonetheless resistant to the NK effect. So, the specificity of NK cells is still unclear. Even in this discussion, data will be presented by others to the effect that a considerable variation in target cell sensitivity is evident in various kinds of NK cell systems.

Rat NK cells are also active against mouse NK-sensitive targets. Using purified mouse NK cells and human tumor targets, Haller has found that human T cell lymphomas also seem to be sensitive. So, it appears as though this kind of NK reactivity is operative across species barriers. There are no H-2 compatibility requirements for NK lysis to occur.

At this point, it would be appropriate to emphasize that it is misleading to refer to *antigens* in connection with NK cell system. Rather, we should refer to sensitive targets and surface structures in preference to antigens. There is no reason to believe that the receptors on NK cells bear any relationship to conventional immunoglobulins. There is a striking age dependence in the time of NK appearance. Virtually no NK killer activity is found in mice until about 22–23 days of age, at which time they emerge rapidly in spleen and peripheral blood. Little activity is manifested in the lymph nodes, and virtually none in thymus or in bone marrow. Peak NK activity occurs in young adult mice three to four months of age, after which reactivity declines.

Organ distribution studies suggest that spleen is very important in NK cell systems since it manifests the highest efficiency or capacity for NK activity. However, if neonatal splenectomy is performed, the emergence of NK cells in peripheral block seems unaffected. Thus, the development of NK cells is spleen independent.

Conversely, NK cells arise at a normal rate in nude mice. In fact, the nude mouse has significantly higher cytolytic capacity in spleen than the corresponding heterozygous littermates. So, the NK cell is spleen independent and thymus independent as well.

Also, as mentioned earlier, ^{89}Sr treatment stops the generation of NK cells. Thus, a functioning bone marrow is essential for maintenance of NK activity in adult mice. However, we do not know whether radioactive strontium directly kills the NK cells, or whether it blocks their recruitment. The fact remains that unlike T and B lymphocytes, NK cells or their precursors are remarkably sensitive to radioactive strontium.

As to surface markers, NK cells are nonadherent and lack any of the structures that are commonly found on T cells, that is, Thy-1, TL, and Lyl, 2, or 3, despite treatment of spleen cells with agents known to provoke the development of T cell markers. Moreover, mouse NK cells lack Fc receptors and do not display complement binding receptors, as opposed to human cells, for instance. The mouse cells actually lack these receptors but do carry H-2 antigens of SD type, and they also carry the Ly8 antigen, an alloantigen present on both T and B lymphocytes. On the basis of a few experiments, NK cells were found to be heterogeneous in size. There is some evidence to suggest that the NK cell might be in rapid turnover. The actual number or frequency of NK cells is not known since there is yet no assay available for enumeration.

Mouse strains were classified as high or low with respect to splenic NK activity. Examples of high and low strains are C57BL, C57L, and CBA vs. A, BALB/c, and AKR, respectively. F_1 hybrids from high and low strains are high. In F_2 mice segregating for H-2 there is striking linkage of NK activity with this marker gene. This is so in segregants from outcrosses with unrelated and congenic mice. In addition, a second gene not associated with H-2, regulates NK activity.

Is there any relationship between the findings of NK cell lysis assays and the capacity of mice to resist the transplantation of Moloney lymphomas? Is there any relationship between NK cell activity in individual animals and their resistance to transplantation of such Moloney lymphomas?

High-responder mouse strains have been subjected to thymectomy, lethal irradiation, and bone marrow repopulation and then studied for NK cell activity. In these animals, removal of the thymus results in enhanced NK cell activity and enhanced resistance *in vivo* to transplants of syngeneic Moloney lymphoma cells. Also nude mice of the appropriate strain are resistant. This does not necessarily mean that cells operative *in vitro* are the very same cells functioning *in vivo*. However, by removing most other cells, we can concentrate on splenic NK cells; such cells, devoid of T and B lymphocytes and macrophages, can be mixed with syngeneic lymphoma cells and transferred *in vivo* in a Winn assay. Such tests yielded a direct correlation between the NK cell activity in the population as measured *in vitro* and the ability to passively transfer protection.

CUDKOWICZ: Does Wigzell have any information concerning the presence of NK cells in the peripheral blood of man?

CHAIRMAN WIGZELL: We have done but few experiments seeking to demonstrate these cells in man. If we remove cells positive for the C3b receptor there might be a tendency for the remaining cells to be lytic against T cell lymphomas more than against other targets.

ELKINS: Is the killer cell in the spleen radiation sensitive, and can Wigzell transfer killer cell activity to a low-responder strain by bone marrow transplant from a high-responder donor?

CHAIRMAN WIGZELL: Elkins's first query will shortly be covered by Shearer and Trentin. As to the second question, Haller has transferred fetal liver cells devoid of NK cells from a high to a low strain and vice versa. The result is that NK reactivity is transferred by fetal liver irrespective of the host genotype. What emerges as high or low NK reactivity is already set at the precursor level of the stem cells in bone marrow.

BORANIC: Wigzell stated there is no way of enumerating NK cells. On the other hand, he also mentioned that the lytic effect is the result of a one-to-one activity. Would he explain this apparent contradiction?

CHAIRMAN WIGZELL: By time lapse cinematography one can actually see a single cell killing a target. I do not remember saying that this is always a one-to-one effect. A test is available to calculate the frequency in the spleen of cells with NK ability, but it still is not enumeration.

HENNEY: Does Wigzell know whether NK cells can kill repeatedly? The answer holds the key to meaningful enumeration. If the NK cell can only kill one target cell, then NK cells can be enumerated. The problems with killer T cell enumeration arise only from the fact that they can recycle.

CHAIRMAN WIGZELL: We have not done careful analysis of recycling. I do not know. My guess would be that the NK cell can act on targets repeatedly.

SPRENT: Wigzell mentioned that the levels of NK cells were higher in nude mice. Do the levels decrease after injecting syngeneic T cells or after a thymus graft?

CHAIRMAN WIGZELL: We do not know in the nude mouse. We know that in adult thymectomized mice added thymus cells reduce NK activity.

FESTENSTEIN: Does Wigzell have any indication of the target determinants that are involved?

CHAIRMAN WIGZELL: I want to emphasize that we have no evidence as to the exact nature of the target structures or what determines sensitivity. There is also no evidence as to the possible role of the M locus.

SHEARER: Since NK reactivity is diminished in older mice, would reactivity be maintained longer in the germ-free state?

CHAIRMAN WIGZELL: NK cell activity in germ-free normal mice appears normal, but aging studies were not done.

METCALF: Does the injection of endotoxin increase NK cell activity?

CHAIRMAN WIGZELL: Freund's adjuvant given locally increases NK cell activity. On the other hand, endotoxin has no such effect.

BACH: Is there any evidence that NK cell activity is effective against targets other than lymphoid tymors?

CHAIRMAN WIGZELL: Not really. We have only found sensitive targets among lymphoid cells, or hematopoietic cells.

BACH: Wigzell mentioned that the nude homozygous mouse has a higher NK activity than the nude heterozygous normals, but I would like to know if the nude heterozygotes are higher than normal mice.

CHAIRMAN WIGZELL: If there is a difference it must be minor. We should now get further information from Cantor, who was able to raise an antiserum specifically reactive with NK cells.

CANTOR: Two of the central questions concerning the NK phenomenon are (1) its importance for antitumor responses *in vivo,* and (2) delineation of the differentiative pathway *in vivo.*

Both of these aims would be facilitated by an antiserum defining a cell surface component selectively expressed on NK cells. We believe we now have such an antiserum. The target for NK killer activity in our system is the RL♂1 tumor of BALB/c mice, which expresses leukemia virus-associated antigen.

NK cells seem to be resistant to treatment with anti-Thy-1 and complement, or anti-Ly2.2 and complement. Therefore, we were quite surprised to find that antisera against Ly1.2 reduced or even eliminated NK activity both in B6 and NZB strains. This was noteworthy because the Ly1 component is considered to be expressed selectively on T cells, yet by every other criterion the NK cell does not conform to a mature T cell. Consequently we considered the possibility of a contaminant antibody that was in fact responsible for elimination of NK activity by Ly1.2 antiserum.

Anti-Ly1.2 is a C3H anti-CE thymocyte antiserum. CE is an $H-2^k$ strain as is C3H, but the two strains differ at non-H-2 loci.

We sought to resolve the problem by testing the C3H anti-CE antiserum against cells of B6 mice and of B6 congenic mice differing at the Ly1 locus. Were the antiserum to abolish NK activity of both B6 strains, one would then conclude that the anti-NK effect was not due to anti-Ly1.2. NK activity of cells from both strains was eliminated after treatment with C3H anti-CE antiserum and complement.

We attempted then to render the antiserum monospecific by absorbing it with Ly1.2-positive but NK-negative cells. To this end we absorbed the serum with BALB/c thymocytes and succeeded in separating anti-Ly1.2 from anti-NK activity.

We then attempted a more direct approach. This was to insert the BALB/c genotype into the mouse used for immunization and thus obviate the need for absorption. So instead of making a C3H anti-CE antiserum, we made the antiserum in (C3H × BALB/c)F$_1$ mice. The antibody produced was selective, for it eliminated NK cells while leaving intact other T and B cell functions. It should be noted that this antiserum lyses less than 5% of splenic lymphocytes and thus is not broadly cytotoxic. This antiserum may be useful for characterizing properties of NK cells since it seems to selectively eliminate this subpopulation of cells from a heterogeneous lymphocyte population.

WARNER: Would Till comment on the relationship of Cantor's serum to the one he described several years ago, which ablated resistance to Hh-positive cells.

TILL: It was a C3H anti-C57BL serum. We were able to show that the activity wasn't directed against H-2 and, in fact, it need not be directed against any donor cell marker. It must have been directed against some specificity in the F_1 recipient, but we haven't a clue as to what it was.

CANTOR: Till's immunization—C3H anti-B6—could produce, in addition to many other antibodies, an antibody to the NK antigen, insofar as B6 is NK-antigen positive and C3H is NK-antigen negative.

SANFORD: Is there any dose of radiation at which you can eliminate NK activity and, if so, can one reconstitute an animal and use Cantor's serum against NK to selectively deplete this population and establish whether resistance to marrow grafts is also eliminated or persists?

CANTOR: We do not know if the antiserum will eliminate natural killer cells *in vivo*. The difficulty is that we have to look very quickly after repopulation of these animals with, for example, spleen cells, because one worries about the possibility that new NK cells will be generated, especially if one is under the impression that these are rather immature cells and can be generated from stem cells in the donor inoculum.

TILL: Is there any information about how fast NK cells return in the irradiated animal?

CHAIRMAN WIGZELL: Three weeks after transplantation of bone marrow cells.

CUDKOWICZ: One problem is that there is not a measurable drop in NK activity for some time after irradiation. Even though transplanted marrow adds further NK activity, one doesn't have a zero base line for its evaluation.

FESTENSTEIN: Could one inhibit the killing of NK targets by adding normal lymphiod cells of differing H-2 types?

CHAIRMAN WIGZELL: No. Normal cells, including embryonic thymocytes from AKR mice, do not compete in the NK assay.

WARNER: I would like to return to several aspects of the NK cell situation that were introduced by Wigzell. I want to emphasize NK performance with a different series of tumors and especially to consider their relationship to *in vivo* mechanisms of serveillance. The data I shall present are from collaborative studies with Burton, Woodruff, Holmes, and Barr.

Concerning the nature of the cell, our data are basically in agreement with that of Wigzell. The one point I would like to add concerns the activity of cells from different types of peritoneal exudates.

The bottom line in Fig. 19, referred to as PPB PEC, is a proteose peptone broth-induced exudate, which is a "classical" mononuclear/macrophage type of exudate, and shows relatively minimal killing activity of the target tumor WEHI-7. This is a radiation-induced BALB/c T lymphoma. In contrast, spleen cells from BALB/c mice show a marked degree of lysis, as in other studies; even greater killing activity is given by an exudate induced by PVP (polyvinylpyrrolidone). This exudate was obtained 18 hr after the first of two injections of PVP and is more than 80% granulocytic in nature, with the remaining 20% mononuclear cells of undetermined type. In our experience, this exudate consistently shows the greatest degree of killing activity. In this exudate the cell that is responsible for lysis is nonadherent. We are now involved in cell fractionation

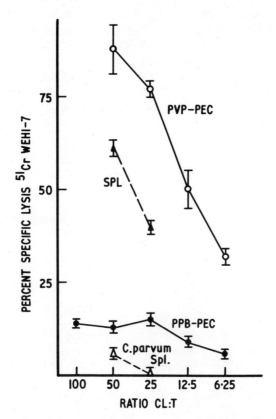

Fig. 19 Comparison of effectiveness of various exudate cells in killing WEHI-7 tumor targets.

studies with this exudate, and I allude to these data primarily to suggest consideration of the NK cell as being in the granulocytic lineage, perhaps at an early stage of differentiation.

An argument against this view however might be that bone marrow cells show no such activity. Again, it could be that it is a reflection of the state of maturity of the cell type involved, or that bone marrow also contains a cell type that suppresses NK-mediated lysis.

Another point to note in Fig. 19 is the considerably reduced activity of spleen cells from *C. parvum*-treated mice. Now, one of our general themes here is the question of the possible relation of the NK cell to the Hh rejection mechanism. In this instance, we find a positive correlation between these systems in that the spleens from *C. parvum*-treated mice, albeit being considerably enlarged in size, have markedly reduced NK lytic activity. This expanded spleen population reflects a massive proliferation of several cellular elements, including lymphoid and certain macrophage types. Clearly, however, none of these are involved in the NK lytic system, and this perhaps parallels the ability of *C. parvum* to abrogate *in vivo* the hybrid histoincompatibility mechanism.

In relation to the specificity of NK cell-mediated lysis, Table 49 indicates that these cells kill many different tumors. In relation to possible genetic control of NK cells, I would emphasize, however, that one must look at a variety of strain combinations for each tumor. The data in Table 49 are all obtained with nude spleen cells. Virtually all of these tumors are killed by spleen cells of at least one nude strain.

There are also some interesting negative results. For example, WEHI-265, which is an Abelson virus-induced myeloid leukemia in the granulocytic series,

TABLE 49

Killing of a Number of Tumor Targets by Nucleated
Spleen Cells from Three Strains of Nude Mice

Tumor targets	Mean specific lysis (%) ± S.E.M. of ^{51}CR tumor targets		
	BALB/c.nu	CBA.nu	C57.nu
ABE-8	14 ± 3	0	0
WEHI-265	0	15 ± 7	6 ± 3
MPC-11	13 ± 2	30 ± 2	9 ± 2
HPC-10	13 ± 1	13 ± 1	17 ± 2
EL4	18 ± 2	19 ± 2	27 ± 3
Cl.18	32 ± 2	34 ± 2	15 ± 2
RILQ	7 ± 2	13 ± 1	n.d.

TABLE 50

Certain Tumor Targets Not Lysed *in vitro* by Nucleated Spleen Cells

Spleen cell source	No. of experiments	EMT-6	No. of experiments	WEHI-164	No. of experiments	P815
			Mean specific lysis (%) ± S.E.M.			
BALB/c.nu	5	0	4	2 ± 1	2	1 ± 1
BALB/c	4	0	2	2 ± 1	2	0
CBA.nu	1	0	1	0	1	0
CBA	2	0	1	0	2	0
C57.nu	1	0	1	3 ± 1	1	0
C57	2	0	2	3 ± 1	2	0

is not killed by BALB/c spleen cells, even though the tumor is of BALB/c origin; it is, however, killed by spleen cells from another strain. All of these tumors are producing C-type virus; indeed some of them were specifically induced by such viruses.

In contrast, Table 50 shows three other tumors also studied with spleen cells from a variety of nude mouse strains. These nonlysable tumors are a carcinoma, a fibrosarcoma, and a mastocytoma. The P-815 data are of particular interest in relation to Henney's data showing that this cell can be killed, however, by certain other types of exudate cells. None of these tumors, to our knowledge, produce C-type virus.

Figure 20 addresses itself to the *in vivo* correlation with NK activity. Initially, to our surprise, we observed the exact opposite of what might have been expected on the basis of classical T-cell-mediated immunosurveillance concepts, namely, that with tumors grafted into syngenetic nude mice, we would expect to find more rapid growth in athymic than in control animals. However, this was not the case with certain tumors. We show in Fig. 20 the *in vivo* growth rates of a plasmacytoma and two B cell lymphomas, which grow at considerably reduced rates in syngeneic BALB/c nude mice.

We have observed three types of growth patterns in doing this experiment with a large number of tumors: (1) reduced growth rate in the nude, (2) similar growth rate in athymic and normal mice, and (3) accelerated growth rate in the nude mouse compared to the normal. Which of these patterns, if any, correlates with susceptibility as determined by the natural killer cell?

A few representative examples of data obtained are shown in Table 51. Tumors that grow either at the same rate in normal and nudes, or even at an accelerated rate in nudes (such as the last three tumors in this table), are not susceptible to NK cell lysis. In contrast, all the tumors that are susceptible to NK lysis grow at a slower rate in the athymic mice than in normals. Hence, this

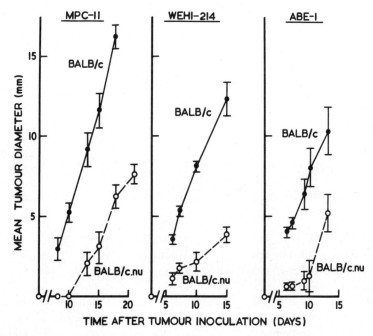

Fig. 20 Correlation of tumor resistance with NK cell lysis: enhanced resistance against a plasmacytoma and B cell lymphomas in athymic mice.

correlation suggests that the NK cell could play an important role in surveillance against tumors.

I would point out, however, that a few of the tumors do grow faster in nudes and accordingly surveillance could involve *both* T cells and the NK cell, perhaps responding to different types of stimuli.

TABLE 51
In vitro Lysis and *in vivo* Growth of BALB/c Tumors

			In vivo tumor growth[b]	
Tumor	Type	*In vitro*[a] lysis	BALB/c	BALB/c. nu
MPC-11	Plasmacytoma	13 ± 2	12.8 ± 1.5	0.5 ± 0.3
WEHI-265	Myeloid tumor	0	10.8 ± 1.3	12.7 ± 1.5
EMT-6	Carcinoma	0	9.4 ± 0.7	9.4 ± 0.3
WEHI-164	Fibrosarcoma	0	6.9 ± 0.3	8.0 ± 0.7

[a] Mean specific lysis (%) ± S.E. by BALB/c. nu spleen cells.

[b] Mean tumor diameter (mm ± S.E.) two weeks after sc inoculation.

CHAIRMAN WIGZELL: Does Warner have any evidence of NK cell activity against tumors that were not of the hemopoietic system?

WARNER: Wigzell has raised an important point. We did not find any such tumors. However, I would not be surprised if such tumors were eventually found. In fact, we started these studies in the athymic mice with Woodruff, who had originally observed that a CBA fibrosarcoma grew at a slower rate in thymectomized CBA mice than in controls. It may well be that one will find such tumors to be susceptible to NK lysis.

O'REILLY: Are there any data on an effect of thymocytes on NK activity, whether this involves active inhibition of effectors or of induction?

WARNER: In general, the greater NK lytic activity of nude spleen cells as contrasted to normals would be accounted for by the absence of the T cells from the spleen, thus affording a twofold enrichment. However, since the relative increase is sometimes up to fourfold, it could be that some active suppression occurs in the normal spleen. We have also found that there is a cell type that can markedly suppress the activity of NK cells in the cytotoxic assay: it appears to be a macrophage type.

O'REILLY: Does Warner think that this explains the *C. parvum* effect?

WARNER: It is a very good possibility. It may also explain the apparent absence of NK lytic activity in the bone marrow. We are currently titrating all of these populations.

TRENTIN: E. Klein reported at the recent Hilton Head meeting that in the system of NK lysis of YAC lymphoma, there was no correlation with leukemia virus antigen or virus-induced antigen. Does Warner have any explanation for that?

WARNER: I think that all are in agreement that there is no absolute correlation of NK target "antigens" with the leukemia virus-associated antigens, as defined either by tumor-specific immunity of T-cell-mediated type or by serology. There does, however, appear to be a general correlation of susceptibility of targets with virus production by the tumor. Though we don't know the exact nature of the determinant, we suspect it is virally determined or associated.

STUTMAN: One of the predictions from the hyperactivity of nude mice would be that tumors arising in nudes should be resistant to natural kill. We tested this prediction with chemically induced fibrosarcomas and we found that of 17 tumors tested only two were susceptible to natural killers (measured using pre-labeled adherent cells in a 12-hr assay).*

CHAIRMAN WIGZELL: We shall now move onto the next topic, which is the relationship of the findings on NK cells to the phenomenon of resistance to bone marrow transplantation and the Hh system.

SHEARER: For more than a year it has been apparent to some of us working with the Hh models that certain striking parallels exist between the conditions for which NK cell activity can be demonstrated and those for which *in vivo* rejection of hemopoietic grafts as well as the generation of Hh CML responses are detected. In collaborative effort between several laboratories, a number of these unusual features associated with Hh reactions that affect NK cell activity have been investigated in detail. A summary of the parameters studied and their effects on marrow graft rejection *in vivo,* F_1 antiparent cytotoxicity *in vitro,* NK cell activity, and allogeneic CML *in vitro* are compared in Table 52. The genes responsible for the expression of the Hh determinants that appear to be recognized in marrow graft rejection and the development of F_1 antiparent cytotoxicity map in or near the H-2D region, although as discussed earlier, the cytotoxic response may display additional requirements. In contrast, the NK cell activity thus far described appears not to be associated with Hh-1. Allogeneic CML reactions mainly recognize products of the K and D regions of H-2, and possibly I region products to some extent.

The ability to react in both the *in vivo* and *in vitro* Hh models develops during the fourth week of life—more precisely between the twenty-first and twenty-fourth days. Published results indicate that NK cell activity in mice develops sometime before two months of age (Herberman *et al., Int. J. Cancer* **16**:216, 1975; Kiessling *et al., Eur. J. Immunol.* **5**:117, 1975). A recent more detailed study indicates that NK cell activity also develops between 21 and 24 days of age. In contrast, allogeneic CML activity is quite pronounced at one week of age.

Another feature that distinguishes both the *in vivo* and *in vitro* Hh models from their allogeneic counterparts is the observation that attempts to preimmunize the F_1 prospective graft recipients or responding cell donors with parental lymphoid cells expressing the Hh-1 determinant results in specific loss of F_1 reactivity against the parental Hh-1 determinant, as indicated in the third line of Table 52. Similarly, the NK cell activity (directed against the H-2^a YAC-1 tumor line) of (A/J × C57BL/6)F_1 mice pretreated with parental A spleen cells was

---

*Editor's comment: Since the target cells were not of hemopoietic origin and the assay conditions differed considerably, the experiment does not constitute a valid test of the prediction made by Stutman.

TABLE 52

Comparison of the Effects of Several Parameters Known to Affect Anti-Hh Reactivity
on Marrow Graft Rejection, F_1 Antiparent and Allogeneic Cytotoxicity, and NK Cell Activity[a]

	Type of reaction under study			
Parameter investigated	Marrow graft rejection *in vivo*	F_1 anti-parent cytotoxicity *in vitro*	NK cell activity *in vitro*	Allogeneic cytotoxicity *in vitro*
Genetic polymorphism	H-2D-Hh-1	H-2D-Hh-1	?	H-2K; H-2D
Response maturation	4th week	4th week	4th week	1st week
Preimmunization	unresponsive	unresponsive	suppresses	priming
Silica particles	suppresses	suppresses	suppresses	no effect
Iota-carrageenan	suppresses	suppresses	suppresses	suppresses
Antimarrow serum	suppresses	suppresses	suppresses	no effect
900 rad γ-irradiation	no effect	abolishes	no effect	abolishes
200 μCi [89]Sr	suppresses	suppresses	suppresses	suppresses
nu/nu mice	enhanced	no response	enhanced	no response
Effected by:	?	Thy-1(+)	Thy-1(−)	Thy-1(+)
Generated by:	?	Thy-1(+)	?	Thy-1(+)

[a]Summary of results from Kiessling, Hochman, Haller, Shearer, Wigzell, and Cudkowicz, *Eur. J. Immunol.* **7:**655, 1977.

reduced when compared with controls injected with allogeneic cells. Similar treatment prior to an allogeneic response results in priming.

Both the *in vivo* resistance to marrow grafts and development of the F_1 antiparental cytotoxic response are susceptible to the antimacrophage agents silica particles and iota-carrageenan. NK cell activity was reduced after *in vivo* treatment with silica or carrageenan. However, only the treatment with silica particles discriminated between the reactions shown in the first three columns of Table 52 and the allogeneic response shown in the fourth column. Treatment with carrageenan appeared to be toxic for all four types of responses.

Rabbit antimouse bone marrow serum abrogates resistance to marrow grafts when prospective recipients are injected one day prior to grafting. The serum also selectively abolishes or reduces the F_1 antiparent cytotoxic response without affecting the allogeneic CLM. Similar to the *in vivo* and *in vitro* Hh reactions, NK cell activity is reduced by injection of this antiserum.

The effects of γ-irradiation, administered to mice either by whole-body exposure or by prolonged and selective irradiation of the bone marrow by injection of the bone-seeking isotope [89]Sr (Bennet, *J. Immunol.* **110:**510, 1973), were compared in the four models studied. Marrow graft rejection and NK cell activity are resistant to the immediate effects of whole-body irradiation. The development of both the F_1 antiparent and allogeneic CML in culture are both sensitive to irradiation. All of the reactions compared here are abrogated by prolonged irradiation of the bone marrow.

The dependence of these reactions on thymus-derived lymphocytes was investigated by using athymic *nu/nu* mice and/or by treating the reactive cells with anti-Thy-1 serum and complement. Both the *in vivo* rejection of marrow grafts and NK cell activity are enhanced in *nu/nu* mice. No responses were generated *in vitro* by culturing spleen cells from F_1 *nu/nu* donors with stimulating cells expressing Hh or allogeneic determinants. The effector cells for Hh and allogeneic cytotoxic reactions are both Thy-1-positive, whereas NK cells reactive against YAC-1 appear to be Thy-1-negative. Furthermore, the generation of Hh and allogeneic CML are likewise sensitive to anti-Thy-1 serum and complement.

These comparisons thus show that there are a number of similarities among the phenomena of marrow graft rejection, NK cell activity, and F_1 antiparental cytotoxicity that distinguish them from classical allogeneic reactions. It would appear that these three reactions are dependent on a late-maturing, silica-sensitive event, which is probably cellular in nature. This cell could be a splenic macrophage-like cell that provides accessory function for these three reactions, but that is not required for developing strong allogeneic responses. It may be that the macrophage-like cell provides accessory function for the *in vitro* generated cytotoxic response and possibly NK cell activity, and is itself the effector for marrow graft rejection. Such a model has been recently considered (Shearer *et al., Cold Spring Harbor Symp.* **41**:511, 1977). However, it is unlikely that the macrophage-like cell is the effector of marrow graft rejection or NK cell activity for two reasons. Both hemopoietic rejection and NK cell function exhibit clear but distinct specificity as illustrated by the observations that (a) F_1 antiparent marrow graft rejection is directed against Hh-1, which is associated with the b haplotype in or near H-2D, whereas the NK cell activity considered here is associated with YAC-1, an H-2^a tumor; and (b) abrogation of marrow resistance by preinjection of parental spleen cells is specific for the H-2^b haplotype, but the reduction of NK cell activity is specific for the H-2^a haplotype. This is not meant to imply that all NK cell populations will in every instance exhibit specificity distinct from resistance to Hh-1, since NK cell activity was reported against RBL-5, an H-2^b tumor cell line (Herberman *et al., Int. J. Cancer* **16**:216, 1975). Nevertheless, the effectors responsible for hemopoietic resistance to Hh-1 and NK cell activity to YAC-1 appear to be of different specificity. It is noteworthy that although the F_1 antiparent CML is effected by a Thy-1-positive cell type, it is specific for Hh-1.

The specificity associated with the unresponsiveness resulting from injection of parental spleen cells also implies that this abrogation directly affects the specific effector cell line—most likely the precommitted precursors. The induction of this type of unresponsiveness probably requires potentially immunocompetent cells, since unirradiated parental cells abrogate F_1 antiparental CML potential.

It should also be noted that NK cell activity is sensitive to cortisone, whereas marrow graft rejection and the development of F_1 antiparental cytotoxic effectors are not reduced by this treatment. In fact, Hh CML response potential is elevated in the spleens of F_1 mice treated with cortisone (Hochman and Cudkowicz, *J. Immunol.*, in press). These differences in cortisone sensitivity (48 hr) of NK cells, hemopoietic resistance, and F_1 antiparent CML imply that these systems are effected by functionally distinct cell populations and assume that all three systems employ a common accessory cell pathway.

Finally, there are, among the four types of reponses compared, distinctions that tend to associate the Hh and allogeneic CML reactions and distinguish them from hemopoietic resistance and NK cell activity. These include the selective sensitivity of the CML reactions to (a) γ-irradiation immediately prior to *in vitro* sensitization, and (b) anti-Thy-1 serum and complement. Such findings imply that the two cytotoxic reactions are effected by and generated from Thy-1-positive lymphocytes, and that sensitization involving proliferation and differentiation is a prerequisite for the appearance of cytotoxic effector cells, irrespective of whether they are generated against Hh or allogeneic determinants. In contrast, it is significant that hemopoietic resistance and NK cell activity do not appear to require any active immunization. A model illustrating the possible relationships among marrow graft rejection, NK cell activity, and T-

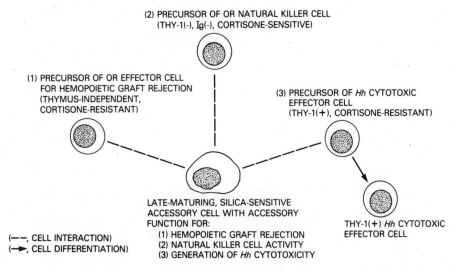

Fig. 21 Model illustrating possible relationships among the cells involved in hemopoietic graft rejection, natural killer activity, and F_1 antiparental cytotoxicity.

cell-mediated cytotoxicity against Hh targets that includes the foregoing considerations is depicted in Fig. 21.

CHAIRMAN WIGZELL: I have two comments before proceeding to Trentin's presentation of further data.

The matter of enhanced NK cell activity *in vitro* after 900 R irradiation to the cell donor only means that the reactivity per unit number of cells recovered is enhanced. This is a relative enrichment despite the possible loss of total NK activity. With respect to ^{89}Sr-induced NK suppression, the effect is not necessarily exerted directly on the NK cells, but may instead involve recruitment or generation of NK cells.

CANTOR: What is the most effective way of eliminating *in vivo* anti-Hh-1 activity? And what is the duration?

CUDKOWICZ: In my opinion this is best achieved with antispecies antibody, which can be selective. For example, anti-bone marrow or antifibroblast sera are devoid of general immunosuppressive activity. Such antisera selectively abrogate Hh-1 and the effect lasts for several weeks.

CHAIRMAN WIGZELL: I would suggest the alternative of ^{89}Sr, because in our experience it is quite selective for NK suppression.

TRENTIN: In recalling the comparison of two *in vitro* systems with *in vivo* resistance to bone marrow transplantation, it would appear from the differential effect of radiation, from the response of nude mice, and from the need for priming in the F_1 antiparent CML, that the NK system is a better *in vitro* correlate of *in vivo* resistance to bone marrow transplantation than is the F_1 antiparent CML response *in vitro*.*

When Kiessling was with us he worked with the system of NK lysis of YAC-1 lymphoma cells that he had brought with him. We, on the other hand, utilized the *in vivo* resistance to C57BL bone marrow transplants in irradiated hybrids. Mice irradiated earlier than 21 days of age were not resistant to parental marrow, but mice irradiated shortly thereafter were resistant. Similarly, unir-

Afterthought by Cudkowicz: A better correlation between the properties of marrow graft rejection and NK system was expected, since the generation of NK cells is an *in vivo* process, like resistance. With regard to the discrepancies with F_1 antiparent CML *in vitro*, these are apparent rather than real. Irradiation of responder cells prevents the establishing of a culture without necessarily interfering with anti-Hh reactivity. Stimulation of F_1 responder cells may not be equivalent to "induction" of a response, and T-cell dependence of CML may be a reflection of the assay's, endpoint which is quite unrelated to cytostasis *in vivo*.

radiated animals of the same litters had no splenic NK cells before 21 days, but did have NK cells shortly thereafter.

Genetic resistance to marrow transplantation is relatively radioresistant, in that it is normally measured after 900–1000 R. The extent of weakening of resistance by doses of radiation from 2200 to 6600 R was comparable to the reduction of NK cells lysis.

Silica, cytoxan, and carrageenan have an inhibitory effect on hybrid resistance, and also on NK cells. Two antisera of known efficacy for suppression of hybrid resistance had comparable effects on the NK system.

So, all these diverse modalities exerted an essentially parallel effect on the NK cell system and on the *in vivo* resistance to parental bone marrow transplants.

O'REILLY: I have a question relative to both Trentin's studies with the anti-bone marrow serum and Cantor's with anti-NK serum.

I would like to know whether the specificities of these antisera are directed against differentiation antigens, and whether the antisera were absorbed with spleen from infant versus adult animals.

TRENTIN: We have not done absorption with young spleen cells.

CANTOR: We do not know whether the antigen can be present on cells that are not capable of mediating NK activity. We cannot block the NK phenomenon *in vitro* by inclusion of the anti-NK antiserum.

CUDKOWICZ: We have absorbed some of the sera that had been used to abrogate marrow graft rejection. These are the same sera that were then used in the NK studies. It turned out that the relevant component is an antispecies antibody, with the antigen being widely distributed among mouse tissues. It is actually a consequence of these studies that we raised antifibroblast, antimacrophage, and antisquamous cell carcinoma sera that were free of antilymphocytic activity, but yet remained active in suppressing anti-Hh reactions and the generation of NK cells.

HENNEY: I want to describe a killer cell that has all the hallmarks of being an NK cell but seems to differ from the one that Wigzell described by two characteristics: its specificity and its distribution in lymphoid tissue. It is a cell that is found in peritoneal exudates following administration of BCG, but not following administration of thioglycollate or proteose peptone (Table 53).

The target cells we use, P815-X2 and EL4, are both cells that Wigzell and Cantor find not to be lysed by NK cells, and yet our effector cell is, like theirs, a "null" cell. It is not an "activated" macrophage, but is in fact a nonadherent

TABLE 53

Lytic Activity of Murine Peritoneal Exudates[a]

Treatment used to induce exudate	Exudate fraction used to assess lytic activity	Specific cytolysis (%)	
		P-815	EL4
None (normal exudate)	Unfractionated	0	1
	G-10 nonadherent	0	1
BCG	Unfractionated	37	28
	G-10 nonadherent	48	39
BCG (heat-killed)	Unfractionated	7	9
	G-10 nonadherent	9	13
Thioglycollate	Unfractioanted	0	3
Proteose peptone	Unfractionated	0	2
	G-10 nonadherent	0	2

[a]C57BL/6 mice, eight weeks old, were injected with 10^8 viable BCG-organisms (Pasteur Strain, Trudeau Institute); 10^8 heat-killed (80° 60 min) BCG; 2 ml 3% (w/v) thioglycollate or 1.5 ml 10% (w/v) proteose peptone. Exudate cells were harvested three or four days later and assayed against 10^4 ^{51}Cr targets at a ratio of 50:1. A 4-hr assay time was used.

cell, with no T cell surface markers, no surface immonoglobulin, no Fc and C3b receptors (*Nature* **262**:584, 1976).

The tissue distribution of this effector cell is rather different from the NK activity described by Wigzell and by Herberman. We do not find activity in the spleen, but we do find it in peritoneal exudates. We do not find it in mesenteric lymph nodes nor in popliteal or inguinal nodes, and it is only induced when BCG is given interperitoneally. When we administer BCG intravenously or in the foot pad, we do not obtain reactivity.

When we give BCG to animals with high (B6C$_3$F$_1$) or low (A/J) NK activity, the cytolytic activity of the peritoneal exudates increases in both cases but the spleen cell reactivities do not change.

I do not know what feature of BCG infection causes the induction of killer cells in this system, but I shall say that we have to date only been able to induce this reactivity with viable BCG organisms. Heat-killed BCG induces only minimal reactivity in the peritoneal exudate. A methanol extract residue (MER) of BCG and a sonicated BCG product (given to us by Minden) were both ineffective.

One further issue is whether the "null" cell-mediated kill described here (and subsequently referred to as NK-mediated lysis) could be modulated by drugs

TABLE 54
Effect of Various Drugs on T-Cell-
and NK-Cell-Mediated Lysis[a]

Drug		Inhibition of specific cytolysis (% mediated by)	
		NK cells	T cells
Cytochalasin A	5 μg	100	98
	1 μg	28	37
Cytochalasin B	5 μg	94	97
	1 μg	12	23
PGE$_1$	$10^{-5}M$	72	62
PGF$_1\alpha$	$10^{-5}M$	2	0
Colchicine	$10^{-4}M$	71	68
	$10^{-5}M$	15	12

[a]T-cell-mediated cytolysis was assayed using spleen cells from eight-week old C57BL/6 mice given 10^7 P-815 cells i.p. ten days previously. NK-mediated lysis of normal C57BL/6 mice was assayed using peritoneal exudates obtained four days after 10^8 viable BCG organisms. In both cases ^{51}Cr P-815 cells were used as targets, and a 50:1 effector:target cell multiplicity was used in a 4-hr assay. Drugs were present throughout the assay period.

known to inhibit T cell kill and ADCC: it could. The NK activity was inhibited and in the same dose range by all of the pharmacologic agents that inhibit T cell killing (Table 54). The cytochalasins A and B, prostaglandin E1, and other cyclic AMP "active" drugs, and colchicine all inhibit lysis, but not the analogs.

CHAIRMAN WIGZELL: Could Henney provide us with more detail about specificity?

HENNEY: We have not found a nucleated cell that our NK cells will not kill. They will kill syngeneic, allogeneic, and xenogeneic cells. They will kill 3T3 as well as 3T6 and 3T12 cells. They will kill teratomas that do not even bear H-2.

Other than making these all or none comparisons, I do not want to comment of the relative susceptibility or resistance of target cells. I think we are all a little lax in the way in which we compare cytolytic activities. We are all aware that the assay systems that we use for measuring either T cell, K cell or NK function do not enumerate killers. We nonetheless have a tendency to imply that they do by making quantitative comparisons of lytic activities. During this discussion several of us mentioned quantitative comparisons between lytic activities. I think this is a very dangerous practice since such comparisons do not take into account any considerations about variations in the efficiency of killer cells.

MOORE: Does Henney assay nonadherent cells?

HENNEY: We routinely assay nonadherent cells. Actually Sephadex G10 passed cells are what we usually use.

MOORE: Do the adherent cells suppress the nonadherent cells if they are mixed together?

HENNEY: I do not know the answer.

STUTMAN: We have been working with another NK cell that is closely related to the one described by Wigzell. This one is a cell that is also obtained from normal animals, but tested against adherent nonlymphoid tumor targets. The assay used is with target cells labeled with tritiated proline. Table 55 shows the strain distribution of reactivity and Table 56 shows that a variety of targets can be killed by normal spleen cells.

   This cytotoxic cell is also a null cell. It has no Fc receptors or T markers, or immunoglobulin. However, it is retained by nylon wool columns and by Sephadex G10 columns. So, it is an *adherent* cell. It is heterogeneous in size and

TABLE 55

Cytotoxicity of Normal Spleen Cells from Various Mouse
Strains against Meth A (BALB/c) Target Cells

Strain	Number of experiments	Cytotoxicity (%)[a]	
		Mean	Range
BALB/c	18	45	18–64
I	4	46	38–62
BALB/c nu/nu	2	45	25–64
CBA/H nu/nu	2	62	53–71
CBA/H	1	49	—
DBA/2	1	49	—
NZB	1	62	—
(C57BL/6 × DBA/2)F$_1$	1	45	—

[a]Mean percentage cytotoxicity (six replicates) at E:T of 100:1 after 24 hr of culture. Cell donors were one to four months old.

TABLE 56

Cytotoxicity of BALB/c Spleen Cells against Various Adherent Target Cells

Target cell	Strain of origin	MuLV surface antigens[a]	MuLV reverse transcriptase[b]	Cytotoxicity (%)[c]	
				Natural	PHA
Meth A	BALB/c	+	+	45[d]	68
Meth 113	BALB/c	+	not tested	−2	74
E4	C57BL/6	−	not tested	20[d]	70
Meth X	CBA/nu/nu	−	−	20[d]	59
Meth Y	CBA/H nu/nu	−	−	15[d]	55
Meth Z	CBA/H	−	not tested	−5	56
B65	C3H/He	−	−	−10	58

[a] Surface antigens were detected by indirect immunofluorescence using antiwhole disrupted MuLV and anti-gp 69/71.

[b] Performed on supernatants of cells.

[c] Mean cytotoxicity (six replicates) of spleen cells from four to eight week old BALB/c females at E:T ratios of 100:1 and 24 hr incubations. "Natural" indicates the effect of spleen cells alone (all results from a single experiment). "PHA" indicates cytotoxicity of spleen cells in the presence of 2 μg of PHA/well after 24 hr incubation at 100:1 ratios. B65 is a mammary adenocarcinoma cell line; the other tumors are chemically induced fibrosarcomas.

[d] Significant cytotoxicity above controls.

in velocity sedimentation at unit gravity it has a range from 3.5 to about 6 mm/hr. The cytotoxic effect is not influenced by removal of macrophages with carbonyl iron, by treatment with silica, or with ammonium chloride *in vitro*. It is present in the spleen, lymph nodes, peritoneal exudate (Freund adjuvant), and thymus, Another distinction is that it is detectable from birth and persists. We have studied mice even up to two years of age, and find it is still present. The response is not related to presence or absense of MuLV (murine leukemia virus antigens) on the surface of the target cells. We still do not know what makes a cell susceptible or resistant to this natural killer.

Sensitive targets can absorb NK cells, while the resistant targets cannot. The natural cytotoxic cell in this system is also present in the nude mouse (Table 56).

CANTOR: There are targets that are resistant to NK activity in given systems, even when one takes into account that there may be different families of NK cells. Does this really reflect a kind of specificity? If one incubates a source of natural killer cells with a so-called resistant target in the presence of Con A (which will bind and allow expression of cytotoxic activity present in other cell populations even though they do not have specificity) will one see NK activity expressed?

CHAIRMAN WIGZELL: There might be two minimum necessary requirements for lysis of target cells. One is that it requires a receptor for the effector
cell to attach. The second is that it would be intrinsically susceptible to lysis.
With regard to the NK cell system that we have been studying, we have found
one BALB/c myeloma cell that is insensitive to lysis but is very good as a blocker
of NK cell activity and can actually be shown to bind to the NK cells. In a
rosetting assay one can sediment the relevant NK cells with these large tumor
cells, yet as far as we can see that tumor cell is completely resistant to NK lysis.
So, in these systems, binding would not necessarily lead to lysis.

In view of the complexities that emerged in this discussion and the variety of
NK systems, I would like to make a few summarizing remarks. It is quite
important in considering NK cells that we really look into the definition of the
cell types. For instance, Henney's system contains an additional element, that is,
the obligatory activation with BCG in order to get full expression of cytolytic
cells, whereas in the NK systems we were using cells that reflect a natural,
unstimulated situation. This difference is basic.

We have been considering the relationship between NK cells, bone marrow
graft resistance, and possible protection against leukemia. The question was put
to me by van Bekkum "What have NK cells to do with bone marrow resistance?" The answer is that at the moment we cannot really say much that is
clear-cut on this matter. All we can say is that these three systems, the genetic
resistance to bone marrow, the NK cell, and the resistance to leukemia, are
intimately related. But we should realize that the data supporting this kind of
relationship do not prove that the very same cell is responsible for all three
phenomena. We have every reason to believe that in these systems, like in
others, complex cellular interactions lead to effector cell functions. Perhaps,
specific reagents, such as the one developed by Cantor, will help us resolve the
issue of the relationship between NK cells and the urgent biological phenomena
dealt with by this conference.

DISTINCTIVE MECHANISMS IN NATURALLY OCCURRING
GENETIC RESISTANCE TO LEUKEMOGENESIS

Discussion Introducer:

Richard A. Steeves

CHAIRMAN STEEVES: In this session we shall first consider genes that control resistance to Friend leukemia virus in mice, and then proceed to studies on T suppressor cells and Hh effects.

The genetics of susceptibility to Friend leukemia virus began in 1962 with Odaka's work in which he found that C57BL mice had a potent resistance gene, where his parameter for measuring virus resistance was splenomegaly. Then in 1965, Odaka followed up these initial studies with a parameter based on spleen focus formation. Axelrad and Lilly soon joined the hunt, using the same assay, and over the next decade a considerable collection to genes was mapped and briefly characterized with respect to the manner in which they control susceptibility to Friend virus (Table 57).

The Rgv-1 and Rfv-1 genes apparently affect late responses in the leukemogenic process, without affecting early responses or virus replication. Instead of detecting an influence on the spleen focus response, mice that have the H-2^b haplotype usually develop the initial signs of Friend disease but recover from it more frequently than H-2^k or H-2^d mice.

The next three genes are responsible for genetic anemias of mice. Cudkowicz, Bennett, and I were interested in the first two of these, the dominant spotting (W) and stell (Sl) genes, the first of which controls the availability of stem cells, the second the environment for stem cells to differentiate along the erythroid pathway. Mice carrying mutations at either locus are resistant to Friend virus-induced spleen focus formation and leukemia, especially if two mutant alleles are present. The third of these anemia-inducing genes, f, was found by Axelrad to confer resistance to Friend virus as well.

The Fv-1 gene is dominant for resistance, the n and b alleles conferring resistance to MuLV of the opposite tropism. That is, the b allele confers resistance to N-tropic viruses and the n allele to B-tropic viruses. Therefore, Fv-1 n/b hybrid mice are resistance to both N-tropic and B-tropic viruses, but they are susceptible to NB-tropic virus because it has been adapted to the resistant strain and has lost its sensitivity to restriction by mice of any Fv-1 genotype.

Fv-1 resistance appears to be directed against the helper virus in Friend virus stocks rather than against the virus directly responsible for spleen focus formation (SFFV). It appears that this gene is involved in a fairly late phase of the virus cycle and, if Friend virus is passaged in Fv-1-restrictive mice with another helper virus that is, let us say, NB-tropic and can escape the Fv-1 restriction, pseudotypes of SFFV will be produced that have the host range and/or the antigenicity of the superinfecting helper virus, and that can escape Fv-1 restriction.

In contrast to Fv-1, the Fv-2 gene is recessive for resistance to Friend virus and prevents spleen focus formation after Friend virus infection. Because C57BL mice are virus resistant at other loci besides Fv-2, Lilly back-crossed (C57BL × DBA/2)F$_1$ hybrid mice with susceptible DBA/2 mice, selecting for Fv-2$^{s/r}$ hetero-

TABLE 57

Mapped Mouse Genes That Control Susceptibility to Friend
Leukemia Virus

Gene	Chromosome	Gene action
Rgv-1 (at H-2K)	17	b haplotype has a stronger immune response
Rfv-1 (at H-2K)	17	b haplotype is associated with more persistent viral antigen expression
W	5	two dominant W alleles severely limit the availability of hemopoietic stem cells
S1	10	two dominant S1 alleles alter the environment to inhibit erythroid differentiation
f	13	f/f homozygotes have limited proliferative capacity of their erythopoietic precursor cells
Fv-1	4	dominant n and b alleles inhibit helper MuLV of opposite tropism
Fv-2	9	r/r homozygotes do not develop spleen foci in response to Friend virus infection

zygotes at each generation. After two back crosses, Fv-2$^{r/r}$ homozygotes
were prepared and we tested them according to several parameters. The results,
summarized in Table 58, show that the Fv-2^r gene was consistently associated
with an inhibitory effect (between 25- and 100-fold) after the mice were infected
with Friend virus, but no inhibition was observed in experiments where Fv-2^r

TABLE 58

Effect of Fv-2 Resistance on Parameters for Evaluating
Friend Leukemia

Parameter	After virus infection	After tumor cell graft
Virus recovery	decreased	—
Tumor cell recovery	decreased	unchanged
^{59}Fe uptake	decreased	unchanged
Recovery of Erythropoietin-independent CFU-E[a]	decreased	unchanged
Focal splenic lesions	no foci	no colonies

[a]Colony-forming units: erythroid, as defined by Axelrad
and McLeod.

mice had been grafted with tumor cells that had already been transformed by Friend virus in susceptible mice.

However, a serious exception to this general rule arose, and it perplexed us greatly. Whereas no spleen foci were observed after virus infection, no spleen colonies were observed after tumor cell grafts either. This is in sharp contrast with the lack of inhibition of other parameters after tumor cell grafts. Although spleen colony formation by Friend virus-infected tumor cells was clearly shown by Thomson and Axelrad to be based on donor cell proliferation in lethally irradiated hosts, recent evidence from our laboratory and from others suggests that a significant number of host cells may by contributing to spleen colony formation, which requires a certain amount of virus synthesis and infection of adjacent host cells. It would then be relatively straightforward to conclude that the Fv-2^r gene interferes with some step in SFFV replication. Current experiments are aimed at resolving this question.

Another unexpected observation with the Fv-2^r gene arose from attempts to recover homozygous mice after 13 back crosses to the DBA/2 strain. Instead of obtaining the expected ratio of 1:2:1 among susceptible homozygotes, heterozygotes, and resistant homozygotes, we observed a 1:2:0 ratio in a significant number of progeny mice. This was so consistent that we are entertaining the possibility that the Fv-2^r gene is lethal. But in the C57BL mouse this lethal effect would not be expressed if there were a protector gene in the C57BL family of mice that could have been eliminated in serial back-crossing to the DBA/2 strain presumably lacking the protector gene. Until now, the Fv-2 gene has been thought to be a gene demonstrable only by the host response to Friend virus, but it may be demonstrable in uninfected mice if it is affecting an essential step in embryogenesis. These studies are still in their early stages and will have to be extended.

Now, recall that Table 57 refers only to genes that have been mapped. C57BL mice are very intriguing animals, and they have a number of other genes that have not yet been mapped, one of which has been investigated by Kumar and Bennett.

Briefly, it would appear that the gene or genes that Bennett is analyzing affect a population of precursor M cells, the so-called marrow-dependent cells, and this in turn may be related to the NK cell, which has already received so much of our attention. It appears that the mature effector M cells are radioresistant and control a population of T suppressor cells. These can restrict mitogen-responsive T and B cells, the host immunocompetent cells. If animals (e.g., C57BL) have a high population of M cells, the number of T suppressor cells will be restricted and the mice will be able to mount good immune responses and resist Friend virus. In contrast, animals such as DBA/2 have apparently smaller numbers of M cells or, in some way, a not particularly good M cell function. Consequently, in the DBA/2, the T suppressor cells would be able to suppress mitogen-responsive immunocompetent cells; as a result these animals would be sensitive to Friend virus infection. Bennett will elaborate on further details in this system, but first Moore will present some recent data regarding Fv-2.

MOORE: I would like to contribute some information concerning the work of Dexter from the Patterson Laboratories in Manchester, which involves a system that he has developed for the continuous maintenance of mouse bone marrow stem cell proliferation and differentiation *in vitro*. I shall describe the basic system first and then mention some of his recent experiments on infection of these cultures with Friend virus. The culture system is very simple and is one that I think many investigators have attempted. It involves inoculating mouse bone marrow into glass bottles or, as we have done, into plastic flasks, and over a period of some two to three weeks the cultures progressively decline in the production of cells, and the content of multipotential stem cells and of committed granulocyte–macrophage precursors. I think at this stage most of us who had attempted continuous marrow culture threw the cultures away, but Dexter reinoculated them with fresh bone marrow. By doing this, he was able to initiate continuous cultures, which at weekly intervals were refed after removal of half the nonadherent cells. There was essentially a weekly doubling of cells, and numbers of CFU-S and CFU-C; this growth was maintained for periods as long as 10–15 weeks.

The differentiation in the culture system was restricted to neutrophil granulocytes, megakaryocytes, and macrophages. There was no erythropoiesis and no detectable maintenance of T or B cell populations. However, even after prolonged periods the cultures contained multipotential stem cells that could reconstitute lethally irradiated mice. These animals by virtue of their prolonged survival were clearly reconstituted both in their lymphiod and myeliod systems.

The requirement for reinoculating the initial cultures of bone marrow related to the need to establish an adherent population of marrow cells that acted as a feeder layer supporting the subsequent proliferation and differentiation of stem cells. This adherent layer was comprised of cells that were morphologically macrophage, epitheloid, and certain cells that were giant lipid-containing cells. This system, the interaction between a microenvironment generated *in vitro* and prolonged stem cell renewal and differentiation, is to my mind a major technical breakthrough that provides an opportunity to investigate cell–cell interactions.

As far as leukemogenesis *in vitro* is concerned, Dexter infected these cultures with Friend virus at either time zero of initial feeding with the bone marrow, or at various periods up to two weeks after the establishment of the continuous bone marrow culture, and followed these cultures for prolonged periods of time. He observed in infected BDF$_1$ bone marrow cultures that the maintenance of stem cells—both multipotential and committed granulocyte—macrophage progenitors—was prolonged to as long as 17–24 weeks after initiation of cultures. This interval is long after the control population has converted to essentially a population of macrophages with no detectable stem cells. Now, a question is whether these stem cells were transformed or abnormal in any way. As far as the CFU-C was concerned, the colony-forming cell retained the requirement for CSF, underwent granulocytic differentiation, and was not leukemic. However, the CFU-S, after about six to nine weeks of culture maintenance, no longer showed evidence of erythroid differentiation in spleens of irradiated recipients. The majority of spleen colonies from the control cultures were erythroid; however, they were predominantly granulocytic from Friend-virus-infected cultures. This is somewhat paradoxical, since we generally think of the Friend virus as inducing an erythroleukemia.

In this instance, it would appear that the Friend virus had induced in culture a disease that corresponded rather to a chronic myeloid leukemia. The mice that were recipients of bone marrow cells from prolonged Friend-virus-infected cultures developed, after two or three weeks of injection of either cells or supernatants, a classic erythroleukemia that was of host origin. However, the myeloid proliferation observed in the irradiated recipients in the first two or three weeks was of donor origin, as determined by sex chromosome marker analysis.

I suspect that we are not observing erythroleukemia in this system because the microenvironment does not support the development of committed erythroid progenitor cells from multipotential stem cells. Of course, we are not adding erythropoietin to maintain erythropoiesis, and so we are seeing what one would see in the mouse if one prevented the development of erythroleukemia.

To briefly turn to the question of the Fv-2 resistance, Dexter infected cultures of bone marrow from the resistant strain C57BL/6, but failed to observe any of these transformation events. The FV-infected B6 cultures showed that same pattern of proliferation, differentiation, and ultimate decline in stem cells, as did the uninfected BDF$_1$ cultures. At no time were the supernatants from the B6 cultures able to induce Friend erythroleukemia in recipient mice. There seems to be clear evidence here of an *in vitro* system that demonstrates resistance in terms of leukemic transformation and resistance with respect to propagation of the Friend virus complex.

CHAIRMAN STEEVES: What was the tropism of the Friend virus used by Dexter?

MOORE: NB-tropic.

CHAIRMAN STEEVES: So, Moore has excluded Fv-1 as the cause of restriction. But there are other unmapped C57BL genes that could have been involved as well.

MOORE: Yes, and I hope that we can resolve that issue when we get the various congenic strains of mice.

TILL: Did Friend virus persist in the cultures throughout?

MOORE: Up to 25 weeks after infection with Friend virus, the cultures were still producing virus, and were capable of inducing classic Friend erythroleukemia in recipients.

PARKMAN: What happens if erythropoietin is added to the cultures?

MOORE: The problem is that erythropoietin preparations are contaminated with CSF and endotoxin. It is rather embarrassing for those of us working in the area that addition of this factor to continuous bone marrow cultures switches off granulopoiesis and converts the culture to macrophages. At present we are repeating these studies with highly purified human urinary erythropoietin (5000–10,000 units per milligram of protein) not contaminated with a lot of exogenous factors that suppress the culture system. I hope we would then see erythroleukemia developing *in vitro*.

BENNETT: A major aim of this conference is to ascertain the role of the cells responsible for the rejection of marrow allografts, not only for its importance in clinical bone marrow transplantation, but also for what it portends for other host defense mechanisms. The first model that we investigated was the Friend virus leukemia model. Eckner, Kumar, and I chose this system because leukemia is a disease of stem cells, and the marrow allograft rejecting system is directed against such cells.

As Steeves has indicated, the strains of mice that are genetically resistant to Friend virus leukemia are also resistant to most bone marrow allografts; that is to say, they are better rejectors of bone marrow allografts, in general, than strains that are not resistant to Friend virus. When we found that mice treated with ^{89}Sr would no longer reject bone marrow allografts, it seemed important to determine whether these mice were still resistant to Friend virus.

In genetically susceptible mice, Friend virus induces a profound immunosuppression, primarily of the humoral response but also of mitogen responsiveness *in vitro*. C57BL/6 mice treated with strontium proved to be very susceptible to Friend virus as they developed erythroleukemia and were immunosuppressed. Using the latter parameter, we decided to explore the mechanism by which M cells function in Friend virus leukemia.

The first major finding was that those strains of mice that are genetically susceptible to Friend virus leukemia *in vivo* also had mitogen-responsive cells that were susceptible to suppression by Friend virus *in vitro*. Conversely, strains of mice such as C57BL/6, which are genetically resistant, have cells that were only marginally or not suppressed *in vitro*. If one filters spleen cells of a susceptible BALB/c mouse through nylon wool columns, the nonadherent spleen cells are no longer susceptible to suppression by Friend virus. This means that the mitogen-responsive cells are not intrinsically suseptible to suppression by Friend virus. In fact, if one mixes normal unfractionated with nonadherent spleen cells, in ratios as low as 1:15, this mixture now becomes fully susceptible to suppression by Friend virus. Hence, genetically susceptible mice have a population of suppressor cells. The evidence that they are T suppressor cells derives from their absence in athymic nude mice. Moreover, these cells are susceptible to lysis by anti-Thy-1 serum and complement.

There is a population of T suppressor cells, which are themselves the targets of Friend virus, and suppress, upon activation, mitogen-responsive cells. We harvested cells from strontium-treated mice and challenged them with Friend virus *in vitro*. Spleen cells from control adult C57BL/6 mice respond to Con A or other mitogens quite well even when 200 focus-forming units of the virus are added to each reaction mixture. However, spleen cells taken from genetically resistant C57BL/6 mice pretreated with strontium became as susceptible to suppression as spleen cells from genetically suseptible mice.

Another condition in which mice cannot reject bone marrow allografts is immaturity as neonates and infants. Up to the age of three weeks mice are incapable of rejecting bone marrow allografts and, as many have pointed out, are lacking in NK cells. Thymus cells taken from such infant C57BL/6 mice also are susceptible to Friend virus suppression *in vitro*. However, an agent known to suppress marrow allograft rejection, silica particles, had no effect in this system. This is not surprising since T suppressor cells have to be generated after M cells, or effectors of marrow allograft rejection, are eliminated.

If one filters spleen cells from strontium-treated C57BL/6 mice through nylon columns, the mitogen-responsive cells are themselves resistant to Friend virus. If one now adds unfractionated normal spleen cells it is possible to fully reconstitute susceptibility. With this model, one studies interaction between mitogen-responsive cells and T suppressor cells. The latter are modulated by the M cells, which are affected by radioactive strontium; whether they are eliminated or their function compromised remains to be determined.

From the work of Chesebro *et al.*, Lilly, Freedman, and Steeves, it appeared that the relevant region of the H-2 complex for the regression of Friend virus leukemia was the D-end of H-2, at or near H-2D. We wondered if the interaction between the T suppressor and the mitogen-responsive cells also might show H-2 restriction, especially for this D region.

The way these experiments are done is to mix 9×10^5 spleen cells containing mitogen-responsive cells, with 1×10^5 spleen cells containing T suppressor cells. Spleen cells from genetically resistant mice, such as C57BL/6, and nonadherent spleen cells from genetically susceptible mice are the source of mitogen-responsive cells. Spleen cells from genetically susceptible mice or from resistant mice given ^{89}Sr are the source of T suppressor cells. B10.A, 2R, 5R, and HTG mice are genetically resistant to Friend virus immunosuppression *in vitro*, whereas A,DBA/2, C3H, and 129 mice are susceptible (Table 59). There was clearly a requirement of identity at H-2D for suppression of mitogen-responsive cells by Friend-virus-activated T suppressors.

These results were surprising to us inasmuch as there was no restriction *in vivo*. When one infects genetically susceptible adult DBA/2 mice, four days prior to irradiation, and transfers genetically resistant, H-2 compatible B10.D2 bone marrow cells, immunosuppression and leukemogenic transformation are obtained. However, when B10.D2 bone marrow cells are allowed to repopulate the infected DBA/2 host, no leukemia cells are found. This is the model we are using to see if we can cure leukemia with a bone marrow transplant by using donors

TABLE 59

H-2 Compatibility Requirements for Friend-Virus-Activated T Suppressor Cells
and Mitogen-Responsive Cells

Exp.	Mitogen-Responsive Cell[a]		T Suppressor Cell[b]		Suppression[c] (%)
	Strain	H-2	Strain	H-2	
1	B10.A	kkk ddd	—	—	10
			A	kkk ddd	76
			DBA/2	ddd ddd	58
			C3H	kkk kkk	12
			129	bbb bbb	5.1
2	B10.A (2 R)	kkk ddb	—	—	11
			DBA/2	ddd ddd	1.3
	B10.A (5 R)	bbb ddd	—	—	4.7
			DBA/2	ddd ddd	54
	HTG	ddd ddb	—	—	−1.8
			DBA/2	ddd ddd	−8.1
			129	bbb bbb	75

[a]Donors resistant to Friend virus *in vivo* and *in vitro*; 9×10^5 spleen cells/well.

[b]Donors susceptible to Friend virus *in vivo* and *in vitro*; 1×10^5 spleen cells/well.

[c]Suppression of Δ blastogenesis statistically significant, $p < 0.01$. Cells were cultured in triplicate in 0.2 ml volume m RPMI 1640 medium with 10% fetal calf serum, with or without 0.5 μg Con A and/or 300 focus-forming units of NB-tropic Friend virus complex, for 72 hr at 37°C, 5% CO_2 in air. ^{3}H-thymidine (0.5 μCi/well) was added 18 hr prior to harvesting cultures. Suppression (%) = Δ blastogenesis (^{3}H-thymidine incorporation, cpm, Con A-no con A: no FV–FV/ no FV × 100.

TABLE 60

Evidence for an "Interfering Cell" Preventing Suppression of Mitogen-Responsive Cells
by T Suppressor Cells

Mitogen-responsive spleen cell population[a]	T Suppressor spleen cell population[b]	Δ Blastogenesis[c]		Suppression[c]	
		−FV	+FV	%	Student t-test
C57BL/6	None	54,693	54,513	0.32	NS
	DBA/2, adult, 0 R	53,584	54,165	−1.0	NS
	DBA/2, adult, 1000 R	55,677	32,192	42	$p < 0.01$
	1:1, 0 R:1000 R	51,473	55,541	−7.9	NS
	DBA/2 infant	48,804	33,629	31	$p < 0.01$
	1:1, adult, 0 R:infant	41,800	53,982	−29	NS
C57BL/6	None	58,353	63,092	−7.0	NS
	DBA/2, vehicle	53,830	59,082	−9.0	NS
	DBA/2, cortisol	34,874	13,569	61	$p < 0.01$
	1:1, vehicle:cortisol	41,794	40,720	2.5	NS

[a,b,c]See Table 59. Adults, 12 weeks old; infants, 3 days old. Spleen cells exposed to 1000 R γ-rays *in vitro;* cortisol (2.5 mg) injected i.p. two days prior to culture.

that are known to be genetically resistant to the virus, but matched at the major histocompatibility complex.

We had noticed that with infant DBA/2 mice infected and transplanted with H-2 incompatible C57BL/10 marrow cells, transformation of such B10 stem cells and immunosuppression were obtained again. Therefore, we considered the notion that the inability of H-2 incompatible T cells to suppress *in vitro* mitogen-responsive cells in the presence of Friend virus involved interference by a third cell. To verify this explanation of the *in vivo* vs. *in vitro* discrepancy, we irradiated DBA/2 spleen cells with 1000 R *in vitro* and determined if they could now suppress B6 mitogen-responsive cells. The irradiated cells did suppress (Table 60).

If one mixes irradiated DBA/2 with unirradiated DBA/2 spleen cells in a 1:1 ratio, the resulting cell suspension does not suppress B6 spleen cells (Table 60). That is to say, that the nonirradiated cells in the suspension prevent the T suppressor cell from inhibiting proliferation of B6 mitogen-responsive cells.

A very similar result was found using infant mice. Three-day-old spleen cells from DBA/2 mice also suppress across the H-2 barrier. A mixture of adult DBA/2 spleen with infant DBA/2 spleen cells likewise results in no suppression. This interfering cell could also be eliminated by treating adult DBA/2 mice with cortisol (Table 60). Spleen cells taken from cortisol-treated mice are able to suppress across the H-2 barrier, but if one mixes spleen cells from cortisol-treated DBA/2 mice with normal DBA/2 cells, the H-2 restriction again applies.

Therefore, the Friend virus model is even more complex than had been suspected. Mitogen-responsive cells are resistant to Friend virus but are the target cells of the T suppressor cells. The T suppressor cells are activated by Friend virus to suppress mitogen-responsive cells. The numbers and/or functions of the suppressors are regulated by M cells. Still another cell, an interfering cell, enters the scheme by interacting with the H-2D gene product of the mitogen-responsive cell. H-2D incompatibility between the interfering and the mitogen-responsive cell prevents T suppressors from functioning. We do not know the nature of this interference, but this could involve the release of receptors for H-2D alloantigens, as has been observed by Ramsaier.

SHEARER: What other immune function is affected beside mitogen-responsiveness?

BENNETT: Because we like to correlate *in vitro* phenomena with *in vivo* situations, we have done a genetic analysis of the control of T suppressor cells. DBA/2 mice are susceptible and B10.D2 mice are resistant. The F_1 hybrids are susceptible. Therefore, it appears that susceptibility is dominant. If one back-crosses these mice to DBA/2, all the animals are susceptible. If one back-crosses to B10.D2, approximately one-half are susceptible, one-half resistant. One can type individual mice for their *in vitro* susceptibility or resistance. We perform a hemisplenectomy for *in vitro* testing after which the animal is infected with Friend virus and tested for the Fv-2 phenotype. Susceptibility or resistance *in vitro* is not linked with Fv-2. Friend virus immunosuppression *in vivo* (antibody to SRBC) follows the *in vitro* pattern with rare exceptions.

MERUELO: Did Bennett imply that the need for H-2D identity between T suppressors and mitogen-responsive cells is related to the mechanism of H-2 control of Friend-virus-induced leukemogenesis?

BENNETT: No. It does not prove it nor does it exclude it.

METCALF: Did I understand Bennett to say the Friend virus infects T suppressor cells? If that is the case, what is the evidence, since suppressors are rather mystical and poorly visualized cells?

BENNETT: I did not mean to say that Friend virus infects suppressor cells, but that it acts via the T suppressors. Replicating virus is required for this phenomenon. But whether the T suppressor cell is productively infected with Friend virus remains to be determined.

WERNET: I am thinking of experiments done by Bubbers and Lilly, where it was shown that the D region controls the expression of antigenicity for a virus-modified MHC product, whereas the K region codes for immune response capacity of T cells. Would experiments in which the H2-D alleles of suppressor and/or mitogen-responsive cells are manipulated disclose a way of turning on or off the function of suppressor cells in Friend virus leukemia?

BENNETT: The H-2 haplotype of the suppressor can be of any known type. We do not know which, if any, of these cells are productively infected with Friend virus. It is conceivable that the mitogen-responsive cell expresses something "new" at H-2D that is recognized by the T suppressor cell. Alternatively the suppressor cell may itself have altered receptors.

CHAIRMAN STEEVES: Golub will now describe for us the features of another suppressor cell in AKR leukemia.

GOLUB: We have been studying immunosuppression in AKR leukemia utilizing a variety of parameters, but I shall also refer briefly to the suppression of normal *in vitro* antibody responses to SRBC by leukemic cells of AKR mice. AKR leukemia is a Gross-virus-associated disease and so it differs from the system used by Bennett.

We found that if we mix leukemic spleen, or thymus and to a variable extent lymph node cells, from AKR mice with normal AKR cells *in vitro,* the ability of the latter cells to generate an anti-SRBC response is shut off. This is a T cell-mediated suppression since this is a T cell tumor. So we are dealing with a T suppressor cell.

All of these experiments are done with spontaneous leukemias; each experiment is done with a different spontaneous tumor from a different leukemic mouse. We find that a great majority (~80%) of spontaneous leukemias we study will only suppress the normal cells of another AKR. When tested on allogeneic normal cells, there is no suppression. If we test, say, a CBA or C3H (AKR is H-2^k) there is still no suppression. When we controlled for genes other than H-2 or genes within the MHC, we found that any incompatibility resulted in no suppression. For example, we used AKR.M, which being kkkkkq only differs at H-2D, and there is no suppression.

We call these *restricted suppressor* cells. The suppression involves cell contact. Supernates of the tumors, or tumors growing on the other side of filters, do not yield suppression. The suppression could be overcome by adding irradiated allogeneic cells to the cultures of normal AKR spleen cells. So if we have leukemic AKR and a normal AKR, we get suppression. But if we add to the system some x-rayed allogeneic cells, say B10, the suppression is then overcome. Furthermore, if we take any two strains and react them for three days, the supernate of this reaction when added to the test system of leukemic AKR plus normal AKR overcomes suppression. When we sought to determine whether this supernate was enhancing the response of the normal cells so that they are not suppressible, or if it was instead affecting the leukemic cell, we found that it was affecting the suppressor cell, i.e., it was blocking the suppressive action of this cell.

We designate 20% of spontaneous leukemia as nonrestricted suppressors. These leukemic cells will suppress all strains. They will suppress cells of any H-2 haplotype. These cells apparently do not suppress by cell contact but rather elaborate a soluble factor. Adding irradiated allogeneic cells or allogeneic supernates to cultures with these cells does not overcome suppression.

Furthermore, we can overcome the restricted suppression by adding submitogenic doses of either LPS or Con A, but these agents are ineffective with the nonrestricted suppressors.

We have also been examining suppression in neonatal mice. We find, wonder of wonders, that neonatal spleen (within the first week of life) contains suppressor T cells, and we determined that these cells suppress by cell contact, not by soluble factors. Also we found that there is genetic restriction. The suppression is overcome by the presence of irradiated allogeneic cells and allogeneic supernates. So there is great similarity between the leukemic and neonatal suppressor systems.

With Potter of the NCI we have been exploring long-established AKR and BALB/c lymphomas. We find that all of them are nonrestricted. Now that we are aware of the restricted/nonrestricted nature of suppression by spontaneous tumors, we examine both spleen and thymus of every mouse developing spontaneous leukemia. We have been finding that in a good proportion of our animals the spleen will be restricted and the thymus nonrestricted, or vice versa. There is no set pattern.

We think that as the tumor develops, suppression is at first restricted and then moves on to a nonrestricted state. The long passage tumors that most workers use are the ones that have gone through this kind of change. We believe that in the neonate we are seeing something analogous to a malignant kind of suppression.

ELKINS: I have recently read some papers by Proffitt stating that leukemic and preleukemic AKR cells killed normal AKR fibroblasts and that this showed a restriction similar to what Golub reported. Would Golub comment on the possibility that his suppression involved a killer cell?

GOLUB: We sought them by the usual means but have been unable to find killer cells. We have used only lymphoid targets.

CAMPBELL: Does Golub have any evidence that the suppressors are really T cells?

GOLUB: Yes. They are thymus-derived, i.e., Thy-1-positive. Now, the interesting thing that I didn't go into is that with the restricted tumors the membranes themselves will suppress.

CANTOR: Is restricted immunosuppression relevant to the growth of the tumor *in situ* and, experimentally does it mean that you can influence the growth of a tumor by injecting allogeneic cells or allogeneic supernatants into the host?

GOLUB: Allogeneic cells injected into AKR mice led to the development of leukemia even in the mice used to produce anti-Thy-1 serum. These leukemias were of both the restricted and nonrestricted type.

METCALF: Just a comment about using the term "leukemic cell suspension," and this also applies to spontaneous leukemias. It should be noted that a tumor mass is not composed entirely of leukemic cells. In lymphomas, particularly T cell lymphomas, it is very characteristic that large numbers of highly activated macrophages are present. It would therefore be worth checking whether Golub could remove reactivity be removing adherent cells.

GOLUB: We have started such experiments but don't have clear results yet. One of the things we have done, though, is velocity sedimentation. In the thymus we find that there are suppressor cells in all sizes of fractions, but, in the leukemic spleen, we find suppressor cells only in fractions that sediment from about 3.5 mm/hr downward.

WARNER: I would like to return to a major area of discussion, namely, the expression of Hh on tumor cells.
     This topic may have some relevance to the NK mechanism, which could operate against tumor cells as well as against allogeneic transplantation of marrow. We have already touched on the problem of whether the NK cell, and its possible interaction with cells expressing Hh antigen, should be considered as an immunological phenomenon or not. Should we use the term "antigen" and "immune" responding cells? If we are going to view the NK cell as a distinct type of mechanism reacting to a tumor (and the parallels have already been considered between NK lysis and mechanism of Hh resistance), should we then consider the possibility that the NK cell is reacting to an Hh-type material on the tumor cell surface? We have indicated before that in various studies the exact nature of the antigen on the tumor cell that is recognized by the NK cell is unknown, but may be viral associated or directed.

TABLE 61
Growth of SJL Tumors in Hybrid Mice

| Tumor line | Splenic tumor growth (ratio tumor injected/control) | | | |
	SJL	(SJL × C57)F$_1$	(SJL × B10.BR)F$_1$	(SJL × B10.D$_2$)F$_1$
WEHI-293	11.3 ± 1.1	3.6 ± 0.1		2.0 ± 0.4
WEHI-289	14.6 ± 2.1	4.1 ± 0.2		1.5 ± 0.3
WEHI-285	7.7 ± 0.8	2.6 ± 0.5		1.8 ± 0.2
WEHI-251		9.2 ± 0.3	3.1 ± 0.2	2.3 ± 0.2
WEHI-244		4.5 ± 0.4	1.5 ± 0.1	1.6 ± 0.2
WEHI-220		4.1 ± 0.3	2.3 ± 0.2	2.3 ± 0.1
WEHI-219		3.9 ± 0.5	1.3 ± 0.1	1.3 ± 0.1
WEHI-201	7.9 ± 0.3	6.0 ± 0.6	3.8 ± 0.5	2.6 ± 0.4
WEHI-175	9.3 ± 0.9	6.6 ± 0.4	4.4 ± 0.6	3.3 ± 0.2
375V		6.1 ± 1.1	2.0 ± 0.4	1.5 ± 0.1
All tumors	10.2 ± 1.3	5.1 ± 0.6	2.6 ± 0.5	2.0 ± 0.2

The following studies are to demonstrate that certain tumor cells do, in fact, express Hh "antigen" on their surface. This study is similar to that done by Cudkowicz several years ago, but in this present system a series of SJL tumors were employed. Table 61 shows data for ten different SJL tumors, with the mean values on the bottom line. The growth of SJL tumors in inbred hosts or in three F$_1$ hybrid strains was measured by splenomegaly indexes. From studies with anti-H-2 sera, it was shown that in the (SJL × C57BL)F$_1$ hybrid virtually all the increase in spleen size is due to tumor cell proliferation. The main point to note is that, consistently throughout these studies, there is a marked reduction is the growth rate of SJL tumors in certain SJL hybrids, exactly correlating with the data given previously in relation to CFU colony formation in SJL hybrids. Furthermore, as in the CFU studies, this distinction in growth rate is also shown in irradiated F$_1$ hybrid mice and, furthermore, this mechanism of resistance can be abrogated by split-dose radiation.

I wish to stress another point made in relation to the CFU studies, namely, that genetic control of hybrid resistance also operates in regard to the F$_1$ response to parental tumors (Fig. 22). The expression of reactivity to Hh-1 antigen is associated with H-2D in the (SJL × B10.D2)F$_1$ hybrid. However, in the (SJL × A.TH)F$_1$ hybrid, which also is heterozygous for s/d alleles at H-2D, a normal type of growth pattern is observed, suggesting that there is Ir type of genetic control operating at the recipient level.

The main point to be made is that there are several different tumor types that express Hh antigen. They include T lymphomas of several both radiation-induced and spontaneous SJL, in the reticulum cell sarcoma type B tumors of

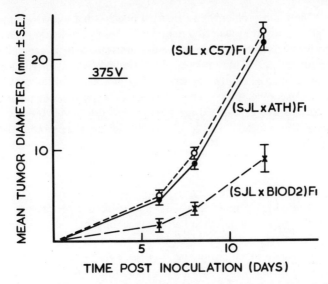

Fig. 22   Manifestation of hybrid resistance in the response of F_1 to parental tumors.

SJL mice, and certain meyloid tumors such as 375V, which we obtained from Haran-Ghera. The next stage of this work is to determine whether the type of "Hh" molecule on the tumor cell surface is, indeed, of the same nature as that expressed on normal SJL cells, and in turn whether the NK mechanism is operating in the response to both tumors and CFU.

CUDKOWICZ: I infer that the major criterion by which Warner regards resistance to SJL as an anti-Hh response is genetic.

WARNER: It is both genetic analysis for resistance to CFU and tumor cells and also correlation of host resistance mechanism to CFU and tumors. The resistance to tumors is operative in irradiated mice but is abrogated by split-dose irradiation. However, silica pretreatment does not abrogate this resistance.

We have considered the possibility that this Hh resistance mechanism may be confined to the spleen. If anti-Hh reactions were operating for tumors, this statement can be denied because the resistance to tumor 375V occurred in the subcutaneous site.

CUDKOWICZ: We have also addressed ourselves to some of these issues and we have analyzed radiation-induced tumors of four different congenic strains. We have chosen two strains that were Hh positive in their normal hemopoietic cells, and then two other strains whose cells do not bear Hh products generating resistance. The main problem is to find parameters that allow one to attribute unequivocally deficient growth of a tumor in F_1 hybrids to natural resistance, as opposed to host immune responses to tumor antigens or to Ir gene effects.

In the limited series of tumors we have studied, whenever Hh alleles were expressed in the normal cells of the tissue of origin, they were also expressed in the tumor; on the other hand, whenever normal cells did not possess alleles generating resistance, neither did the tumors (Table 62). As to our criteria for attributing deficient tumor growth to anti-Hh reactions they were the genetic control by the D region of H-2 where Hh-1 maps, relative radioresistance, abrogation by silica, and the behavior of athymic nude mice (Table 63).

The use of nude mice is not always possible because their genetic background must be such that the tumor cells grow progressively in the euthymic littermates. The athymic mice are usually not permissive for Hh-positive tumor cells because of the strength of their anti-Hh reactions, but nude mice are permissive for Hh-negative cells, even of allogeneic origin.

I would like to stress again the need to satisfy stringent criteria before assigning Hh antigenicity to tumors. It may be useful to remember the work that Oth and Burg did several years ago showing how a situation that resembled very

TABLE 62
Resistance of Irradiated Mice to Allogeneic Lymphoma Grafts.
Requirement for Incompatibility at the H-2D/Hh-1 Region[a]

Lymphoma[b]	Host strain	MHC differences	Classification
L5MF-22	B10.A(2R)	K,I(A-C),S,G	Susceptible
(H-2[b])	B10.A(5R)	I(J-C),S,G,D	Resistant
	B10.A	K through D	Resistant
LAF-17	B10.D2	K,I(A-J)	Susceptible
(H-2[a])	B10.BR	I-C,S,G,D	Resistant
	B10.A(2R)	D	Resistant
	B10	K through D	Resistant
LHM-14	B10	K,I(A-C)S,G	Susceptible
(H-2[h2])	B10.A	D	Resistant
LIM-65	B10.D2	K,I(A-J)	Susceptible
(H-2[15])	B10	I(J-C),S,G,D	Resistant

[a] 10^5–10^6 lymphoma cells were injected i.v. into irradiated mice (800–850 rads of γ-rays). [125]IUdR was injected i.p. five to seven days later to evaluate synthesis of DNA in the spleen by transplanted cells.

[b] Lymphomas were radiation induced in mice of strains congenic with B10. Since the recipients were also congenic with B10, tumor–host differences were restricted to the MHC or regions thereof. Differences at regions other than D never resulted in allogeneic resistance.

TABLE 63

Macrophage Dependence and Thymus Independence of Resistance to Allogeneic Lymphoma Grafts[a]

Lymphoma	No. of cells grafted	Host strain[b]	Experimental variable	Splenic uptake of [125]IUdR (% ± S.E.)
L5MF-22	10^5	B10.D2	No treatment	0.04 ± 0.01
		B10.D2	Silica	0.95 ± 0.17
LAF-17	10^4	B10.BR	No treatment	0.07 ± 0.01
		B10.BR	Silica	0.68 ± 0.11
L5MF-22	10^6	B10	Compatible host	5.06 ± 0.59
		BALB/c	nu/+ (euthymic)	4.76 ± 1.08
		BALB/c	nu/nu(athymic)	0.66 ± 0.14
LHM-14	10^6	C57BL/6	Compatible host	1.30 ± 0.15
		BALB/c	nu/+	0.12 ± 0.02
		BALB/c	nu/nu	0.09 ± 0.01

[a]Lymphoma cells were injected i.v. into irradiated mice (800–850 rads of γ-rays). 2 or 3 mg of silica particles were given i.v. a few hours before or after transplantation. Uptake of [125]IUdR was measured five to seven days later.

[b]Genetically resistant according to Table 62 or preliminary tests.

much hybrid resistance was, in fact, due to hyperreactivity to tumor antigens due to hybrid vigor.

WARNER: Cudkowicz's point, applied to the carcinomas, then correlates with the type of work that we were discussing earlier, namely, that there are many tumors that are not susceptible to NK cells and these grow at the same rate in normal and in nude mice. It therefore again looks as if this correlation is appearing with the use of tumors in regard to NK susceptibility and Hh-type genetic resistance. I think we need to know more about possible cell types that express Hh for both normal and malignant populations.

VAN BEKKUM: Is there any relation between the splenomegaly in the SJL mice and the invasion of bone marrow by tumor cells?

WARNER: We have not examined bone marrow. Some of the tumors are very metastatic and grow in liver, ovary, and a variety of other sites. In studying the weights of all of these organs following tumor inoculation, it appears that the resistance mechanism is operating in all such sites.

TRENTIN: What is the natural biologic function of genetic resistance to bone marrow transplantation? Genetic resistance is strongly expressed in the C57BL strain and its F_1 hybrids. The C57BL strain is a low cancer strain, and spontaneous leukemia is virtually nonexistent in it, even though these mice harbor RadLV. The strong resistance of C57BL mice to leukemogenesis can be abrogated by four weekly exposures to 225 rads of whole-body irradiation, which results in a high incidence of leukemia that is virus-mediated (Kaplan, *Cancer Res.* **27**:1325, 1957). We have found that this same irradiation procedure also abrogates genetic resistance to marrow transplantation (Rauchwerger *et al.*, *Biomedicine* **24**:20, 1976). Kumar *et al.* have reported that treatment of mice with ^{89}Sr abrogates both genetic resistance to marrow transplantation and to spleen focus formation by Friend leukemia virus (Kumar *et al.*, *J. Exp. Med.* **139**:1093, 1974). It is possible that genetic resistance to marrow transplantation represents a manifestation of a leukemia "surveillance" mechanism. To test this hypothesis, experiments were set up comparing the ability of resistant and nonresistant strains of mice to recognize and reject malignant lymphiod cells, as compared to normal narrow cells of the same strain.

Resistant (C57BL × AKR)F_1 hybrid mice show genetic resistance to C57BL parental, but not to AKR parental bone marrow cells. Nonresistant (C3H × AKR)F_1 hybrids show no genetic resistance to bone marrow transplantation from either parental strain (Table 64). Transplantation of AKR lymphoma cells into lethally irradiated resistant (C57BL × AKR)F_1 and nonresistant (C3H × AKR)F_1 hybrids produced lymphomatous spleen colonies in nonresistant hybrids but *not* in resistant hybrids (Table 65). Thus, resistant (C57BL × AKR)F_1 hybrids can recognize and reject AKR lymphoma cells, but *not* normal AKR bone marrow cells.

TABLE 64

Gross Spleen Colony Formation in Recipients Exposed to
γ Irradiation and Injected with Bone Marrow
from Various Donors

Number of mice	Recipient[a]	Donor	Number of colonies per spleen[b]
12	(C57 × AKR)F_1	C57	0
12	C57	C57	confluent[c]
12	(C57 × AKR)F_1	AKR	confluent
10	AKR	AKR	confluent
12	(C3H × AKR)F_1	C3H	confluent
12	C3H	C3H	confluent
12	(C3H × AKR)F_1	AKR	confluent
12	AKR	AKR	confluent

[a]5×10^5 bone marrow cells were inoculated.

[b]Mice receiving irradiation alone (950 R) showed no colonies.

[c]>20 colonies.

TABLE 65

Lymphoma Spleen Colony Formation in Recipients Exposed to
γ Irradiation and Injected with AKR Lymphoma Cells

Number of mice	Recipient	AKR lymphoma cell dose	Average number of colonies per spleen[a]
6	AKR	10^3	14.3
12	AKR	10^4	confluent[b]
6	(C3H × AKR)F$_1$	10^3	8.5
11	(C3H × AKR)F$_1$	10^4	confluent
6	(C57 × AKR)F$_1$	10^3	0.0
10	(C57 × AKR)F$_1$	10^4	1.8

[a]Mice receiving irradiation alone showed no colonies.
[b]>20 colonies.

A titration of AKR lymphoma cells in nonirradiated hybrids indicates the strength of the resistance phenomenon (Table 66) without preimmunization. (C57BL × AKR)F$_1$ mice survive a challenge of 10^6 AKR lymphoma cells, in contrast to less than 10^2 for AKR and the susceptible (C3H × AKR)F$_1$ hybrid. So, it looks very much as though what has been known for a good many years as hybrid resistance to bone marrow transplantation is a manifestation of lymphoma resistance.

CUDKOWICZ: I want to ask Trentin about these nonirradiated hybrids, the ones that survived. Has he had a chance to rechallenge them and observe any-

TABLE 66

Mortality in Unirradiated AKR and Hybrids Challenged
with AKR Lymphoma Cells

Mouse strains	Number of AKR lymphoma cells given i.v.	Mortality at 90 days
AKR	10^2	12/12
	10^4	12/12
	10^6	12/12
(C3H × AKR)F$_1$	10^2	12/12
	10^4	12/12
	10^6	12/12
(C57 × AKR)F$_1$	10^2	0/12
	10^4	0/12
	10^6	2/12
	10^7	12/12

thing like a second set response? I ask that since in that event Trentin might have in addition to hybrid resistance also a response to a viral antigen or something analogous.

TRENTIN: No, we have not done that. Yes, I suspect that in the unirradiated survivors one would also see conventional T cell immunity coming in, superimposed.

TILL: On the same point raised by Cudkowicz, how long has Trentin followed those animals that got the low-dose challenge? That was a 90-day assay. Do they die subsequently with lymphoma?

TRENTIN: They have not, except for a few of the ones we have kept as 90-day survivors of the 10^6 tumor cell inoculum.

CANTOR: I am not familiar with some of the genetics of the Hh alleles. Is Trentin implying that the AKR lymphomas are now expressing the B6-type Hh gene product?

TRENTIN: No. AKR lymphoma cells express an AKR specificity not present on normal AKR hemopoietic cells.

CANTOR: The specificites get to be important because one direct test of this hypothesis is to see whether in animals that have been given the AKR leukemia, you find subsequent decreasing resistance to appropriate bone marrow cells as though you had induced unresponsiveness with an Hh antigen.

SHEARER: The answer to Cantor's query involves the work of Zatz and Schmitt-Verhulst in my laboratory. They have studied this issue in the five-day *in vitro* F_1 antiparent sensitization system described earlier. They were able to demonstrate the generation of F_1 antiparental cytotoxic effector cells specific for the AKR haplotype using normal stimulating cells. It was not restricted to tumor system as far as stimulation is concerned.

TRENTIN: One of the characteristics of genetic resistance to bone marrow transplantation is that it can be overriden acutely by a large inoculum of either bone marrow itself or standard inoculum of bone marrow plus a large inoculum of some other tissue, e.g., normal thymus, which apparently shares the same Hh antigenicity and which allows a smaller dose of bone marrow to break through.

SANFORD: It seems to me that Trentin may have got two things mixed. As Cudkowicz pointed out before, we have long known about a "hybrid effect," which appears to be restricted to the response to tumors and which differs in many ways from "hybrid resistance" as we are discussing it. The hybrid effect, which is an F_1 response to parental line tumors, really is an immunologic response, probably due to a T-cell-dependent reaction to tumor antigens. It appears that the reaction is more effective in the F_1 animal than in the parental strain in which the tumor arose. Whether this is due to a specific Ir gene or to a polygenic effect is not yet know. This is what Oth and Burg called "hybrid hyperractivity" and what we call "hybrid vigor."

I think that both hybrid resistance and hybrid vigor are probably involved in Trentin's system, and I am having difficulty distinguishing between the two.

TRENTIN: Well, some of the F_1 hybrid effect that has been described is apparently a reflection of hybrid resistance to marrow transplantation. Cudkowicz has spent much time on this and could answer this better than I can.

CUDKOWICZ: There are really several mechanisms by which a tumor grows deficiently in F_1 hosts. Only in some cases is this due to a response of the Hh type. In addition to hybrid hyperactivity or vigor, there could be an Ir gene that prevents the response in the strain of origin of the tumor, not in F_1 hybrids if the strain of origin has the recessive allele. By outcrossing one might confer to the F_1 the dominant allele for responsiveness. This situation superficially mimics hybrid resistance, but it can be discriminated.

So there are several possibilities, and there may be even more. It is really up to the investigator to decide each time what he is dealing with. We have a good example now in the data Trentin has shown. Because of the deficient growth in the irradiated animal, it is very likely that he is dealing with an anti-Hh response. But had we only seen the data in the nonirradiated animal, we could not have said that, because in that case most likely there would also be involved an immune host response to tumor antigen.

ELKINS: My query is on xenogeneic resistance. Is this conditioned by the strain of rat?

TRENTIN: Yes. (C57BL × A)F_1 mice are strongly resistant to Lewis, Fisher, and Brown Norway rat marrow and less resistant to Buffalo rat marrow.

ELKINS: Are there murine lines resistant to one strain of rat and not to another?

TRENTIN: Yes.

ELKINS: Can this resistance be related to the AGB determinants in the rat?

TRENTIN: That analysis remains to be done, but there are strains of mice that will respond to one strain of rat and not another. We know of some strains of mice that have responded to none of the four strains of rats, and for either allogeneic donors or xenogeneic donors, one can categorize the irradiated mouse strains as good responders, weak responders, and nonresponders. In xenogeneic resistance, as in allogeneic resistance, there is genetic specificity, as a result of both Hh-like genes and immune regulation genes.

MERUELO: I am going to show the results of studies with AKR hybrids utilizing AKR × C3H, AKR × B10.BR, and other AKR × C57BL/10-derived strains. Injection of AKR thymoma cells into these F_1s will result in death within 20–35 days. There is very little difference in survival among any of them. This is in contrast to Trentin's results, but then the AKR tumor cells I use are different from those used by Trentin, having been maintained in tissue culture for 22 years. The system I am dealing with is probably affected by an Ir gene rather than by an anti-Hh response, primarily because secondary responses are readily detected and the pattern of responsiveness observed is different from the one just presented by Trentin.

These studies derive from the work of Lilly and others suggesting that H-2 control of susceptibility to virus-induced leukemia operated via Ir gene(s) specific for tumor or virus-associated antigens. AKR cells in culture were injected into a number of hybrid strains and immune responsiveness was measured by cell-mediated cytotoxicity *in vitro*. The optimum cytotoxic response occurred between 10 and 15 days after tumor cell injection. No cytotoxic response was elicited by spleen cells, whereas good responses were obtained from lymph node and PEC (peritoneal exudate). Lymph node cells were used routinely because they were always highly specific in contrast to PEC. Tumor cells such as EL-4 or normal cells were never killed by effector lymph node cells attactking AKR tumor targets.

(CKB × AKR)F_1 or (B10.BR × AKR)F_1, both of which are H-2$^{k/k}$, gave a very good CML response against AKR tumor cells (Fig. 23). On the other hand (C3H.Q × AKR)F_1 or (B10.G × AKR)F_1 mice, both of which are H-2$^{q/k}$, gave very poor CML responses, if any. These same results were obtained when irradiated AKR lymphoma cells were used for primary immunization (3000 rads).

Although the use of congenic mice strongly suggested that genetic control was H-2 linked, a segregation analysis was done by back-crossing nonresponder (AKR × B10.G)F_1 to AKR mice. The expected result is 50% H-2$^{k/k}$ responders and 50% H-2$^{q/k}$ nonresponders. In fact, none of H-2$^{q/k}$ mice responded, whereas 8 of 11 H-2$^{k/k}$ animals responded. It is surprising that homozygous animals are able to respond, whereas heterozygotes are unable. Either a recessive trait confers

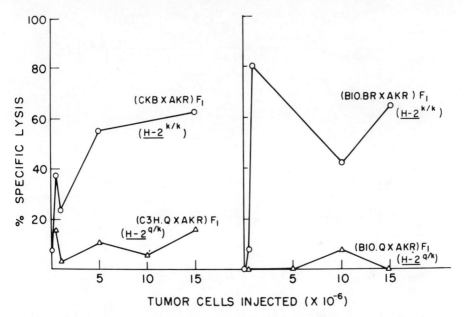

Fig. 23   Differential responsiveness of selected F_1 hybrids to antigens of parental AKR lymphoma cells. Primary immunization *in vivo,* secondary challenge *in vitro.*

responsiveness, or a dominant suppressor mechaniam is operating. Should some other H-2^k heterozygote be able to respond, the hypothesis of suppression would be more plausible. The only heterozygote capable of responding was the AKR $\times$ B10.S, which is H-2$^{s/k}$. The fact that these mice responded suggests, but does not prove, that one is *not* dealing with a recessive Ir gene.

Figure 24 shows the CML response of various H-2 recombinant F_1 mice to two doses of injected tumor cells. When 5×10^6 AKR tumor cells are injected, animals having the H-2^k allele in the I-J subregion respond, whereas those having H-2^b allele do not. At the higher dose of tumor cells (10^7), animals having the I-J^b allele respond when high lymph node:target ratios are used. (5R $\times$ AKR)F_1 differ from (3R $\times$ AKR)F_1 mice only at the I-J subregion. The former F_1 animals have the genotype I-J^k and give a reasonable cell-mediated response, whereas the latter F_1 mice are I-J^b and show significantly poorer cell-mediated responses.

These data tentatively map gene(s) regulating CML responsiveness to AKR tumor cells to the I-J subregion. In light of the fact that most presently known genes associated with the I-J subregion appear to code for antigenic determinants present on suppressor cells and their soluble factors, such mapping provides circumstantial evidence for considering the cell-mediated unresponsiveness to the tumor the result of a mechanism operating via supporessor lymphocytes.

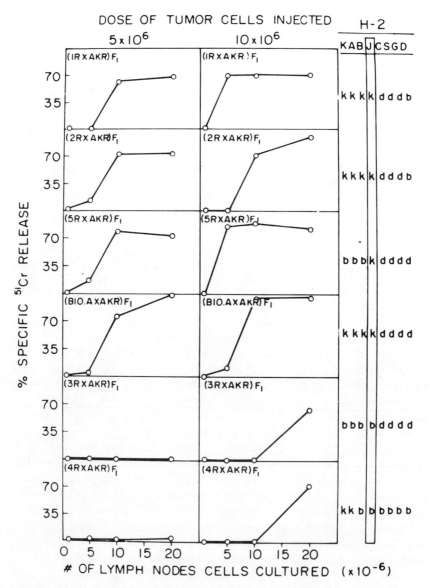

Fig. 24 Differential responsiveness of selected F₁ hybrids to antigens of parental AKR lymphoma cells. Primary immunization *in vivo,* secondary challenge *in vitro.*

Editors' comment: While this volume was in press, we learned of work that would place a quite different interpretation on some of Festenstein's experiments (L. Flaherty and E. Rinchik, No evidence for foreign H-2 specificity on the EL-4 mouse lymphoma, *Nature,* in press).

SHEARER: It should be pointed out that there is no activity in the spleens of Meruelo's animals, whereas this organ is the primary site of anti-Hh reactivity. In these tumor reactions both T cell and non-T cell mechanisms may be operative.

PARKMAN: In view of the diversity between the experiments and results of the two last presentations, is Trentin's AKR cell also a long-term tissue culture line?

TRENTIN: No, ours was a recently arisen AKR spontaneous thymoma serially transplanted in AKR mice.

PARKMAN: The question with respect to Meruelo's studies is what antigens have been acquired while AKR cells have been in culture for 22 years. Are these the targets of the specific immune response described by Meruelo?

MERUELO: We were led to approach the issue of immunity to AKR leukemias in our way by the mapping of resistance genes to Gross virus in the K end of the H-2 complex, and by the data of Aoki *et al.* and Sato *et al.*, indicating that there was more antivirus antibody produced by resistant mice. This is the evidence for genes mapping in the K end of the complex, which comprises the I region, affecting immune responsiveness and resistance to leukemogenesis.

FESTENSTEIN: We have had a fair amount of discussion concerning the cells that participate in alloimmune reactions. I propose now to give some indication as to what targets might be involved in rejection and GVH reactions. The data I shall present are collaborative work in my laboratory with Garrido, Schirrmacher, Schmidt, Matossian-Rogers, Di Giorgi, and Biasi. *

In the course of tissue typing tumor cells propagated *in vivo* we found to our surprise *extra* specificities that are normally present only on cells from mice of foreign genotype. There was, however, no change in the representation of the regular H-2 specificities of the original host strain.

We developed an assay specially suited to type tumor cells. Living cells were assayed by measuring their capacity to take up radiolabeled thymidine and/or uridine. There is a vast difference between the capacity of tumor cells and normal cells to take up these nucleic acid precursors; so for all practical purposes this constitutes a measure of tumor cell viability.

After treating the tumor cells with specific antibody and complement there is substantial reduction in the radio thyidine uptake, so we measure the percentage reduction of isotope incorporation in the test cultures compared to the controls, which are treated only with normal serum and complement. Thus if the antigen is present, there is a low count and there is a large percentage reduction compared to the controls and vice versa. The results of typing the Garnder (H-2^k) and SL2 (H-2^d) tumors are shown in Table 67. There is variation in the expression of H-2 antigenic specificities on these two cells, when assayed in this instance by ^{14}C-uridine uptake after pretreatment with various sera. One would expect to find the H-2K.23 and H-2D.32 specificities on the Gardner tumor since these are the normal private specificities of the H-2^k haplotype and the Gardner tumor was derived from an H-2^k mouse. Surprisingly however, the Gardner tumor expressed only one of these—the H-2D.32—and consistent with expectation, does not express H-2K.31 and H-2D.4, the private specificities of the H-2^d haplotype. Turning to the SL2 tumor, which is derived from an H-2^d mouse, we find that in addition to the regular H-2D.4 and the H-2K.31 specificities, which we would expect it to have, it also has the H-2D.32 specificity. This specificity normally belongs to the H-2^k haplotype. So not only does this tumor have its regular expression of private specificities of the K and D end of H-2^d, but it also has an extra specificity, which belongs to the H-2D locus of H-2^k. Thus, the Gardner tumor (H-2^k) has the normal H-2D^k specificity but is missing the H-2K^k specificity. It has not extra specificities. The SL2 tumor (H-2^d) has both its normal private specificities but in addition has the H-2D^k as an extra specificity.

Not only were inappropriate H-2 specificities found on *in vivo* propagated tumor cell lines but changes in the H-2 profile were also brought about by passaging the tumor *in vivo* together with vaccinia virus. H-2 typing of sarcoma "Meth.A" passaged in BALB/c mice with and without vaccinia are shown in Table 68. In these experiments with Meth.A tumor, cells typed as expected for an H-2^d cell, but Meth.A-vaccinia cells had, *in addition,* a whole variety of extra private and public specificities normally found on cells of *non* H-2^d haplotypes such as H-2K.19, H-2K.23, and H-2D.32. This phenomenon is selective, since it

TABLE 67

Variation in the Expression of H-2 Specificities on Tumor Cells

Pretreatment with antiserum and complement against	^{14}C-Uridine uptake after pretreatment			
	by Gardner (H-2^k) H-2K.23, H-2D.32		by SL2 (H-2^d) H-2K.31, H-2D.4	
	cpm	(%) Reduction	cpm	(%) Reduction
−	8109		6248	
+	5559		6091	
H-2K.23 +	5461	0	6232	0
H-2K.31 +	5601	0	122	98
H-2D.4 +	5790	0	548	91
H-2D.32 +	778	86	1472	75

TABLE 68

Cytotoxic Activity of Anti H-2 Sera against Meth.A Sarcoma Cells Grown
in Syngeneic Mice in the Presence of Vaccinia Virus

Sera used to pretreat tumor cells	C	Meth.A control	(%) Reduction	Meth.A vacc.	(%) Reduction
Private					
anti H-2D.4	+	176 ± 50	96	131 ± 28	97
anti H-2K.19	+	3614 ± 451	0	833 ± 115	78
anti H-2K.23	+	3660 ± 81	0	1326 ± 381	65
anti H-2K.31	+	423 ± 171	90	141 ± 14	96
anti H-2D.32	+	3648 ± 280	0	638 ± 77	82
Public					
anti H-2.13	+	112 ± 37	98	121 ± 38	97
anti H-2.25	+	3622 ± 431	0	3947 ± 428	0
Others					
anti-Ia (A.TH anti A.TL)	+	3042 ± 201	15	3127 ± 414	27

involves some but not all H-2 specificities, the particular "extra set" of specificities dependent to some extent on the original haplotype. Just as an illustration of this situation, H-2.25 was present neither on the Meth.A control nor on Meth.A vaccinia.

What is the nature of the extra specificities? Are they really H-2 or something else that mimics H-2? We tried to answer these questions by absorption analysis in two ways. First, we absorbed the sera (which react inappropriately with the tumor cells) with *normal* cells positive and negative for that particular specificity and retested them on the tumor cells and the tumor cells passaged with virus. Second, we did the opposite, i.e., we used the cell expressing the inappropriate specificity to absorb the serum and retested on chromium-labeled normal lymphoid cells. The results of the first kind of test are shown in Table 69. The H-2D.4 specificity of the H-2^d haplotype is normally present both on Meth.A and Meth.A vaccinia but not on Gardner (H-2^k). When the antiserum was absorbed with B10.BR, which is H-2D.4 negative, there was no effect, but when absorbed with B10.A, which is H-2D.4 positive, the activity was specifically removed. Likewise, when the anti H-2D.32 serum was absorbed with a normal H-2D.32 positive cell (B10.BR), it no longer reacted with Meth.A-vaccinia while absorption with H-2D.32 negative cells had no effect. (Meth.A-vaccinia expressed this inappropriate H-2^k antigenic specificity.) Similar results were obtained with other antisera.

The reciprocal way of absorbing was to expose the serum to cells containing the *inappropriate specificities* and testing such absorbed serum on target cells

TABLE 69

Reactions against Meth.A Vacc. after Absorption
of H-2 Antisera with Normal Lymphocytes[a]

Pretreatment		^{14}C-uridine uptake after pretreatment		
Antisera	Absorption with	Meth.A(H-2^d) H-2K.31,H-2D.4	Meth.A vacc. H-2K.31,H-2D.4, H-2D.32,H-2.1	Gardner[b] H-2D.32,H-2.1
		cpm, reduction (%) (3114 ± 251)	cpm, reduction (%) (2296 ± 132)	cpm, reduction (%) (2316 ± 613)
Private				
H-2D.4	—	96	95	2
H-2D.4	B10.BR (H-2D.4 neg.)	96	93	0
H-2D.4	B10.A (H-2D.4 pos.)	6*	0*	0
H-2D.32	—	0	82	89
H-2D.32	B10.A (H-2D.32 neg.)	0	75	87
H-2D.32	B10.BR (H-2D.32 pos.)	0	9**	4*
Public				
H-2.1	—	0	88	89
H-2.1	B10 (1 neg.)	0	87	91
H-2.1	B10.A (1 pos.)	0	18**	14*

[a]Garrido, Schirrmacher, and Festenstein, *Nature* **259**:228 (1976).

[b]Gardner reacts appropriately with these sera. Absorption of anti-H-2 antisera with normal cells removes the normal* and the atypical** reaction of the sera.

labeled with chromium 51 (Table 70). H-2D.32 was an inappropriate H-2^k specificity that was present on Meth.A-vaccinia. B10.BR lymphoid cells (H-2D.32 positive) were used as the target cells. They were labeled with chromium-51 and tested with the absorbed serum. 32-positive normal control cells absorbed out anti-32 activity so that the antiserum was 68% less effective than the unabsorbed serum. Absorption with a 32-negative cell also reduced the efficacy of the antiserum, but only by 18%. Meth.A, which was H-2D.32-negative, behaved like the normal 32-negative cell and there ws also 8% inhibition. But absorption with Meth.A-vaccinia, which was 32-positive, produced 36% inhibition. This was not as good as the inhibition obtained with the normal 32-positive cells. There may be a technical problem or "32" may be heterogenous and only part of what we call 32 is present on Meth.A-vaccinia. Absorption of anti-H-2.25, which was absent from both Meth.A and Meth.A-vaccinia, with either

TABLE 70
Removal of Specific Anti-H-2 Activity from H-2 Antisera
by Absorption with Meth.A Vacc. Tumor Cells[a]

Pretreatment of tumors			
Antisera and complement	Absorption with	Inhibition (%) (cpm ^{51}Cr release)	Labeled target lymphocyte
H-2D.32	—	(1423 ± 27)	B10.BR
H-2D.32	B10.BR (H-2D.32 pos.)	68	(H-2D.32)
H-2D.32	B10.HTT (H-2D.32 neg.)	17	(H-2.25)
H-2D.32	Meth.A (H-2D.32 neg.)	18	
H-2D.32	Meth.A vacc. (H-2D.32 pos.)	35[b]	
H-2.25	—	(1471 ± 140)	
H-2.25	B10.BR (H-2.25 pos.)	75	
H-2.25	B10.HTT (H-2.25 neg.)	14	
H-2.25	Meth.A (H-2.25 neg.)	12	
H-2.25	Meth.A vacc. (H-2.25 neg.)	12	
H-2.5	—	(1229 ± 116)	B10.HTT
H-2.5	B10.HTT (H-2.5 pos.)	83	(H-2.5)
H-2.5	Meth.A (H-2.5 neg.)	28	
H-2.5	Meth.A vacc. (H-2.5 pos.)	48[b]	

[a]Garrido, Schmidt, and Festenstein, *J. Immunogenetics* **4:**115, 1977.
[b]Significant and specific reduction in cytotoxicity by absorption with Meth.A vacc. carrying the inappropriate specificity.

Meth.A or Meth.A-vaccinia had not effect. Thus, the modifications of the H-2 encoded profile (as tested serologically) of Meth.A cells passaged with virus and other tumor cells passaged *in vivo* are such that the ragular specificities remained unaltered except in one case where a private specificity was lost. Extra specificities of foreign haplotypes were found and by absorption analysis behaved, for the most part, like regular H-2 specificities but of the 'wrong' kind.

Inappropriate reactions were also found by *in vitro* tests of cell-mediated immunity. Mixed lymphocyte reactions, cell-mediated lympholysis, and a cytos-

TABLE 71

Cytotoxic Reactions against Meth.A and Meth.A-Moloney Tumor
Cells by Effector Cells Produced after Congenic H-2
Sensitisation *in vitro*

Responding cells	Stimulating cells	Target cells	Specific lysys (%) 40:1
B10.BR kkkkkk	B10.D2 dddddd	B10.D2	31.9
		Meth.A	−0.4
		Meth.A-Moloney	−2.8
B10.D2 dddddd	B10 bbbbbb	B10	47.4
		Meth.A	0.24
		Meth.A-Moloney	22.9
B10.D2 dddddd	B10.BR kkkkkk	B10.BR	34.7
		Meth.A	−3.4
		Meth.A-Moloney	−5.4
B10.BR (kkkkkk)	B10.D2 (dddddd)	B10.D2(PHA Blast)	31.9
		Meth.A	−0.4
		Meth.A vacc.	26.8

tasis assay were employed. An *inappropriate specificity* was disclosed in MLC by reacting lymph node cells from vaccinia-virus-infected mice with normal spleen cells of the same strain. The lymphoid cells from vaccinia infected mice incorporated very little isotope on their own, indicating that the virus infection of itself did not account for this result. It is noteworthy that not only does Meth.A-vaccinia have an atypical H-2 profile but so does Meth.A-Moloney. In Table 71 are the results of experiments using Meth.A-Moloney as targets. The H-2 congenic sensitization was effected by culturing B10.BR lymph node cells with B10.D2 lymph node cells. Appropriate killing of B10.D2 targets was obtained (32%) but neither Meth.A nor Meth.A-Moloney was killed. So it seems in this case, even though the Meth.A tumor has the normal expression of the H-2^d antigenic specificities, it did not express a cytotoxicity target.

We see that B10.D2 (H-2^d) sensitized to B10 (H-2^b) appropriately killed B10 targets (47% chromium release) and again failed to kill Meth.A—this time according to genetic expectation (since the responding cell is also H-2^d)—but surprisingly there was inappropriate killing of Meth.A-Moloney. Meth.A-Moloney must therefore in this instance be expressing an inappropriate target, which is being attacked by this H-2-identical B10.D2 killer cell. It must be an H-2 or H-2-like determinant because only congenic (H-2) incompatible strains were employed. It is also unlikely that the reactivity is directed against the virus itself or caused by the virus in some nonspecific way, because Meth.A-vaccinia or Meth.A-Moloney was not killed by B10.BR anti B10.D2 sensitization nor was there inappropriate killing of Meth.A-Moloney with B10.D2 sensitized against B10.BR, while there was appropriate killing of B10.BR PHA blasts.

The cytotoxicity targets are therefore absent from the Meth.A tumor but both appropriate and inappropriate targets emerge when the tumor was passaged with virus. This former situation is also shown in the bottom portion of Table 70.

There is appropriate killing of B10.D2 targets by B10.BR cells sensitized against B10.D2 antigens (32% chromium release), no killing of the Meth.A target, but a very good reaction against Meth.A-vaccinia. The appropriate target on Meth.A thus seems to be hidden or repressed and is brought out only when the Meth.A tumor cell is passaged with vaccinia. This is in contrast to the results obtained with Meth.A-Moloney, which brings out only an inappropriate target. Thus, Meth.A-vaccinia brought out the appropriate target while Meth.A-Moloney the inappropriate one. B10.D2 sensitized against B10 killed B10 cells in an appropriate manner, and did not kill Meth.A but killed Meth.A-vaccina with a small amount of chromium release. The same held for B10.D2 (H-2^d) sensitized against B10.BR, which killed Meth.A (H-2^d) inappropriately with a small amount of chromium release (5.4%) while the appropriate killing against B10.BR caused 35% chromium release.

Passaging the tumor together with virus caused inhibition of tumor growth. This effect held for both Moloney and vaccinia. When Meth.A was injected without virus, the tumor grew and killed the host in all cases (Fig. 25). If Meth.A was passaged with Moloney virus on day 0, the tumors grew less well. If the tumor-bearing mice were given repeated injections on days 7 and 14 there was progressively less growth with almost none in those mice given three injections. So merely by repeating the injections of virus, the growth of the Meth.A tumor was halted. When vaccinia was injected with Meth.A, a similar effect was observed except that following the third injection with Meth.A tumor grew better. The mice in which the tumor regressed were then repeatedly challenged with 10^6 Meth.A cells and observed for up to 200 days. So the administration of the virus induced a resistance to the growth of the tumor, which was directed against the tumor rather than the virus. This implies that there could already have occurred a partial expression of an inappropriate transplantation antigen on Meth.A itself that is completed and rendered much more immunogenic by passage together with the virus. Evidence of the inappropriate H-2-like antigens on Meth.A as opposed to Meth-A-vaccinia were in fact found by means of a fluorescent antibody technique. The possibility that the virus itself could destroy the tumor was also considered but thought unlikely because of *improved* tumor growth after the third injection of vaccinia. Moreover, the use of virus induced a regressor state specific for antigens on the tumor and not for the virus.

H-2 and H-2-like antigens can newly arise in several ways:

1. Alteration of the H-2 antigens by virus, as postulated by Zinkernagel and co-workers.

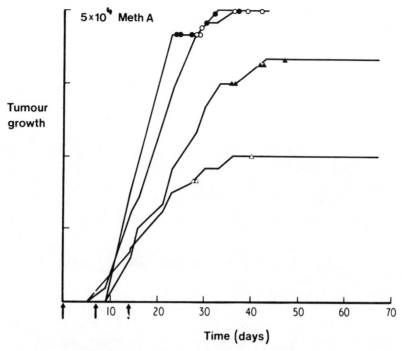

Fig. 25 Meth.A tumor growing in BALB/c control mice (●) and with vaccinia virus, given on days 0 (▲), days 0 + 7 (△), and days 0, 7, and 14 (O——O).

2. Products of derepressed genes: (a) major histocompatibility system genes, (b) other genes of the cell genome.

3. Products of viral origin—either through activated endogenous virus or superinfection: (a) viral genome encoding H-2-like structures, (b) virion envelope antigens cross-reacting with H-2.

The first of these possibilities was discussed earlier in connection with an altered H-2. If the new specificities were to arise out of the old ones, then one would expect the appropriate specificites to be altered. The fact is we could find no evidence of this. Then, if they were the result of altered H-2, why should the new specificities resemble the regular specificities of different haplotypes? It is difficult to formally distinguish between the two remaining possibilities, i.e., between a viral gene product that is similar to H-2, and a gene product of the cell genome that is normally silent and becomes derepressed. The latter explanation would imply that we do not have alleles in the ordinary sense but that we inherit a whole family of MHC genes. Regulatory genes would allow only some of these to be expressed at any given time. This explanation was first offered for the inappropriate expression of Tla antigens in leukemic mice and subsequently for inappropriate allotypes in rabbit and man, most recently in a model for the HLA polymorphism by Amos and Bodmer and others. The genes encoding the extra specificities are normally repressed; occasionally when the cell is damaged or has its metabolism altered in some way they become derepressed and the inappropriate antigen is expressed on the surface.

Although it is formally difficult to distinguish between a viral and cell genome encoded product, from an operational point of view it would not matter; the host would still react against it as if it were an H-2 transplantation antigen. If such a determinant were to be present on transplanted bone marrow, the graft would be rejected even if it were matched for its regular antigens.

SPRENT: Can Festenstein demonstrate that the extradeterminants are immunogenic? For example, can he inject mice with irradiated tumor cells and produce antibody or skin graft rejection?

FESTENSTEIN: We are seeking such antibodies now. So far, we have not found them. Skin graft experiments are also being done.

Recently Oldstone and his colleagues (*Transpl. Rev.* **31**) studied the interaction of measles virus envelope and the expression of HLA antigens. It seems that with measles virus there is no alteration in HLA, but a quantitative reduction in its expression.

STUTMAN: The Moloney data are very interesting, but Meth.A already expresses MuLV antigens. So Festenstein is in effect superinfecting with Moloney and finding changes. It is something to keep in mind.

FESTENSTEIN: As I said earlier, Meth.A passaged *in vivo* does express inappropriate specificities detectable by immunofluorescent techniques, but not with the postlabeling assay. Superinfection with Moloney virus would then presumably convert a partial effect into a complete one.

GOLUB: I gather from Festenstein's comments that there is no way of predicting in any situation what is going to emerge or what is going to be deleted. Is that so?

FESTENSTEIN: Well, we have studied about eight tumor lines thus far, and find that there seems to be about 50% concordance of extra specificities according to the haplotype.

What I mean is, if you have, say, an H-2^d series of tumors, these will tend to express the same type of extra specificity, whether the tumor is induced by chemical means or virus, or even if it was spontaneous. So this extra batch of specificities seems to be more hapoltype-dependent than inducing-agent dependent, although it is not absolute. There are obviously cases where it does not occur.

TILL: If the tumor has a missing specificity and then it is infected with vaccinia, does that missing specificity reappear?

FESTENSTEIN: This didn't happen with the *in vivo* passaged tumors, but Anderson and Garrido in my laboratory were examining Sendai virus from this point of view. Sendai virus was used to infect the L929 cell line *in vitro;* this cell line is missing specificity 11, which is a public specificity of the H-2^k haplotype. When the line was infected with Sendai virus, the 11 specificity came back together with a group of extraspecificities.

MECHANISM OF NATURAL RESISTANCE TO INTRACELLULAR BACTERIA. MANIPULATIONS WEAKENING RESISTANCE SYSTEMS

Discussion Introducer:

Michael Bennett

CHAIRMAN BENNETT: This session is concerned with the means by which engraftment can be enhanced in incompatible bone marrow transplants. I would begin with the effects of ^{89}Sr on mice, since this is one of the most potent agents known for suppression of marrow allograft reactivity. But it should be emphasized that in addition to suppressing the capacity to reject bone marrow allografts, ^{89}Sr has other multiple effects on host defense systems and on other key cellular functions.

If one assumes that the marrow is equivalent to the bursa or thymus and that when it is destroyed selectively by the bone-seeking isotope ^{89}Sr, one can by assays for various immunological or quasi-immunological cell types ascertain whether it is obligatory that these cell types spend a part of their life cycle in the bone marrow for a critical stage in differentiation.

As mentioned earlier, our initial finding with strontium was that the capacity to reject bone marrow allografts was abrogated; later Kumar, Eckner, and I observed that genetically resistant mice became susceptible to the leukemogenic and immunosuppresssive effects of Friend leukemia virus.

Another host defense system that is suppressed severely is ^{89}Sr-treated mice is resistance to the facultative intracellular bacterium *Listeria monocytogenes*. That work was actually stimulated by Campbell's demonstration that in lethally irradiated mice, bone-marrow-derived cells are responsible for restoring host resistance to *Listeria* proliferation. She will summarize that work for us later.

Mice treated with ^{89}Sr retain a variety of immunocompetent cell types perfectly intact. These include, in the B cell system, precursor B cells that give rise to antibody-forming cells, 19S EAC rosette-forming cells (complement receptor lymphocytes), cells responsive to the mitogens dextran sulfate and LPS, and cells responsible for antibody-dependent cellular cytotoxicity against burro RBC. In the T cell line, helper cells for antibody formation, the so-called amplifier cell for CML, and the MLC and GVH reactive cell are likewise quite intact in strontium-treated mice. Finally, the cells that respond to the mitogens Con A and PHA are also functional despite ^{89}Sr.

We are aware that macrophages are involved in marrow allograft rejection. However, many macrophage functions remain entirely intact in strontium-treated mice. These include the accessory function for antibody formation to thymus-dependent antigens, the 7S EA rosette-forming cells (primarily macrophages in mice) and the cells responsible for antibody-dependent cellular cytotoxicity against chicken RBC. Gurney and his colleagues showed several years ago that both skin graft rejection and antibody formation *in vivo* were also operative in strontium-treated mice. Resistance to infection with an extracellular pathogen such as *Pasteurella pestis* is also quite normal in strontium-treated mice.

What then, are some of the defects that develop in mice treated with the strontium isotope? We have already learned from Cudkowicz and Shearer that the *in vitro* F_1 antiparent reactivity is abolished and even the allogeneic CML response is ablated. The mitogen response to Friend virus is likewise affected by ^{89}Sr.

Wigzell mentioned previously that the NK cell is absent in the spleen of strontium-treated mice. Yonkosky of our laboratory has recently found that another cell type is likewise absent or reduced, namely, the cell responsible for mitogen-induced cellular cytotoxicity against chicken RBC (MICC). In this assay, one mixes ^{51}Cr-labeled chicken RBC, lymphoid cells, and PHA. The cells are cultured for one or two days and one measures ^{51}Cr release.

The MICC cell is present in the spleen and bone marrow (Table 72). Indeed, bone marrow is more active than the spleen, but MICC activity is absent in the thymus and lymph nodes. Marrow and spleen, but not thymus or lymph nodes, contain the precursors of MICC effector cells. This tissue distribution is different from that of NK cells.

After ^{89}Sr, MICC activity is dimished (Table 73), without there being evidence for suppressor cells in this particular system. However, it is still possible that a suppressor cell was extremely active in this assay, even at a 1:1 ratio of effector to target cells. These data, taken together with those mentioned previously by Wigzell, suggest that ^{89}Sr suppresses not only cells of the lymphoid series, but also cells of the myeloid series.

Baker and I did experiments with *Listeria,* assessing the growth of this microorganism in the spleen and liver of mice. The organisms grow exponentially for three days, tend to grow slowly for another day or two, and then they are rapidly eliminated. It is thought that by days 3 to 4, T cell-mediated immunity

TABLE 72

Mitogen-Induced Cellular Cytotoxicity (MICC) by Lymphoid Cells from
Various Tissues of (C57BL/6 × DBA/2)F$_1$ Mice

	Mean cytotoxicity (%),[a] No. of lymphoid cells ($\times$ 10^6)						
Tissue	0.5	1.0	2.0	4.0	8.0	10.0	20.0
Marrow	11	21	33	70	68	73	—
Spleen	4	5	10	20	31	34	36
Lymph node	5	3	4	6	7	0	4
Thymus	0	4	0	1	3	3	1

[a]For the MICC assay, 0.5–2.0 × 10^6 lymphoid cells, 10^5 ^{51}Cr-labeled chicken red blood cells, and 10^7 unlabeled sheep red blood cells were cultured in individual test tubes in a volume of 1.4 ml with 0.1 ml of 1/100 dilution of PHA or medium. After 48 hr incubation, cultures were centrifuged and supernatants were removed. The ^{51}Cr release from cells was measured. Percentage specific cytotoxicity, ^{51}Cr; cpm, [(cells + PHA)] − [(cells + medium)]/(total releasable − (cells + medium).

TABLE 73

Depressed MICC Activity in BDF$_1$ Mice Treated with ^{89}Sr

Exp.	Number of spleen cells ($\times$ 10^6)		Mean $\pm$ S.E. (%), cytotoxicity[a]	Number of cells ($\times$ 10^6) per spleen
	^{89}Sr	Control		
1	0	5	45 $\pm$ 3	^{89}Sr: 229
	5	0	16 $\pm$ 2[b]	Control: 208
2	0	5	35 $\pm$ 2	^{89}Sr: 200
	5	0	5 $\pm$ 1[b]	Control: 237
	0	10	48 $\pm$ 3	
	10	0	13 $\pm$ 1[b]	
	0.5	5	33 $\pm$ 2	
	1.5	5	36 $\pm$ 1	
	1.0	10	55 $\pm$ 6	
	3.0	10	60 $\pm$ 4	

[a]As in Table 72. Mice were treated with 100 μCi ^{89}Sr i.v. twice at a monthly interval. Cells were harvested for assay one month after second injection.

[b]Mean values significantly different from controls, $p < 0.05$.

becomes operative, and by days 5 to 8, activated macrophages have been generated that eliminate the organisms. But Campbell showed that early in the infective process (first two days) bone-marrow-derived cells are responsible for limiting *Listeria* proliferation. Accordingly, our studies focused on the first two days of *Listeria* infection; ^{89}Sr markedly increased the susceptibility of mice to *Listeria,* which now can proliferate in spleen and liver essentially unimpeded.

The literature contains interesting information concerning genetic resistance to *Listeria*. C57BL/6 mice are resistant whereas A-strain mice are susceptible. This resistance to *Listeria* could be analogous to the well-documented resistance to Friend virus and marrow allografts. Moreover, agents other than ^{89}Sr known to suppress marrow allograft reactivity, e.g., silica, likewise suppress this early resistance to *Listeria* infection.

In examination of the spleen of strontium-treated mice, the extreme degree of hemopoiesis is impressive. Myeloid cells, including macrophage-like cells and granulocytes are abundant. It is noteworthy that while the resistance to *Listeria* is markedly suppressed, that to *P. pestis* is quite unaffected. Thus, cells of the myelo-monocytic differentiation pathway do not all come from a common precursor cell. Indeed, these cells may prove to be just as heterogeneous as lymphocytes.

Strontium-89 is not the only agent that affects marrow allograft rejection, and I have compared a variety of agents with respect to their effects on resistance to marrow allografts and *Listeria*. For example, agents known to be active against lymphocytes and to suppress marrow allograft rejection include cyclophosphamide, horse or rabbit antimouse bone marrow or thymocyte serum, antispleen cell cerum, and split-dose irradiation. But other antilymphocyte agents do not affect marrow allograft rejection, including azothioprine, cytosine arabinoside, cortisol, and thymectomy. As has been stated repeatedly, the macrophage poisons silica and carageenan effectively suppress marrow allograft reactivity. However, azothioprine, another agent van Furth had shown to be particularly effective against the monocyte differentiation pathway in the bone marrow, has no effect on resistance.

One can also stimulate macrophages *in vivo* with heat-killed *C. parvum* so as to generate suppressor function by these cells. Such stimulated mice lose the ability to reject bone marrow allografts. The tumor-bearing state has been shown repeatedly to stimulate the RES in general and to generate suppressor macrophages, in particular. Kumar and I observed that this state of tumor bearing also suppresses the ability of mice and rats to reject bone marrow allografts.

To continue the analysis of myelotoxic agents, one has to mention cyclophosphamide, because it is very toxic to the cells of the myeloid series and suppresses marrow allograft rejection. However, other agents that are likewise myelotoxic do not suppress marrow allograft rejection. The drugs dimethylmyleran, myleran, and cytosine arabinoside are an example in point, since they have no effect on marrow allograft reactivity.

Another approach to abrogate marrow allograft rejection would be to act on the stem cell itself. Golub and Till have been investigating anti-stem cell sera and may contribute further information.

Finally, other modalities for suppressing marrow allograft rejection include administration of a larger cell inoculum. Storb indicated earlier that in man the cell inoculum size is very important for engraftment. Induction of spleen amylodosis in CBA mice by repeated injections of casein, renders the mice incapable of rejecting foreign marrow cells.*

---

*Editor's comment: Bennett's analysis of the agents and procedures that influence the function of cells involved in "natural" resistance to foreign cells, tumors, bacteria, viruses, etc., disclosed that these agents defy simple categorization. Thus, not all antimacrophage agents weakened resistance nor did macrophage stimulation necessarily strengthen it; moreover, few myelotoxic agents weakened resistance, but one of the most powerful of them did; finally, an array of lymphocytotoxic agents also yielded variable effects. This seeming confusion can be resolved when it is appreciated that resistance phenomena are mediated by no less than three interacting cell types: lymphoid effectors, macrophage-like accessory cells, and lymphoid suppressors. There is compelling evidence that each of these three represents a small specialized subpopulation, which is moreover functionally heterogeneous, e.g., distinctive effector cells engaged in NK-type kill, in Hh-type kill, and in microbial kill. It follows then that an analysis of the agents influencing these systems is not a productive approach to an understanding of the mechanisms of natural resistance.

UHR: What is the effect of splenectomy?

CHAIRMAN BENNETT: The spleen is not essential, even though it represents the richest source of effector cells. Warner emphasized earlier that one reason the spleen appears to be more effective than bone marrow could be the presence in the latter organ of suppressor cells.

ELKINS: This is a question concerning Bennett's statement that the CTL precursor was sensitive to strontium. Is he referring to the conventional anti-H-2 killer cell?

CHAIRMAN BENNETT: Yes, I was, but I pointed out that the CML reactivity was lost probably as the result of the acquisition of suppressor cells.

HENNEY: Bennett referred repeatedly to mitogen-induced cellular cytotoxic reactions. Could he tell us whether the assay system detects a single effector cell.

CHAIRMAN BENNETT: This is still a matter of debate. The original experiments by Perlmann indicated that the effector cell was thymus independent and present in a variety of tissues. Blaese and his colleagues did a very extensive study with this cell and found that the effector cell was not a T cell, a B cell, or a macrophage by the same criteria Wigzell employed for NK cells.

SHEARER: I am not convinced that there is hard evidence for the cytotoxic precursor cell itself being sensitive to ^{89}Sr. We know that in the F_1 antiparent CML response an accessory cell is necessary and this cell may be sensitive to ^{89}Sr. Should there be a helper cell required for the generation of allogeneic CMLs it could also be that this cell rather than the effector is depleted or suppressed.

CUDKOWICZ: The question Elkins asked was whether the CML responsiveness was abrogated in strontium-treated mice regardless of whether one would assay for F_1 antiparent or allogeneic anti-H-2 responses. The answer to this question is that both reactivities are indeed abrogated in the spleen of such mice.
    Now, if one examines the cellular basis of this deficiency, I agree with Shearer. It is far from my mind to say that the T effector cell line is depleted by strontium treatment. Rather, a non-T accessory cell is involved in both responses. As Moore also pointed out earlier, it doesn't necessarily follow that, because the strontium-treated mouse has an acellular bone marrow, the CML deficit is due to a missing cell. We have evidence for a suppressor cell in the spleen of strontium-treated mice, which when added to cultures of normal cells, will suppress CML responses, both F_1 antiparent and allogeneic (Table 27).

WIGZELL: When Haller and I examined strontium-treated mice we failed to detect decreased reactivity of T cells to H-2 antigens. However, we had removed the adherent subpopulation from spleen cells.

CUDKOWICZ: The suppressor cells are actually part of the nylon adherent subpopulation.

MOORE: Bennett earlier cited work that implies concepts that are difficult to accept. The fact is that somehow the macrophage–granulocyte stem cell *can* transmit specific information to its progeny, allowing them to recognize a particular tumor to which the animal had been exposed. We have repeated similar studies rather extensively employing the Meth.A fibrosarcoma as our model, and generating macrophages in methycellulose culture from the bone marrow of tumor-bearing mice vs. control mice or mice bearing an unrelated tumor. We have observed that the *in vitro* generated macrophages can suppress the proliferation of the tumor cells and possibly kill the tumor when they are in contact with it, but there is no specificity. In other words, macrophages from the bone marrow of non-tumor-bearing mice were as effective as were those from the tumor-bearing mice.

I think there is a big question mark here as to whether there really can be any specificity to the suppressive macrophage–tumor interaction, but there is a nonspecific suppressive component that is generated *in vitro.*

PARKMAN: Is the kinetics of cell regeneration after bone marrow grafts different for cells inhibitory to *Listeria* and regular T or B lymphocytes?

CHAIRMAN BENNETT: Cells responsible for resistance to *Listeria* were generated within eight days. Precursor B cells are also generated within this time.

Now Till will describe for us another agent that suppresses marrow allograft reactivity.

TILL: In our laboratory, Gregory made a C3H anti-C57BL spleen antiserum, which has been referred to earlier. The test for activity was to determine if it would permit spleen colony formation by C57BL calls in irradiated (C57BL × C3H)F_1 hybrids. It did so. The antiserum also permitted more rapid regeneration of C57BL CFU-S in the irradiated F_1 hybrid after transplantation. Under these conditions, there is usually a lag of about a week before parental CFU-S increase, but when the antiserum was given prior to transplantation, the lag period was shortened to a couple of days. Gregory attempted to characterize the antiserum. Anti-H-2^b activity could be removed by absorption, but not the activity against resistance.

A C3H anti-B10.BR ($H2^k/H2^k$) spleen cell serum was prepared that should not have had anti-H-2 activity; this serum was also active in abrogating resistance in a number of parent–hybrid combinations. The conclusion of this work was that the activity of the serum was not directed against parental donor cell determinants, but against something in the F_1. Since we were unable to absorb the activity, we have no idea of the mechanisms involved.

CHAIRMAN BENNETT: I believe Cantor reported earlier that he could produce certain types of Ly antisera in one of the strain combinations Gregory employed.

CANTOR: The first of Till's antisera was C3H anti-B6. Clearly, this serum has many specificities, including some Ly specificities, and also anti-NK activity, since C3H is NK antigen-negative and B6 is positive.

CHAIRMAN BENNETT: I would like Trentin to describe to us the properties of the antisera he has worked with.

TRENTIN: Many but not all antithymocyte sera abrogate genetic resistance to bone marrow transplantation, yet thymectomy does not. So obviously the reactivity of these sera must be directed at cells other than those of thymic origin. Since many antimacrophage agents abrogate genetic resistance, we thought an antimacrophage activity could be present in antithymocyte sera.

In a comparative study of activities in various lymphoid antisera, we prepared rabbit antisera against thymus, spleen, bone marrow, peripheral lymph nodes, mesenteric lymph nodes, Peyer's patches, and peritoneal exudate cells of mice. They were tested for ability to prolong the survival of cardiac allografts, to inhibit SRBC plaque-forming cells, to inhibit acute GVH, and to abrogate genetic resistance to marrow transplantation. Clearly, the most effective antiserum for abrogating resistance was that directed against bone marrow. Next, and comparably effective, were antithymus and antiperipheral lymph node sera. Next was antiperitoneal exudate cell serum. Surprisingly, antispleen serum was the least effective of the active antisera. Totally ineffective were antimesenteric lymph node, and anti-Peyer's patch sera. The relative effectiveness of these various sera in abrogating genetic resistance to marrow transplantation did not appear to be correlated with their activity for prolonging heart allografts, inhibiting hemolytic plaque-forming cells, or inhibiting acute GVH.

CAMPBELL: Before reporting on our studies of resistance to *Listeria,* I would like to summarize a bit of the history of studies on resistance to intracellular bacteria in general. As the conferees know well, the dogma that has developed over the years is roughly as follows: resistance to *Listeria* and to other intracellular parasites is thought to involve stimulation of specific T cells by microbial antigens. T cells then release lymphokines, which in turn activate macrophages, which then kill or inactivate *Listeria*. This has long been described as *the* mechanism of resistance to all intracellular parasites. We became interested in looking more carefully at the cells involved in resistance. Not having read the literature very well, we were unencumbered by knowledge, and consequently did some rather naive experiments. These gave us findings easily interpreted, but entirely at odds with establishment views.

The system we used employed BDF_1 mice lethally irradiated (1000–1100 rads of ^{60}Co γ-rays) and reconstituted intravenously with 10^7 of the cells under study. These were usually bone marrow, spleen, or thymus from syngeneic donors. Eight days later the mice were challenged with *Listeria* and sacrificed 48 hr thereafter. Serum, liver, and spleen were taken for enumeration of *Listeria* by standard bacteriological plating techniques. In this manner, we could accurately determine the numbers of organisms per liver and spleen of the recipient mice. The data for cell transfer reconstitution experiments were obtained by subtracting the number of *Listeria* per organ in the reconstituted animals from the number of *Listeria* per organ in controls.

So, in the course of many such experiments we explored the transfer of immunocompetent vs. hemopoietic cells and cell combinations (Table 74). This table is actually a compilation of many individual experiments. The number of

TABLE 74

Restoration of Resistance to Listeria Infection in Irradiated
Mice by Passive Transfer of Immunocompetent
vs. Hemapoietic Cells

Cells injected	Number of surviving mice	Mean $\log_{10}$ *Listeria* per organ (control minus experimental)	
		Liver	Spleen
B + T	72	4.95	3.61
Bone marrow	70	3.31	2.28
Thymocytes	27	0.83	−1.22
PEC	19	0.24	0.30
PC	14	0.64	0.81
Spl	5	−0.02	0.39
Spl (anti-Thy 1)	5	0.05	1.39
Immune T	10	0.36	0.77
Immune T + PC	10	0.89	1.04
T + PEC	8	1.30	0.54

mice indicated is the total number of mice that survived irradiation. A proportion of animals died because of infection or inadequate reconstitution.

Bone marrow plus thymus cells effectively reconstituted the animals, since they yielded four to five logs fewer *Listeria* in liver and spleen than did the irradiated controls. That means that there was a 10,000–100,000-fold reduction. Bone marrow alone gave essentially the same result. But thymocytes provided no protection, presumably because they contributed no hemopoietic cells.

At this point, the simplest interpretation would be that by giving bone marrow we had provided hemopoietic cells, including the precursors of macrophages, which in the irradiated environment became activated macrophages (perhaps by intestinal microbial flora or by radiation) and in turn actually provided the resistance.

But it seemed to us that, if that were the case, one ought to be able to induce resistance by passively transferring macrophages as such, possibly in the presence of immune T cells, so as to mimic the postulated classical model of cellular immunity. However, transfer of peritoneal exudate cells was found to provide no resistance.

It was first rationalized that this failure was because the peritoneal exudate cells induced by either thioglycollate or proteose peptone were so preoccupied handling agar, thioglycollate medium, or proteose peptone that they could not deal with the *Listeria*. But when we gave 10^8 nonexudate peritoneal cells on days -8, -2, and -1, we likewise failed to induce resistance. This is a huge population of peritoneal cells; nevertheless, giving 10^8 cells on three different days, and even giving them immediately prior to challenge, so as to minimize migration, peritoneal cells did not enable the mice to resist *Listeria* challenge.

We then explored immunocompetent cell populations including normal and immune spleen cells; these were also ineffective. We then sought to duplicate the classical model by injecting immune T cells with either exudate or normal peritoneal cells; still no significant resistance was transferred.

A further cell population gave surprising results. We could not transfer resistance into the irradiated animal with either 10^7 or 10^8 "immune" spleen cells from mice immunized with live *Listeria* six days previously. Consequently, we have come to the conclusion that a bone-marrow-derived cell is essential in addition to macrophages in order to confer host resistance to infection by intracellular bacteria.

SPRENT: Did Campbell take into consideration the difference between number of stem cells in marrow as opposed to spleen?

CAMPBELL: Yes. That is why we gave 10^8 spleen cells instead of 10^7, but that number still did not confer resistance. Although we routinely give 10^7 marrow cells, the fact is, we could also get this effect with only 10^6.

STUTMAN: Our studies on transfer of *Listeria* resistance with immune bone marrow also showed that there was a requirement for a marrow-derived cell, but one for a small increment of T cells as well. However, our concern was with a *late* response to *Listeria*.

CAMPBELL: We treated marrow with a great excess of anti-Thy-1 serum plus complement to eliminate T cells. But such treated marrow restored resistance even better.

   We then removed all but 1% of the Ig-positive cells from bone marrow, but such processed cells worked as well. It should be remembered that eight days after grafting, both Thy-1 and Ig-positive cells would have been regenerated anyway.

WARNER: A point on the genetics of this resistance. Cheers, in Australia, has shown that the genetic control is associated with neither Ig allotype nor H-2 genes. I think it would be of considerable interest to establish if there is a relationship of the anti-Ly8 and anti-NK alloantisera to the genetics of resistance to *Listeria*.

SHEARER: Since Hh resistance can be overridden with a large inoculum of cells, is Campbell's resistance overcome by increased doses of *Listeria?*

CAMPBELL: If one injects enough *Listeria,* say 100 LD_{50} or so, neither bone marrow transplantation into irradiated animals nor immunization of conventiioal animals will protect mice. The effect we have described holds over a rather wide dose range, which is a challenge inoculum including a range of 10^4–10^5 *Listeria*.

CUDKOWICZ: Has Campbell tried other variations of her experiment, like using nude mice, or antilymphocyte serum? Or, if she has not, could she integrate such literature reports with her own findings?

CAMPBELL: Cheers and Waller have examined resistance to *Listeria* in nude mice. They find that spleen cells of nude mice are more resistant to *Listeria in vitro* than are normal spleen cells. Unfortunately, Finger *et. al.* in Germany very recently reported opposite results.

STUTMAN: In our hands, nude mice with BALB/c and CBA backgrounds are highly susceptible to *Listeria* in our *in vivo* model.

MOORE: We considered in the discussion on macrophages the existance of a compartment of macrophage percursors, particularly common in the peritoneal exudate. Such cells give rise to macrophage colonies in agar culture. The intriguing thing about this compartment of cells is the very prolonged lag period that they exhibit before they initiate colony formation. We score our cultures as late as three to four weeks after the cells are plated and they do not commence proliferation for at least 10–14 days.

I wonder whether in Campbell's experiments, where large numbers of peritoneal exudate cells were transferred, a rather dramatic effect would have occurred a few days later.

CAMPBELL: In some experiments we did wait as long as 11 and 12 days after irradiation before challenging the mice. When we challenged at 12 days, and assayed at 14 or 15 days, the results were essentially the same.

CHAIRMAN BENNETT: It appears that the analysis of the cell types responsible for natural resistance phenomena and of the manipulations to weaken such resistance has implications that go far beyond the study of bone marrow transplantation as such. These cells seem to be central to a variety of host defense systems as has been brought out during this conference. It is also becoming evident that the present classification of T cell, B cell, and macrophage lineages is far too restrictive to accommodate the natural host defenses we have been discussing, especially since the latter represent situations quite apart from specific acquired immunity.*

DAUSSET: I have in mind a hypothesis that may be relevant to the subject of this discussion. Though the hypothesis hasn't yet been finalized, I want to outline here the major features.

---

*Editor's comment: As Bennett indicates, the findings with Friend leukemia virus and *L. monocytogenes* establish striking, certainly nonfortuitous correlations between the host systems responsible for resistance to foreign, altered, and neoplastic cells on the one hand and resistance to microbial pathogens on the other. In our view these two infectious agents are but examples of what must be a far larger, pervasive situation in biology.

It is hardly likely that evolution preserved a system such as anti-Hh reactivity merely to resist marrow grafts. The fact is that natural resistance of mice to *Herpes simplex* virus has been found recently by O'Reilly and co-workers (personal communication, 1977) to resemble closely resistance to hemopoietic grafts with respect to the array of distinctive properties emphasized repeatedly during this conference. Indeed their analysis of viral natural resistance was initially based on the attributes that characterize the Hh system. The notable property of bing not induced and radioresistant, the late maturation and thymus independence, and the unusual manipulations that diminish such resistance all point toward a mechanism that is similar or possibly common to that of Hh and NK systems. Genetic control by a single locus of resistance to Herpes virus was recently described by Lopez (*Nature* **258**:152, 1975).

In the large accumlated literature on infection and immunity are any number of host resistance situations involving viral, microbial, and protozoan agents that are inexplicable in terms of acquired immunity. These concurrent developments suggest to us that the noninduced cellular mechanisms debated in this conference could very well account for at least some of the resistance phenomena that have thus far defied analysis.

One important observation is that certain HLA haplotypes are in strong linkage disequilibrium. The A1 B8 DW3 haplotype is the best known example, since it is observed with a frequency of 0.05 instead of the expected 0.006. A second haplotype, A3 B7 DW2, is also in linkage disequilibrium in caucasian populations, where these two haplotypes seem to be in opposition. For example, the association of B8 with A1 is more frequent than expected, but not that of B8 with A3. The same can be said about the association of B7 with A3 and A1.

A second important observation is the frequent association of A1 B8 DW3 haplotype or the B8 DW3 portion, with autoimmune disorders. Myasthenia gravis, Addison's disease, and systhemic lupus erythematosus (SLE) are a few examples of such disorders. The association is closest with the DW3 gene(s), which may be the equivalent of the murine I-region genes. In contrast, the A3 B7 DW2 haplotype is primarily associated with multiple sclerosis (*Transplant. Proc.* **9**:523, 1977).

Now, in examining the ability of patients with these syndromes to produce specific antibody, one notes that B8 DW3 individuals are usually high responders, since they develop high titers of antibody to a variety of antigens and rapidly clear the Australia antigen. In contrast, B7 DW2 individuals are low responders. It follows that there is an opposition of these haplotypes not only with respect to population genetics and disease associations but also with respect to potential or competence for antibody responses. The opposition goes as far as to result in protective effect when the opposite allele is present. For example, for diseases associated with B8, the B7 allele is protective since it reduces the diseases' frequency in heterozygotes.

The opposition with respect to antibody responses reminds me of the pairs of mouse lines developed by Biozzi, characterized by the ability to develop high titers of antibody, as opposed to very low titers, when stimulated by an array of antigens. These mice are high or low responders without regard to antigen specificity. The lines differ by about ten genes, one of which is linked to the MHC and seems to be responsible for 20% of the total effect. When tested for resistance against *extracellular* bacteria (e.g., pneumococci) high responders are strongly resistant, as expected, and low responders are not. The situation becomes more complex when the mice are tested for resistance to *intracellular* bacteria. In this case, high responders can't even be vaccinated (e.g., against *Salmonella typhimurium* and *Yersenia pestis*) upon injection of nonvirulent bacteria. Low-responder mice are resistant even without vaccination. Biozzi's explanation is that high-responder mice, but not low responders, produce blocking or facilitating antibodies interfering with the handling of intracellular bacteria by sensitized cells and/or macrophages.

My explanation for the failure of high-responder mice to develop immunity to intracellular bacteria would focus on a subpopulation of macrophages (similar to those participating in anti-Hh responses and derived from M cells), taking into account the demonstration by Biozzi and his co-workers that macrophages of low-responder mice are abnormal, i.e., hyperactive in catabolizing antigens.

By tying these various facts together, I am hypothesizing that the A1 B8 DW3 individuals are equivalent to mice of Biozzi's high-responder lines, and that they would possess a nonspecific MHC-linked immune response (Ir) gene that is advantageous and selects positively when such individuals must handle *extracellular* bacteria.

On the contrary, A3 B7 DW2 individuals would possess a nonspecific Ir gene that is advantageous and selective for defense against *intracellular* bacteria. This hypothesis is easily testable: one kind of test I am thinking about in the context of this conference is to verify if A3 B7 DW2 individuals are more prone to reject bone marrow than A1 B8 DW3 individuals.

DUPONT: I wonder if this hypothesis would not be more likely to be correct in diseases that cause selective increase in their haplotype. I think all data so far indicate that one actually does not see a selective haplotype increase for the diseases mentioned.

DAUSSET: There are possibilities other than selective haplotype increase to explain linkage disequilibrium. Degos and I proposed the fusion of populations as an explanation of the disequilibrium. If there is an HLA-linked Ir gene conferring advantage, this would help to select the haplotype and the two mechanisms may work additively.

MANIPULATIONS TO CONTROL THE ALLOGRAFT RESPONSE AND GVH DISEASE

Discussion Introducer:

Harvey Cantor

CHAIRMAN CANTOR: This segment of the conference is concerned with manipulation of the homograft response. I propose that we first consider homograft reactions across both major and minor histocompatibility barriers, and then go on to the graft-versus-host response. Here too, we shall distinguish between reactions across major and minor histocompatibility barriers. The latter is especially important since it is now apparent that homograft and GVH reactions across minor barriers pose the most clinically relevant difficulties. It is a pity that most of the experimental systems that have been studied have produced evidence for cellular mechanisms involving reactions across MHC barriers. We are only now beginning to investigate in animal systems mechanisms that involve cells responding to minor incompatibilities.

To start with, I think it is appropriate to analyze, as a prototype, the classical skin graft rejection model and the cell types involved in this response. One can categorize T cells according to the selective expression of gene products, in this case, Ly gene products. I shall summarize the characteristics of the three major subclasses of T cells defined *in vitro,* and then consider their functional contribution to the homograft response. We have used enriched peripheral T cells obtained after passage of splenic and peripheral lymph node cells through nylon wool columns.

One subclass of T cells expresses the Ly-1 marker and represents about one-third of the peripheral T cell population. These cells appear to be relatively mature, both by the criteria of their ability to recirculate and homing to lymph nodes, their relatively late appearance in in ontogeny, and their resistance to the short-term efffcts of adult thymectomy. These cells seem to be programmed to amplify various effector cells engaged in immune response. They can stimulate B cells to produce antibody, enhance prekiller cell differentiation into killer cells, and stimulate macrophages and monocytes to induce delayed-type hypersensitivity responses.

Now, the common theme of the activities of this subclass of Ly-1 positive cells is that they recognize antigen in association with I region components of the MHC, and respond by production of factors that amplify other subclasses of lymphocytes. We term these cells T_H (T helper cells).

A second subclass bearing the Ly-2 and Ly-3 markers represents less than 10% of the peripheral pool of T lymphocytes. These cells also appear to be relatively mature by the criteria already indicated. However, in contrast to helper cells, these cells are programmed to develop killer reactivity on contact with alloantigen. These cells are the killer effector cells, both after induction with allogeneic lymphocytes as well as after exposure to modified autologous cells. In addition, these cells can also suppress various kinds of immune responses. Ly-2,3 suppressive activity has been documented after polyclonal activation with con A, indicating that this suppressor activity need not be antigen specific. Ly-2,3 cells also suppress the production of Ig allotypes in mice exposed during

251

perinatal life to antiallotype antibody. Finally, Ly-2,3 cells also suppress cell-mediated responses. We designate these cells $T_{c/s}$ cells (cytotoxic/suppressor).

A third major T cell subclass expresses all three Ly antigens. These cells seem to have characteristics of relative immaturity. They appear first in ontogeny: Ly-1,2,3 cells are seen in the first week of life when all Thy-1 positive cells express the Ly-1,2,3 phenotype. So, we designate these as early-appearing cells (T_E).

Ly-1,2,3 cells are sensitive to the short-term effects of adult thymectomy. Within a month one notes a 50% depletion of this population in the spleen. In addition, a portion of Ly-1,2,3 cells don't recirculate and appear to share properties previously attributed to T-1 cells.

The immunologic functions of T_E cells are just beginning to be understood, primarily because it has been technically difficult to separate this subclass from the preceding two. We know that they are essential for the generation of killer cells after stimulation with modified autologous cells. Another intriguing feature is a pronounced deficit of these cells in aged normal mice and in young NZB mice.

Ly-1 (T_H) cells respond very well in MLC to I region differences, whereas Ly-2,3 ($T_{c/s}$) cells do not. This has been shown by the criteria of thymidine incorporation in mixed lymphocyte culture and of antigen binding. That is, Ly-1 cells will bind allogeneic I region, but not K or D region products. On the other hand Ly-2,3 cytotoxic suppressor cells will bind K or D region, but not I region products. So, one is led to believe that T_H and $T_{c/s}$ cells have selective reactivities for products of different portions of the MHC. One also would suspect that their different reactivities reflect a screening capacity whereby the T_H subclass monitors and responds to alterations of MHC central region products. This type of stimulation induces a programmed series of reactions resulting in amplification of various other cells. The $T_{c/s}$ subscreens for alterations of H-2K/D products. Activation of these cells results in a completely different series of immune responses reflected in immunoregulatory and killer activities.

Do T_H and $T_{c/s}$ cells represent different stages along the same line of T cell differentiation and maturation, or do they represent different branches of this differentiation? Repopulation studies of B mice with one or the other separated category have shown that the subclasses are stable. That is, they do not give rise to one another in terms of cell surface phenotype and function.

What kind of *in vivo* reactions do these cells perform? We have examined first the skin allograft responses. To this end, immunologically crippled animals, that is, thymectomized irradiated mice, were given bone marrow cells and then grafted with allogeneic skin. These mice were then reconstituted with selected subclasses of T cells. Unselected T cell recipients promptly reject skin grafts, whereas $T_{c/s}$ cells did not, even though they can generate killer activity to allogeneic antigens *in vitro*. Reconstitution with T_H and $T_{c/s}$ cells results in fairly prompt rejection, but not as effective as that achieved with unselected T cells.

We would suggest that one of two mechanisms is operative. Either, as seen *in vitro*, a cooperative interaction is required between T_H and prekiller cells to achieve efficient homograft rejection, or T_H cells are required to attract Ly-2,3 cytotoxic effectors to the site of the skin graft.

We have repeated the experiment with sensitized cells and here too one needs both sensitized Ly-1 (T_H) cells as well as sensitized killer cells for optimal skin graft rejection.

Another system we have studied involves the attack of T cells against hemopoietic targets. To this end, lethally irradiated F_1 mice were repopulated with small numbers of syngeneic bone marrow cells. One day later, unsensitized or sensitized parental T cells were inoculated into these mice, and seven days thereafter, uptake of an iron isotope by the spleen was determined. Uptake of ^{59}Fe is a direct quantitative measure of hemopoietic activity in the spleen. The parental cells that had been sensitized *in vitro* against F_1 alloantigens were fractionated into cytotoxic Ly-2,3 cells and DTH competent Ly-1 cells before injection into the F_1 mice. We found that activated Ly-2,3 cells were necessary and sufficient, as effector cells, for rejecting the F_1 hemopoietic graft. On the other hand, if one injects nonsensitized parental T cells, one finds that the generation of the cytotoxic effector cell requires an interaction between Ly-1 helper and prekiller cells. Immature T_E cells play a small but significant role in this response.

To sum up, all three T cell subclasses are interacting *in vivo* for optimal generation of the cytotoxic effector cell. In the hemopoietic experiment, we did not need an Ly-1 helper cell. This is consistent with the idea that the DTH competent Ly-1 helper cell is required to attract a cell to the site of a skin graft, but is not required for killing hemopoietic targets, since $T_{c/s}$ effector cells may lodge in the spleen without any assistance.

As for manipulation of this response, it is a general principle that maximum effectiveness requires selectivity. Since elimination of a subclass of cells entails partial incompetence, ideally one would like to eliminate only T cells that specifically recognize a given allograft. One approach that seems expecially promising is that suggested by the antiidiotype work of Wigzell and Binz. I would like Wigzell to delineate this system for us.

WIGZELL: The work I shall briefly recapitulate originally begun as an analysis of the antigen-binding receptors of T lymphocytes involved in transplantation reactions. This eventually led to some approaches that we consider promising for inducing specific transplantation tolerance against antigens in adult immunocompetent individuals.

B and T cells recognize the major histocompatibility antigens via specific receptors with partly identical polypeptide chains. T cell receptors for major histocompatibility antigens contain the same variable part as found on the heavy chain of immunoglobulin molecules of the same specificity. We have not been able, however, to demonstrate the presence of conventional light chains on such T cells. Antiidiotypic antibodies to receptors (and complement) selectively eliminate idiotype-positive cells from lymphocyte populations, irrespective of whether they are normal or immune.

Cells from inbred rats treated with specific antiidiotype antibodies are selectively depleted of specific reactivity for GVH, MLC, and CML. It is not implied that cells responding in the MLC and CML necessarily have the same idiotype, but rather that these reactions are deleted by these antibodies. Reactivity against cells of unrelated rat strains remains unaffected.

Whenever an immunocompetent individual reacts to antigens there are several kinds of specificities involved. There is the antigen itself, the genetically preformed antibody against it, and as it turns out, the potential to make antiidiotypic antibodies, a form of autoantibody. Idiotypic receptors with specificity for MHC antigens of the species are normally present in inbred rats or mice but do not induce tolerance. Accordingly, such animals can produce autoantiidiotypic antibodies against their *own* receptors specific for MHC antigens.

The first experiment we did was to demonstrate that in the rat there is a sufficient number of naturally occurring genetically precommitted cells with receptors for a given MLC determinant, i.e., several percent of the T cell population with preexisting specificity. Turnover of receptors is such that one can isolate them from normal serum, or degraded products from the urine. One can remove such molecules from serum or urine with an antiidiotype immunoabsorbent. For example, an anti-Lewis anti-DA immunoabsorbent will purify the normally occurring Lewis anti-DA receptors. This receptor preparation is polymerized and administered to normal Lewis rats with adjuvant. These rats are able to produce an anti (Lewis anti-DA)-antiserum that is an autoantiidiotypic antibody.

Sera from these autoimmunized rats are incubated with normal Lewis T cells in the presence of complement. These cells are then tested for MLC reactivity against DA and unrelated BN stimulator cells. All but 7% of the reactivity against DA is eliminated, whereas 97% of the reactivity against BN is retained.

T cells of the autoimmunized rats were evaluated for the ability to provoke GVHR. It turned out that these cells are specifically deviod of GVH reactivity in (Lewis × DA)F$_1$ rats, but retain normal reactivity for (Lewis × BN)F$_1$ rats (popliteal node assay). Likewise, there is significant prolongation of DA skin graft survival, but not of BN. Deletion of anti-DA reactivity is therefore incomplete; since there are many histocompatibility loci involved in skin graft rejection, all would not be "covered" by this procedure.

Lewis T cell blasts induced in MLC against a relevant MLC determinant carry on their surface a high density of idiotype-positive receptors. So Anderson and I tried the following: Lewis T cells were stimulated by irradiated DA cells; in the mouse: CBA/H T cells against irradiated DBA/2 cells, C57BL/6 anti-CBA/ H, and CBA/H anti-C57BL in a conventional MLC. The specific cells respond by blast transformation. That provides a population enriched for receptor-positive blasts, which in turn bear a higher concentration of receptors. The blasts were separated by 1 g velocity sedimentation and inoculated with Freund complete adjuvant back into adult animals of the strain that served as donor of responder cells.

Such a procedure generally leads to specific hyporeactivity in MLC, and in some strain combinations, to total lack of MLC responsiveness against the relevant cells, leaving other reactivities intact.

We have been able to show that rats and mice produce autoantiidiotypic antibody after autoblast immunization. This is not to imply that the mechanism by which this blast immunization is leading to the specific unresponsiveness be necessarily caused by the autoantiidiotypic antibody, but thus far results support that view. A single administration of 10^7 blasts results in MLC unresponsiveness in the mouse for up to 180 days. Such lengthy unresponsiveness might well become self-perpetuating.

There are still many parameters that will have to be worked out to determine optimal conditions for achieving specific unresponsiveness. Accordingly, it is still premature to consider this approach for clinical situations. However, the principle is entirely valid.

DUPONT: Has Wigzell examined the MLC supernatants for the presence of receptors and antigen? And what happens when the culture is restimulated?

WIGZELL: Supernates contain both antigen and receptors. Which one is in excess depends on the time of sampling. We have not examined restimulated cultures.

WARNER: Is there any evidence for either natural or induced autoantiidiotypic antibodies against non-H-2 specificities?

WIGZELL: To apply this approach to GVHD in marrow transplant patients, one would be forced to immunize the marrow donor with autologous blasts to eliminate GVH reactivity against the recipient. This maneuver might well be considered unethical at this time.

WARNER: What about heteroantiidiotypic antibodies? Wouldn't they be effective?

WIGZELL: I do not think so, for the reason that different individuals may have different antiidiotypes as to their receptors for the same antigens.

CHAIRMAN CANTOR: The approach involving injection of MLC blasts into prospective recipients of organ grafts may be feasible clincially, but is applicable only when the grafts are made across the MHC. Since one does not obtain MLC responses across non-MHC barriers, one cannot make antiidiotypic antibody against non-MHC antigens.

In addition, the use of heteroantisera to treat bone marrow before transplantation could not be as effective an approach as is active immunization of the host, since it does not preclude the reappearance of the same idiotype-positive cells from stem cells in the transplanted marrow.

ELKINS: We should not lose sight of the fact that antiidiotype responses, although primarily directed against the idiotype of receptors for MHC products, also seem to be controlling the responsiveness to all the minor locus antigens that would have caused skin graft rejection in some of Wigzell's experiments.

CHAIRMAN CANTOR: I don't agree. I recall that Wigzell's autoantiidiotypic immunized animals accepted skin grafts only for 16–20 days. This would be consistent with the idea that the minor H loci incompatibilities were still operative.

GORDON: Would not Wigzell expect this type of antiidiotype responsiveness to ultimately become self-defeating in a sort of network fashion? If one is immunizing against one idiotype and thus expanding another cell that itself would have an idiotype, why ultimately wouldn't the whole system become compromised?

WIGZELL: What we are doing in effect is to shift a balance rather than to immunize. All these cell types are naturally occurring in the individual, both idiotype positive and the so-called antiidiotype. Homeostasis has to be interrupted, which we achieve by introducing Freund's complete adjuvant with the blasts.

CHAIRMAN CANTOR: Now we turn to homograft rejection across minor histocompatibilitiy barriers. This topic merits emphasis in view of advances in HLA and MLC typing. It should be noted that patients receiving organ grafts that are compatible by these criteria experience chronic rejection, presumably because of reaction to non-MHC antigens.

One approach that has been suggested in animal systems involves the passive administration of antibody directed against Ia or H-2 components of the graft, which in certain circumstances enhances it. Therefore, we would like to develop ways of actively immunizing the recipient to produce antibody (rather than a cellular response) against either major or minor histocompatibility products of the organ graft. This has been difficult because non-H-2 alloantigens are notoriously poor at inducing antibody responses.

There is, however, a newly developed reagent that might assist in the selective production of antibody against such weak determinants while leaving the T cell system unaffected. This is an antiserum that specifically recognizes a structure on a subclass of B cells. The interaction between this antibody and that B-cell structure induces the cell to produce specific antibody to small or subimmunogenic amounts of antigen. The antiserum is produced in CBA/N mice, a mutant strain of CBA/Harwell. The phenotype of this mutation is expressed exclusively in B cells as an arrest of maturation, so that the mice have a normal set of immature B cells, but lack the mature subset.

One can then use CBA/N mice to produce an antibody that might react selectively with a subclass of mature B cells. The approach that Huber has taken in our laboratory involves crossing CBA/N females with BALB/c males, and since the X-linked mutation is recessive, the offspring include F_1 females that are heterozygous and phenotypically normal, and F_1 males that are defective. So one can use both F_1s to make a test and control serum, respectively, after immunization with BALB/c spleen cells.

We found that this antiserum, although not cytotoxic, reacted selectively with about 50% of B lymphocytes in all strains of mice that we tested. We also found that the appearance of the antigen on B lymphocytes was late in ontogeny, not before the third week of life.

We then asked whether the interaction of the antibody with this B cell structure would influence the ability of these cells to respond to antigen. To this end, we administered the antibody along with a subimmunogenic dose of antigen.

Adminstration of a very small number of SRBC results in a very feeble antibody response in terms of plaque-forming cells (PFC). Administration of the same amount of antigen along with optimal amounts of this antibody (anti-LyB3), results in a 20-fold increase in the number of PFC. The only cells that could absorb the serum's activity were B cells. Therefore, one can conclude that the enhancement effect is due to an interaction between this antibody and a structure on B lymphocytes. The enhancement is antigen-specific, and requires both the interaction of the antibody with the B cell surface and the triggering of B cells by antigen.

The action of the anti-LyB3 antibody replaces the requirement for T cells in B mice. Moreover, upon transfer of immune B cells to an irradiated host, one can induce a secondary response (indirect PFC) in the presence of this antiserum. We can use this antibody to obtain humoral responses to weak non-H-2 antigens. Unlike other "adjuvants," no concomitant T cell activity is produced.

So, it is conceivable that administration of this antiserum with a graft that differs at minor H loci would induce early production of antibody against these minor H gene products. Such antibody should enhance the survival, perhaps even permanently, of such grafts. Since this is an active immunization, it would not be necessary to continue to passively administer enhancing antibody to graft recipients over a long period of time.

GORDON: Is the antibody equally effective in different strains of mice? Is there a species restriction?

CHAIRMAN CANTOR: The LyB3 antibody is effective in recognizing and enhancing B cell responses of all strains of mice so far tested. As you might expect from the tactics of immunization, we are presumably recognizing the constant portion of a B cell structure common to all mouse strains. We are seeking to determine whether this antibody is also absorbed by human B cells.

WARNER: Does Cantor know whether his antibody affects cells producing all classes of immunoglobulin?

CHAIRMAN CANTOR: I don't know whether LyB3 antisera promote production of all classes and subclasses of immunoglobulin.

BENNETT: Does Cantor's anti-B cell antiserum activate B cells or does it kill B suppressor cells?

CHAIRMAN CANTOR: The antibody is a γ_1 immunoglobulin. It is possible that it could opsonize a subclass of B suppressor cells, if such cells exist, but the dose–response curves indicate that optimal enhancement is achieved at relatively low doses of antiserum. Were opsonization the mechanism, higher concentrations of antiserum would be required.

SPRENT: Do other types of anti-B cell reagents, such as anti-Ia or anti-Ig antisera, have the same enhancing activity *in vivo*?

CHAIRMAN CANTOR: We have tried anti-Ig serum and failed to enhance *in vivo*.

MERUELO: Is there an overlap for Ia, Ig, and LyB3 specificities on individual B cells?

CHAIRMAN CANTOR: Stripping B cell surfaces with anti-μ does not interfere with precipitation of the LyB3 product from the B cell surface.

ELKINS: In raising this antiserum Cantor is starting out with a B-cell deficient male, is injecting B cells into it, and is asking for antibody to these B cells. The fact is, however, that this animal does not have much machinery to make that antibody. So, what are we seeing here? Does he have a weak antibody response that is extraordinarily effective?

CHAIRMAN CANTOR: This is probably the case. The CBA/N mouse is abnormal in that it cannot respond to low amounts of antigen, but it can make antibody of low affinity after immunization with large amounts of antigen. The antibody we have raised was made after a series of 5–10 immunizations with normal spleen cells. This resulted in the development of an antibody of the γ_1 class. It probably is not a high-affinity antibody.

Now we shall move on to discussing the GVH response and consider the categories induced across MHC and across non-MHC barriers.

I might say that most of the current GVH studies are not clinically relevant because with recent advances in HLA and MLC typing, acute GVHR have been prevented. The major problem now is dealing with a chronic type of GVH, not reflected in most conventional experimental models, and with acute GVH in MHC identical combinations.

As Elkins has already stated, the nature of the GVH effector cells is not clear, but we know that donor T cells are necessary and sufficient to initiate a GVHR. One may then ask which subclasses are particularly involved. If one fractionates the T cells with respect to Ly phenotype, one finds that the Ly-1 cells are ineffective. On the other hand, the prekiller cells expressing the Ly-2 phenotype are somewhat more effective, although less so than unselected T cells. Mixtures of these two populations do not provide synergy, but it is possible that there is such a synergy with the immature Ly-1,2,3 cell, lacking in this mixture. In fact, Ly-2,3 cells (prekiller cells) combined with thymocytes, which are mainly Ly-1,2,3 cells, do yield a marked synergistic effect.

The two major advances in the area of GVH involving minor histocompatibility barriers are the use of bone marrow stem cell concentrates as inocula, and improvements of MLC and HLA typing. Nonetheless, it seems that MLC/HLA matched patients infused with stem cell concentrates do develop GVHD. One important point is the separation of pluripotent stem cells from those that have only the lymphocyte option. These are observations from Fialcow's group in female patients with chronic myelogenous leukemia heterozygous for G6PD. According to Lyon's theory, normal cells from these patients should be chimeric, some cells expressing one G6PD allele and other cells expressing the alternate allele. In contrast, clonal populations would be hemizygous for G6PD. Since chronic myeloid leukemia cells are hemizygous, whereas normal lymphocytes are heterozygous, it is believed that in man there is a stem cell capable of generating megakaryocytes, red cells, and granulocytes but not lymphocytes, and a separate stem cell restricted to lymphocytes. Maturation of these cells in an allogeneic environment can often result in "chronic" GVHD.

Now Van Bekkum will assess his group's experience with the clinical problem of GVHD.

VAN BEKKUM: With regard to the nature of the GVHD, it is customary to distinguish two different clinical syndromes, the acute and the delayed form of GVHD. In the context of marrow transplantation we usually employ recipients that are *conditioned* with a lethal dose of whole-body irradiation, and the GVHD that develops after grafting of allogeneic cells is also termed secondary disease (SD).

SD has been reported to occur under certain exceptional conditions (very high dose of irradiation) following syngeneic bone marrow transplantation. This can obviously not be attributed to a GVH reaction: we provided evidence for an autoimmune mechanism related to a radiation-induced autoimmune dysfunction of the recipient's thymus. This particular syndrome could well be comparable to the "autoaggression" mechanism proposed by Parkman. After irradiation and transplantation of bone marrow from H-2 identical donors differing at minor histocompatibility loci there is either no SD or a mild nonlethal form of delayed SD. After transplantation of H-2 incompatilbe bone marrow, characteristic de-layed SD develops starting between the third and fourth week after grafting and mice die from it between 30 and 90 days after transplantation. In certain host–donor combinations this delayed SD results in 100% mortality; in other combina-tions some mice survive 90 days and seem to recover, although they exhibit immune suppression for many months thereafter. To induce acute SD in mice the allogeneic bone marrow graft has to be supplemented with lymph node or spleen cells.

In the clinical situation, aplastic and leukemic patients are being conditioned with a comparable regimen, either whole-body irradiation or cyclophosphamide, or a combination. These patients are presently grafted with bone marrow from HLA identical sibling donors; this involves minor histocompatibility differences. In contrast to the mouse experiments, one does observe in some patients *acute* GVHD, which begins as early as day 14 and may run a very severe course. Other patients develop *later* GVHD still rather severe; there is doubt whether this *subacute* complication involves the same mechanism as the delayed-type SD in mice. The important difference between mouse and human bone marrow is that the former contains relatively small numbers of mature T cells, while human (and monkey) marrow is relatively rich in T lymphocytes, as judged by PHA re-sponses. We have postulated that the acute form of SD in *mice* is caused by a direct reaction of T lymphocytes present in the graft (or in the added lymph node or spleen cells), while the delayed type of GVHD in mice is induced by T lymphocytes that develop from primitive precursor cells—perhaps even from the

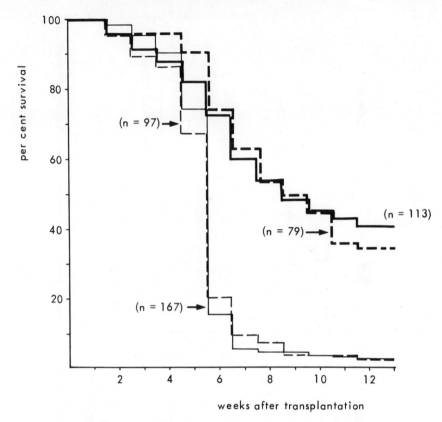

Fig. 26 Survival after allotransplantation of fetal liver and bone marrow cells. C57BL → CBA (900 rads). Transplants (1200–3500 CFU-S): ——, bone marrow; – –, bone marrow stem cell fraction; —, fetal liver; --, fetal liver stem cell fraction.

hemopoietic stem cells under influence of thymus factors. The most recent evidence for these postulates comes from experiments with lethally irradiated mouse recipients that are treated with (a) unmodified bone marrow or fetal liver of an H-2 incompatible strain, (b) purified stem cell fraction from marrow, and (c) purified stem cell fraction from fetal liver. In all these groups, the donor strain was C57BL/Rij and the recipient CBA/Rij. Stem cell purification was performed with the discontinuous albumin density centrifugation technique and the number of CFU-S in the various grafts were kept about similar. The results shown in Fig. 26 demonstrate that there is no difference between unseparated marrow and marrow stem cells, or between fetal liver cells and purified fetal liver stem cells with regard to mortality due to delayed-type SD. This indicates that mouse bone marrow does not contain sufficient T lymphocytes to influence the course and

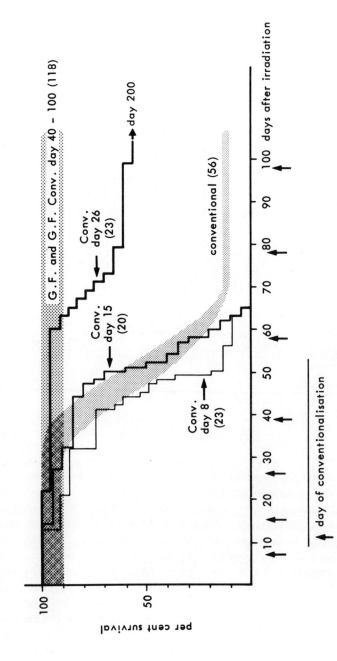

Fig. 27 Mortality of conventionalized GF mice after lethal irradiation and allogeneic bone marrow transplantation. C57BL BM → CBA 900 rads.

262

severity of the GVH reaction. The same applies to fetal liver cells, but both unfractionated and purified stem cells from fetal liver induce less SD than bone marrow. This finding suggests that during the development of mature T cells from primitive precursor cells of fetal liver, immunological tolerance is more likely to occur than when this development originates from precursors present in bone marrow.

In monkeys, the (hyperacute) SD that results from transplantation of bone marrow from nonmatched random donors kills the recipients in 5–25 days (average 13 days). Removal of T lymphocytes, i.e., transplantation of a purified stem cell fraction, prevents the acute SD. However, the animals die from a delayed-type SD that is somewhat more severe than the syndrome seen following allogeneic H-2 incompatible bone marrow transplantation in mice.

When the monkeys treated with stem cell fractions are bacteriologically decontaminated, their survival is further prolonged, which suggests a role for endogenous infections comparable to that in mice. Mortality due to delayed-type SD can be completely prevented by bacteriological decontamination of mice or by keeping them in the germ-free state (Fig. 27). Moreover, if the mice are recontaminated with intestinal microflora at about one month after transplantation, the GVHD no longer develops. We were intrigued by the magnitude of the effect of decontamination, which seemed to exceed the effect of a mere prevention of infectious complications. To investigate that issue further, we employed a model that allow the observation of the GVH reaction in a normal (with microflora) and germ-free intestine in the same radiation chimera.

We used F_1 hybrids between CBA and C57BL as recipients. The F_1 hybrid mouse is transplanted with two pieces of fetal gut, one from the F_1 hybrid strain (the same strain as the host) and the other from CBA (bone marrow donor type). The gut implants grow out into structures that resemble the adult gut, and can be considered as a germ-free intestinal tract (Fig. 28). The F_1 mouse is subsequently irradiated and transplanted with CBA bone marrow and spleen, so that it develops acute GVHD. The gut lesions characteristic of the disease can be scored quantitatively by counting the number of degenerated crypts in the gut implants. We could then measure the effect of the presence of microflora in the intestine on the GVHR in these sterile gut implants by comparing conventional carriers with similarly prepared animals that had been decontaminated before the experiment. The results can be summarized as follows. In the conventional mice we scored 43% of damaged crypts in the F_1 implant and 23% in the CBA implant. In the decontaminated animals, we scored 23% in the F_1 implant and zero in the CBA implant. These data indicate, first, that the presence of microflora in the intestine can influence the GVH reactions at a distance in sterile gut implants, and second, that sterile gut implants of the marrow donor develop significant GVH lesions when microflora are present at a distant site.

One last word about the applicability of these measures to clinical situa-

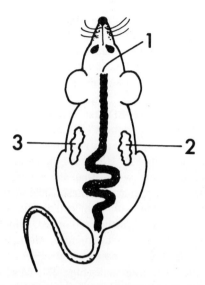

Fig. 28   F$_1$ hybrid host with two fetal gut implants. (1) The host's own intestinal tract *with* micro-flora; (2) CBA fetal implant, no microflora; (3) F$_1$ hybrid fetal implant, no microflora.

tions. Stem cell separation is practical, but there is an indication that the engraft-ment of stem cell fractions in aplastic patients is more difficult to achieve than that of unfractioned bone marrow. Accordingly, we have not systematically employed stem cell grafts in aplastics, but only in patients with combined im-mune deficiency disease. In the latter situation, we have obtained reconstitution with stem cell fractions from HLA-identical siblings. The results with stem cell grafts from nonmatched donors were encouraging in that acute GVHD did not develop. The patients did show a delayed-type GVH syndrome and died with infections. These infants had not been decontaminated.

Complete decontamination has so far been achieved in but few patients and our experience does not warrant conclusions about its effect on the control of GVH.

CHAIRMAN CANTOR: When Van Bekkum refers to problems of engraft-ment with stem cell concentrates, does he mean stem cell concentrates as op-posed to unfractionated marrow, or is he alluding to histocompatibility mis-match?

VAN BEKKUM: We certainly have the impression that stem cell concentrates will not engraft as well as unfractionated marrow. For instance, to get engraft-ment of the stem cell concentrates in monkeys, we have to raise the dose of irradiation.

HIBBS: Has Van Bekkum administered small amounts of endotoxin to germ-free mice to determine whether this microbial product would exacerbate clinical GVHD?

VAN BEKKUM: Yes, we did that and other things such as feeding of bacteria, but we haven't yet found an effect.

O'REILLY: I would like to comment on Van Bekkum's last point. I refer to a child with combined immune deficiency disease who received a marrow transplant from an unrelated D-locus-compatible donor. We considered this case earlier.

The participation of enteric flora might be emphasized in this case. The child was completely decontaminated for a period of one year and a half, and, during that time, no more than ten single isolates of relatively apathogenic organisms were made. Marrow transplantation was successful and the patient developed chronic GVHD involving skin but not gut, without any evidence of hemopoietic suppression. At the time when PHA responsiveness was positive and 100% of the lymphocytes were of donor karyotype, we felt that it would be appropriate to recontaminate the child and maintain him on gamma globulin.

The critical point to be raised is as follows: In the recontamination process, we initially used predominantly gram-positive anerobic microflora of low pathogenicity. For the first month and a half of that particular introduction of flora into the gut, the patient did exceedingly well and was completely stable hematologically and immunologically.

However, when we introduced a nonpathogenic strain of *E. coli,* without any evidence of infection, the patient developed florid GVHD and aplasia of the bone marrow.

ELKINS: Has O'Reilly reasons to say GVHD-induced aplasia? Why wouldn't it be endotoxin-induced aplasia?

O'REILLY: The thought that it might be endotoxin-induced aplasia is worth considering; however, in the case we would have expected fever and other evidences characteristic of endotoxemia, none of which were seen in the child.*

*Editors' comment: The interchange between van Bekkum and conferees regarding a microbial pathogenesis of GVHD points up the confusion of immunologists and the lack of awareness that much of the GVH syndrome seen is attributable to enteric flora and their toxic components. Since the mid 1960s there has accumulated a considerable literature, based largely on experiments in germ-free mice, that implicates the gut flora and their endotoxic components in the development of this postradiation syndrome.

In the context of this conference, special attention is directed to a causative role for the conditioning regimen used in bone marrow transplantation. The fact is that the lethal dose of whole-body

PARKMAN: From Van Bekkum's own data, it seems clear that giving stem cell concentrates to monkeys decreased the severity of GVH; decontamination decreased mortality even more. However, I assume the animals probably died nevertheless.

VAN BEKKUM: In man, even histocompatible sibling marrow grafts do not aviod acute GVHD.

CHAIRMAN CANTOR: But we were referring to stem cells.

---

irradiation employed (900–1000 R) not only causes obvious lesions in the intestinal epithelium, but also leads to the loss of natural host defense against gut contents, i.e., normal enteric flora and their toxic products. Fifteen years ago W. W. Smith observed (*Proc. Soc.* **113**:778, 1963) that exposure to x-irradiation, especially in the lethal range, led to a profound susceptibility of mice to the lethal action of bacterial endotoxin. This susceptibility was most pronounced on the third day after irradiation, at which time the endotoxin LD_{50} for mice exposed to 1000 R was $0.5\mu g$, whereas the value for unirradiated controls was about $500\mu g$. Almost complete protection was afforded by shielding the abdomen. It is noteworthy that comparable protection against death from acute intestinal radiation damage was observed by Swift and Taketa (*Am. J. Physiol.* **185**:85, 1956) where only a small segment of duodenum or ileum was shielded. Since man is exquisitely sensitive to endotoxin, fever and shock being elicited by parenteral administration of doses in the order of 1 ng/kg, the susceptibility seen clinically should be even more drastic. This toxic, postradiation syndrome mimics—really duplicates—many of the clinical features ascribed to GVHD. Yet GVHR and GVHD continue to be attributed to the reaction of the transplanted lymphocytes against the recipient. Actually, much of what is seen reflects the direct consequences of the conditioning regimen. It follows that the lack of engraftment of incompatible marrow compounds the problem, for where engraftment is successful, normal antibacterial and antiendotoxic resistance is restored. The consistent findings of investigators working with germ-free rodents has been that lethally irradiated recipients, challenged with allogeneic bone marrow, do not manifest GVHD.

Indeed Pollard and associates at the Lobund Institute have based their strategy of immuno-prophylactic and therapeutic treatment of neoplasms via allogeneic bone marrow on the fact that lethally irradiated germ-free mice will accept allogeneic marrow, become chimeric, and manifest no GVHD. They found that bone marrow chimerism, thus induced with DBA/2 marrow, prevented spontaneous leukemia in germ-free AKR mice (*Proc. Soc.* **144**:659, 1973); germ-free SJL/J mice made chimeric with marrow from germ-free C3H mice did not develop reticulum cell sarcomas (*Proc. Soc.* **145**:488, 1974); moreover in *therapeutic* experiments, germ-free leukemic AKR mice with advanced neoplasia, irradiated and transplanted with marrow cells from germ-free DBA/2 mice, survived for many months symptom free, whereas controls receiving syngeneic AKR marrow died of leukemia on the average 43 days after transplantation (*Proc. Soc.* **146**:153, 1974). Pollard's experiments, which should have been verified (but to date no reports have appeared) in view of the important implications for tumor immunotherapy, are referred to primarily to emphasize the key factor of the *endogenous* threat and to dramatize what maneuvers become possible when that threat is aviod or controlled. The significant component that continues to be underestimated is the gut contents of the conventional recipient, which, while perfectly managed under normal circumstances, becomes a highly toxic and lethal threat following the conditioning regimen. No small part of the problem is that clinically, attention has been focused on the infectious sequellae of conditioning, primarily because they can be readily monitored by microbiologic means. The fact is however, that bacterial endotoxin exerts by far the more pervasive effect, but this component, so highly toxic to man in submicrogram amounts, is virtually impossible to monitor.

VAN BEKKUM: We cannot prevent *chronic* GVHD by using purified stem cells. We can, however, prevent the acute GVH by removing T cells.

CHAIRMAN CANTOR: Van Bekkum has stated that in the situation of MHC-compatible siblings, infusion of stem cell concentrates results in neither chronic GVHD nor mortality nor morbidity due to infection.

VAN BEKKUM: I was referring only to SCID patients, where that has been our experience.

SPRENT: Van Bekkum asserted that chronic GVHD is due to the emergence of newly formed T cells reactive against the host. In his mouse model there would be an alternative explanation, namely, that there develops a radioresistant chronic host-vs.-graft reaction. Unless one uses a semiallogeneic combination, one can't exclude this. It is conceivable that the dose of irradiation (900 rads) did not abolish completely the capacity of the host to react against the graft. The only way to overcome this objection is to use F_1 mice as recipients.

VAN BEKKUM: We have typed all the long-standing chimeras for the presence of donor cells

SPRENT: But host cells could escape detection if they were present in very small numbers.

TRENTIN: I think some of our data published many years ago give an answer to this issue. We did analyze secondary disease after supralethal irradiation by transplantation of marrow from parent into F_1, or from F_1 into parent. We similarly analyzed the mortality in the second week after "midlethal irradiation" and marrow transplantation. With a high sublethal or midlethal dose of irradiation, one gets a temporary engraftment and then, in about two weeks, a flushing out of the graft, and the animals (which would have lived without a marrow graft) also die in the process. We were analyzing this secondary disease to determine whether it represented host-vs.-graft or graft-vs.-host reactions.

The answers came out clearly by the approach Sprent suggested. The midlethal zone mortality was host-vs.-graft, but the secondary disease in the second month after supralethal irradiation was graft-vs.-host.

SPRENT: But that could have been due to T cells contaminating donor marrow.

TRENTIN: I do not believe so, in that as Van Bekkum showed, secondary disease is not related to the quantitative input of bone marrow cells. In contrast, acute GVH is correlated with the number of spleen or lymph node cells.

CHAIRMAN CANTOR: It seems then that there occurs chronic GVH disease in many patients despite receiving purified bone marrow stem cells from HLA and MLC matched donors.

Now, the possibilities are that the cells causing the disease are T cells, as Van Bekkum suggests, in which case one would think of the Bevan phenomenon with respect to cytotoxic T cells generated against minor antigens. The other possibility is that it is not a T cell at all, but some type of NK cell as was described earlier by Parkman. Perhaps Parkman would comment on this point.

PARKMAN: When we established that there were naturally occurring autocytotoxic cells in man, we looked for its counterpart in mice. When mouse spleen cells are separated on BSA gradients, we isolate a subpopulation that is cytotoxic for syngeneic fibroblasts *in vitro*. Injected into either neonatal or nine-month-old mice conditioned with sublethal irradiation or cytoxan, these cells produces a disease identical to allogeneic GVH and characterized by splenomegaly and wasting.

A lighter fraction of the BSA gradient contains cells that counteract the autocytotoxic cells and reverse wasting. If administration of suppressor cells is started shortly after the injection of the autocytotoxic cells, there is only a slight weight loss and within a week the weight of the mice returns to that of the irradiated controls.

If administration of suppressor cells is delayed one week the animals still recover.

In this mouse model, we have been able to produce a syndrome that mimics secondary disease by the administration of autocytotoxic cells to either neonatal or conditioned adult animals. We have also been able to reverse this syndrome by the administration of a second subpopulation of lymphoctyes that we designate as regulator or suppressor cells.

CHAIRMAN CANTOR: Is Parkman implying that chronic GVH might be mediated by a null-type cell in the NK family and that T cells are actually *suppressing* this type of GVH?

PARKMAN: Yes.

CHAIRMAN CANTOR: In contrast to the hypothesis of van Bekkum?

PARKMAN: Yes. The general T cell deficiency of a transplant recipient with its concomitant decrease in suppressor T cells may produce an unbalanced situation with a relative excess of autocytotoxic cells. These would be the cells that produce the clinical syndrome that is chronic GVHD. We have an approved protocol in which we plan to give patients with chronic GVHD donor regulator cells.

CHAIRMAN CANTOR: Are these "regulator" cells T cells?

PARKMAN: Yes.

STUTMAN: Has Parkman actually tried to correct allogeneic GVHD with the suppressor cells?

PARKMAN: We are now undertaking experiments to determine what are the histocompatibility restrictions between suppressor and autocytotoxic cells. In the human situation especially, with small children, it may be important to be able to use a donor of suppressor cells other than the transplant donor.

CHAIRMAN CANTOR: The major message of these discussions is that there are several approaches to controlling the homograft response: passive administration of enhancing or antiidiotypic antibodies. With respect to chronic GVHD, we are still somewhat uncertain as to the type of cell that induces and mediates chronic GVHD. Until we learn more about the cellular mechanism underlying this disease, it will be very difficult to avoid this problem.

The other issue that has not been emphasized is that we do not know whether further refinements in MHC typing will reveal gene products significant for the induction of chronic GVHD or whether the more pessimistic view will be sustained: that *any* difference between donor and recipient can induce chronic GVHD. After all, differences as minor as the H-Y antigen can induce syndromes that resemble chronic GVHD.

CONFERENCE OVERVIEW AND ASSESSMENT

Discussion Introducers:

Donald Metcalf
Jonathan W. Uhr

CHAIRMAN METCALF: Despite the wide-ranging character of this conference, there are certain aspects of marrow grafting that did not emerge in our discussions. It may be useful to open this general discussion by identifying two of these issues. Mostly, the establishment has tended to focus on the immunological problems of putting marrow grafts into patients with emphasis on tissue typing and avoidance of GVH. However, this procedure also involves hemopoietic considerations. The type of patients that presently are receiving transplants reflects a variety of diseases involving hemopoietic tissues. In the future, more and more patients who have normal hemopoietic tissue will recieve transplants, that is, patients with solid tumors.

Now, one of the problems that merits attention is what permits a hemopoietic cell population to seed and proliferate in a particular site. We really know little about such permissive or nonpermissive conditions, but many of the diseases we seek to treat obviously involve abnormalities in the microenvironment for hemopoiesis. Some of our clinical failures are not really ascribable either to a poor match or to GVH, but rather represent failures stemming from a basic inability of particular patients to support a hemopoietic cell population.

I would illustrate this situation with two examples. If one takes a femur and physically scrapes out the bone marrow rather vigorously with a curette so that the stromal tissue is also removed, that particular bone, no matter how many marrow cells are transferred, will no longer support hemopoiesis. Indeed, it will not support hemopoiesis until and unless a stromal framework regrows and recreates a microenvironment that is capable of supporting hemopoiesis.

Now, there are certain diseases such as myelofibrosis where this constitutes a serious problem. In such diseases the marrow cavity is occupied by fibrous or osteoid tissue. It has often been discussed whether such patients could be transfused or grafted with marrow, but the absence of normal stromal tissue prevents this.

Another example of the role of microenvironment is that of the spleen graft in the mouse. The growth of the spleen graft is determined by the age of the organ grafted, i.e., better engraftment is obtained with neonatal donors. However, the growth of the graft is also greatly influenced by the presence of host spleen. If one desires a good-sized graft, it is essential to remove the host spleen. There is clearly some restriction on the total amount of spleen tissue that is to be present in an animal. If one performs multiple spleen grafts, the total graft mass attained quickly plateaus out at just about the weight of a normal spleen.

These are but two examples of the fact that hemopoietic microenvironments will determine the quantitative amount of engrafted marrow in a particular patient, even assuming a perfect match and no GVH problems. Accordingly, it seems to me that one of the issues the transplantationists had better pay close attention to is whether the laws governing transplantation of hemopoietic populations also apply to hemopoietic stromal grafts.

We tend to make our comparisons between skin grafts and bone marrow grafts, but it is just about as easy to work with a spleen graft as a skin graft, and it carries the important advantage that questions can be posed about hemopoietic stroma. My guess is that the rules governing skin graft transplantation are probably going to be about the same for spleen or bone grafts. However, since the latter have not been exhaustively studied, I think we need to start looking into this because in some diseases stromal grafts may be the way to achieve good marrow engraftment.

Another comment I would make for the record is the fact that the clinician is faced with a series of unsatisfactory compromises. Prospective transplant patients, even if they do not have severe disease such as leukemia (which is a problem in itself), have to be pretreated with irradiation or cytotoxic drugs, which is a less than satisfactory situation for obtaining engraftment. Furthermore, typing will rarely achieve the selection of a perfectly matched donor and again compromises must be accepted.

Earlier in the conference I found myself becoming increasingly concerned by the character of the discussions on tissue typing. I felt that we were beginning to make life a little too complicated for the clinician faced with realities. We were getting to the stage where the new typing and subtyping procedures were producing internally conflicting results. If we are seeking procedures that will have wide applicability in small hospital centers, we should not try to achieve perfection, but rather seek answers that are really more meaningful compromises, a satisfactory rather than a perfect match.

On the biological side, I found the data on NK cells and resistance fascinating for many reasons. A very interesting point for me was the element of localization of reactivity, that one organ would yield cells exhibiting high reactivity and other organs cells with very little reactivity. I share Van Bekkum's concern. If resistance can be shown in one organ and yet not in other sites, what are we really talking about? However, this phenomenon of local reactivity makes me wonder whether it might account for some of the phenomenology that people in cancer research are familiar with. Does the fact that the spleen has a high concentration of naturally reactive cells explain why this organ almost never is the site of metastases? This is really a curious phenomenon, expecially as it is an organ with a good vascular circulation. Nobody has ever explained this; perhaps we are now beginning to get an answer. On the other hand, why is the spleen a frequent site of T lymphomas if the T lymphoma is the cell most susceptible to such NK cells? Again, a rather curious situation. On the positive side, why is the thymus so often the site of development of lymphomas in mice? Is it because the thymus has few, if any, of these NK cells?

I have asked O'Reilly to evaluate the overall results being achieved with the use of present typing methods.

O'REILLY: I think that the typing procedures discussed during this conference will be applicalbe in the clinical setting of marrow transplantation for establishing larger donor pools, currently restricted to family members. The systems that were discussed, such as PLT, D locus, and Ia typing, certainly offer us means for further characterizing the phenotypic, and possibly the genotypic, MHC determinants of the donor and recipient. However, when one comes down to a choice of means for selecting a marrow donor with the present state of the art, it can be stated unequivocally that D locus compatibility determined by MLC is the method of choice.

I think the area of major concern is that the MLC, as currently used, provides insufficient discriminatory evidence for identifying, prior to transplant, specificities that may promote GVH or graft rejection.

I think Metcalf's concern that the clinician facing marrow transplantation is usually compromising is very real. Rarely is there more than one donor available in the family. Were more donors the rule, then the question of which tests to employ would be pertinent. As the genetic determinants of engraftment and GVH are established, transplantation from unrelated donors will become more of a practical reality. One can appreciate that in certain situations an unrelated donor might offer advantages over a related donor. Given the means for averting GVH and assuring engraftment, immune reconstitution with a genotypically different marrow should potentiate antineoplastic responses.

DUPONT: I think we are dealing with two separate problems: the first is GVHD in up to 30–50% of HLA genotypically identical siblings. This is a problem we do not know how to deal with at present. The second is how to handle patients who do not have an HLA-identical sibling donor. Sibling availability is limited and the statistical probability for HLA identity is only 25%. To address this problem we are developing a series of different assays for rapid screening of large blood donor populations. The most recent development is the typing for the human Ia-like antigens. We know that at least one set of B-lymphocyte alloantigens is strongly associated with the HLA-D region. Developments in this area should allow us to select unrelated donor candidates, on the basis of the best match in terms of HLA-A, B, C antigens, initial MLC-testing, and Ia-antigen typing.

VAN BEKKUM: In my experience, the patient with an HLA-identical sibling is as great a problem as the patient without it. One still finds an incidence of 50% GVHD in aplastics and even more in leukemics given HLA-identical marrow grafts. The urgency in the HLA-identical sibling combinations is to identify the cases that will develop GVHD and differentiate them from the cases that will not.

Then we can really reserve all the therapeutic procedures to mitigate GVHD for the latter patients and not endanger the former.

Finally, I disagree with O'Reilly concerning unrelated donors because in my opinion chances are that these unrelated donors, however one matches them, will induce more severe GVH.

O'REILLY: I do not take issue with the fact that present matching techniques give better long-term survival in leukemia patients grafted with identical twin marrow.

But even with twins, we are dealing only with about a 30% long-term survival, and most of the patients who die do so either acutely or with recurrent leukemia. It is noteworthy that in 20% of twins in the population at large, leukemia occurs in both. So, what I was saying is that immune reconstitution via bone marrow grafts to be *truly* effective must change the host reactivity to his own tumor.

CHAIRMAN METCALF: I would like to suggest a quite different approach to selecting donor populations. In principle, *in vitro* cloning could be applied to determine whether prospective donor cells, particularly marrow cells, would be either killed or damaged or in some way modified by the cells of the recipients. To my knowledge, no one has yet done mixed cultures of this type and posed the question of damage to the granulopoietic and lymphoid cell populations. The other potential use of these cloning methods, of course, is to monitor the viability of stored marrow.

VAN BEKKUM: How would one go about doing mixed cultures with cells of aplastic patients?

MOORE: We now have data on some 43 patients with aplastic anemia who have a mean colony incidence of 2.2 colonies per 10^5 bone marrow cells. This has proved to be extremely constant over a period of five years. We have indeed done co-cultures of aplastic anemia bone marrow with normal bone marrow for the purpose of investigating suppressor cells present in the marrow. In three cases, there were suppressor cells present in aplastic bone marrow capable of suppressing colony formation by normal bone marrow. We have not, however, mixed cells from the actual aplastic recipient with those of the potential donor. This would constitute one of the experimental studies that should be done in the future, especially since we are aware of this sort of phenomenon.

CHARIMAN UHR: I would like to consider the discussions during this conference that dealt with the generation or functioning of the cells involved in resistance phenomena.

Let us first consider the MHC. This complex is important in the stimulation of T cells and in the recognition of antigen on target cells by effector T cells. For me, one of the most intriguing developments we were exposed to was the series of observations by Festenstein. His studies, if confirmed and extended both in mice and man, would be pivotal in reshaping our thinking concerning the MHC. The simplest interpretation is that our present understanding of the organization and evolution of the MHC is incomplete. In the mouse, it is not composed of two genes per haploid set of chromosomes with an extraordinary number of alleles accounting for the polymorphism; rather, there is a series of genes in tandem, each one of which codes for a different H-2 antigen, and there is a regulatory mechanism that mimics Mendelian inheritance. Festenstein has shown that virus infection can lead to expression of some genes that presumably had been previously repressed.

Theoretically, this interpretation raises the specter of having MHC incompatibilities arise in a situation where typing has revealed MHC compatibility. As important as these practical implications, the interpretation of Festenstein's findings could change our thinking about genetic organization in general. For example, the situation with regard to other multigene families, such as immunoglobulin genes, has analogies. Thus, there are reports of ''inappropriate'' expression of immunoglobulin allotypes in the rabbit. Also, the studies of primary structure of immunoglobulins reveal multiple amino acid differences between immunoglobulin allotypes, differences beyond those predicted for alleles.

I would like to have Festenstein comment further on his remarkable observations. I would like him and perhaps others to comment on the potential problems suggested by these findings for transplantation of bone marrow and other tissues in man.

FESTENSTEIN: On the basis of the evidence, we cannot really be sure at this time whether the interpretation that Uhr has put on this work is the correct one or whether we have some mechanism that can be attributed directly to virus. This is clearly of great importance from a basic point of view, as Uhr has pointed out.

From a practical standpoint, the implications are operationally similar. The phenomenon could be preduced by a virus that has been activated and is elaborating a product cross-reacting so extensively as to be indistinguishable from the gene product. Alternatively, the effect could involve derepression of a cell antigen. The fact is that, if such mechanisms are induced by ubiquitous viruses or by traumatic situations in patients subjected to irradiation or immunosuppressive therapy, then the probability is rather high that such extradeterminants would actually appear during transplantation.

If this should prove to be the case, then the emphasis will be placed on looking at the reactive cell rather than at the target determinant.

I want to comment briefly on the implications of all this for immune surveillance. If the findings are correct, we would, I believe, understand better why so many cells are potentially reactive to histocompatibility antigens rather then to other, ordinary antigens. This particular issue has posed a major intellectual problem and has been discussed for many years. It has not really been understood why the host should possess such a preponderance of cells potentially reactive against histocompatibility antigens. It could be that if cells are constantly expressing these determinants, then we never have anything like a primary reaction in the mature adult, but instead experience only secondary reactions. It would then make for a different view of transplantation immunology; the superabundance of reactive cells would be part of a very fundamental process essential for survival.

DUPONT: In leukemia patients we find positive MLC stimulation of the patient's cells in 15–20% of the cases. These positive reactions disappear when the patients go into remission. Some of them have been blocked by anti-Ia antibodies selected on the basis of family studies.

So, these extrareactions are caused by abnormalities in peripheral blood leukocytes of leukemia patients, since blast cells express Ia antigens. Festenstein's phenomenon, although interesting, has no relevance for clinical transplantation, because we do not pick up such changes in testing.

We also find no positive MLC or CML in aplastic anemia patients, yet that is where rejections occur.

O'REILLY: One relevant comment should be raised here. I refer to the unusual frequency with which viral infections, particularly CMV (cytomegalovirus), are associated with the development of GVHR in marrow transplantation. Simmons has demonstrated the extraordinary frequency of CMV infections one to two days before the onset of rejection crisis in kidney transplantation. The correlation between these two events is extraordinarily high, and the question should be raised whether virus infection may somehow alter surface determinants. This could occur either on a given host tissue in marrow transplantation, such that it might function as a target for GVH, or in cells of the graft.

CHAIRMAN METCALF: At least two groups have shown syngeneic reactivity that could have been due to Festenstein's extraspecificities. Some years ago we showed that AKR cells from preleukemic and, to a lesser degree, leukemic mice were cytotoxic for AKR embryo monolayer cells, and so were C3H cells from mice infected with the Moloney virus. A group in Boston have reported essentially the same phenomenon, except for details.

PARKMAN: The viral agents found primarily in the transplantation patients (*Herpes simplex* and *zoster*, CMV), are not easily eradicated. The possibility exists that a viremic patient before transplantation is somehow "tolerized" to the virus-induced extrahistocompatibility antigens. After the new but "non-tolerized" cells are engrafted, the extraalloantigens may become the targets of GVH.

CANTOR: A number of mechanisms can be invoked to explain reactions against virus-altered cells. One of them, advanced by Zinkernagel and his colleagues, does *not* involve an unorthodox new expression of inappropriate genes; the other is the one advanced by Festenstein.

The most appealing part of the hypothesis of Festenstein involves the way it accounts for the high degree of alloreactivity found in most mouse strains. The difficulty with the hypothesis is that one can see this high degree of alloreactivity in mice at birth. It is difficult to visualize how this can occur if, as Festenstein suggests, alloreactivity is simply a sum of responses to inappropriate expression of H-2 products in the course of the animal's life span.

FESTENSTEIN: I think that if one were dealing with a large number of mutations occurring in the course of prenatal development, one might under these circumstances also have an expression of inappropriate antigens. This need not arise only from infection.

CHAIRMAN UHR: It is interesting how quickly so many permutations of this idea have been generated. I think this indicates that, as was suggested, there are considerable inferences of Festenstein's findings.

I think it would be inadvisable at this stage to set boundaries on the potential implications of the findings. It is also important to confirm these observations and extend them to a molecular level. We want to know whether the new specificities are carried on H-2 antigens as determined *biochemically*. This would exclude an alternative interpretation that a viral antigen is cross-reacting with MHC antigens.

Now we should move on to another issue that has been touched upon in our discussion and in much greater detail during the conference: what are the underlying machanisms responsible for chronic secondary homologous disease? How does one determine the contributions of GVHR, host-versus-graft, infection, etc.?

I invite Sprent to comment on this problem

SPRENT: I think it is perhaps unfortunate that the disease state that one sees in recipients of marrow transplants is referred to by the all-embracing term graft-vs.-host disease. In theory, the disease state that one does see could arise, as Uhr has pointed out, either from an attack by the graft against the host—a graft-vs.-host reaction—or vice versa—a host-vs.-graft reaction.

A third possibility is that many of the symptoms are simply a reflection of the state of prolonged severe immunodepression that follows irradiation and protracted treatment with cytotoxic drugs. In particular, there is a marked deficiency of T cells and here one might bear in mind the example of the neonatally thymectomized mouse. It is important to emphasize that such mice manifest many of the clinical symptoms of patients sustaining what has been referred to as GVHD. For example, they may show either lymphoid atrophy or lymphoid hyperplasia and they may have severe gut damage.

So, for these reasons I would suggest using a *nonspecific* term to describe the disease state that follows marrow transplantation. For example, one might consider the old term of homologous disease or perhaps, to be more modern, allogeneic disease. Once the etiology of the condition had been established, a more precise term (e.g., GVHR or HVGR) could be applied.

My own objection to the term graft-vs.-host disease is that it perpetuates the notion that the disease is due in part to a reaction against the host by the progeny of stem cells differentiating into T cells. I would like to emphasize that to my knowledge there is really no convincing evidence that this is the case. In my own experience, irradiated mice given H-2 incompatible marrow cells do not develop overt symptoms of GVH disease unless the marrow cells are contamined with mature T cells.

BORANIC: I would like to call attention to the fact that soon after transplantation there is certainly attack by grafted cells on the host. This graft-vs.-host *reaction* may or may not be lethal. Even if it is not, this reaction seems to be self-limiting. The graft attack expires soon, so that approximately three weeks after transplantation this reaction comes to an end. However, during the attack the host has apparently suffered damage to many tissues including the hemopoietic and lymphatic tissues.

Later, however, a syndrome develops that we term graft-vs.-host *disease*. I completely agree with Sprent that this might be an inappropriate term. In many instances, indeed this is a GVH reaction that has stirred up again. However, at times it is only lymphatic atrophy consequent to host-vs.-graft-reaction taking place in an animal that has been damaged severely in the acute phase, and all this together may result in a syndrome that is lethal.

VAN BEKKUM: Sprent may be adding confusion to a situation that is really not so confusing. All one needs for clarification is histology. It is perfectly possible to distinguish, for instance, the very common GVH skin symptoms that we encounter in patients that have been grafted. By doing skin biopsies and histology, one can perfectly well distinguish between GVH and any other kind of disease.

SPRENT: I am willing to accept that in the majority of the situations in which one does see skin lesions, these are indeed the result of a GVH reaction. I would argue, however, that for the most part such lesions are caused (or controlled by) T cells that originally contaminated the marrow graft.

O'REILLY: I would like to point out a consistent clinical observation that has been difficult to explain. One of the principal manifestations of GVHD in the reconstituted patient with marrow aplasia is thrombocytopenia and leukopenia. This is a situation where cells of the same genotype are effectors (T lymphocytes) and targets for suppression (myeloid and megakaryocytic precursors).

Parkman's observations on autoreactivity may explain these findings. However, it must also be considered that cells in the host milieu, such as macrophages or histiocytes, may actually mediate host-against-graft reactions, possibly facilitated by factors of donor cell origin.

CANTOR: There is experimental evidence for host-vs.-graft reactions as part of what we call GVH disease. Despite Van Bekkum's plea, I think morphology can be very misleading. There are several observations suggesting that after an initial period of donor cell activity, there is considerable host reaction in the course of the wasting syndrome.

According to Billingham and Silvers, GVHD could be abrogated by the administration of antisera directed against the donor cells up to 14 days after initiation, after which the GVHD proceeded.

Moreover, when parental thymocytes were administered to F_1 recipients, the latter developed several autoantibodies, one of which was directed against red cells. This antibody was produced by host cells at a time when there was little, if any, morphologic evidence of an active lymphoid system. So, in a number of situations GVHD, at least in the chronic form, may be a manifestation of host autoimmune reactions.

WARNER: I would just like to emphasize the importance of this issue. At this conference we have been considering some very imaginative and far-reaching approaches to resolving the issue of GVH in relation to clinical transplantation. These are not going to be of much point if the predominant component disease is host-vs.-graft reaction.

TRENTIN: I get a distinct feeling of *deja vu,* in that I thought we fought and resolved some of these battles of host-vs.-graft and graft-vs.-host almost 20 years ago. We now have methods that can resolve this issue, and one of the obvious approaches is parent-into-F_1 and F_1-into-parent transplants, for discrimination. We used and reported those methods long ago. What they say is that except for the early midlethal radiation dose mortality (where the dose of irradiation is not high enough to preclude recovery of host immune responsiveness against the donor), the secondary disease mortality, which comes in the second month, is graft-vs.-host-disease.

Since then, we have learned that there is another element of host-vs.-graft that is more radioresistant. This is what we have dealth with during this conference, the genetic resistance to hemopoietic cell transplantation. But even this, while present for the week or so after 800–1000 R or rads in which we measure it, dissipates as a late result of the irradiation. Furthermore, nutritional runts, viral infections, thymectomy wasting, cortisone-induced wasting, and the like are all conditions resembling GVHD. But this is not to deny the GVH nature of secondary disease in supralethally irradiated allogeneic mouse chimeras. We have come much too far to revert to that.

ELKINS: The terminology GVHD tends to perpetuate the concept that a patient or animal that is displaying the secondary disease syndrome after receiving a lympho-hematopoietic graft is necessarily undergoing an alloimmune attack at the time when the syndrome develops. As has come out during this conference, there are other possibilities. That is why I define GVHR as the alloimmune response itself, and use the term GVHD for the clinically evident sequellae whether or not these be the direct, immediate result of the GVHR. I would be happy to use the term allogeneic disease instead, but we shall not affect the usage in the world outside even if all of us here could agree.

In this connection I would also like to point out the inability both of Snell's immunogenetic laws and histopathologic studies to help us decipher the mechanisms of GVH (allogeneic) disease. Consider the "big spleen disease" described by Simpson and others recently. In this case the lesions of GVHD appear in BALB/c mice injected at birth with (BALB/c $\times$ C57BL)F_1 cells. There are several possibilities:

(1) An F_1 antiparent immune response based upon an antiidiotypic reaction or an Hh phenomenon that is unusually potent in the strain combination employed.

(2) An immunogenetically conventional host-vs.-graft reaction at the level of recognition. Thus host parental cells recognizing the F_1 as allogeneic generate a back stimulus for F_1 cells to proliferate, presumably via lymphokines.

(3) Simpson showed that there is MuLV activation in this system. The GVH syndrome may be a direct consequence of virus activation and antiviral immunity. Nevertheless, it is also a consequence of triggering the alloimmune reaction.

Obviously, the application of conventional immunogenetic principles does not help us unravel the pathogenesis. We seem to encounter similar problems of interpretation with chronic GVHD.

Most of the GVH research in mice and rats has been confined to studies of H-2 and AgB different combinations. It is generally said that there is no good laboratory model for GVHD of HLA-matched sibs. That may be, but one can obtain strains of mice matched for the MHC but differing in background genes. Furthermore, by immunization of the donor, one could reproduce MHC-matched chimeras that will manifest GVHD. Storb has been working with a suitable model in dogs for many years, so there *are* laboratory models wherein one can study what goes on in the allogeneic chimera in the absence of major incompatibilities.

Since virus infection is such a problem in human radiation chimeras, it seems to me that we should test lymphocytes from human and murine chimeras for their capacity to recognize altered-self MHC antigens in the systems worked out by Shearer, Dougherty and Zinkernagel, Gordon, Schrader, etc. What happens to haplotype-restricted surveillance after chimerism is induced across minor locus barriers in the presence or absence of GVHD? In parallel one could also study the effects of the various kinds of treatments that are used to control GVHR to determine how this therapy might influence these surveillance mechanisms.

I have developed during the course of this conference a tremendous appreciation for the potential role of NK cells in control of leukemia. In some cases at least, the NK mechanism is under genetic control linked to H-2. Thus, as the organizers of this conference were aware, if we really want to control leukemia by bone marrow transplantation, it might be a serious mistake to use MHC-matched sibling donors in each case. Rather one might scan a variety of candidates for NK activity against the patient's leukemia in order to choose the most active donor irrespective of HLA matching. Such an approach would require an effective treatment to control the GVHR, perhaps along the lines suggested by Wigzell. While the clinical potential of the antiidiotypic control of GVHD is being worked out, there is much to be done on animal models concerning our capacity to transplant NK cell activity with bone marrow grafting.

PARKMAN: The three possibilities that are being considered for the pathogenesis of GVHD (virus-induced extraantigens in the host, host-vs.-graft, and classical graft-vs.-host reactions) lead to a persisting decrease of T cell function in the recipient. This decreased function would render the recipient cells unable to eradicate viral infected cells, the donor cells unable to eradicate residual immunocompetent host cells, and T precursors unable to generate adequate numbers of suppressor T cells. Other problems in the graft recipient are the inability to make specific antibody, due to decreased T helper activity, the prevalence of viral and fungal infections, which requite adequate T cell functions for their termination. Furthermore, many of the agents used in the transplantation regimes, besdies being lympholtic, also damage the thymic stroma, aggravating the posttransplant hypotymic state. Thus, there may be a common basis for the many defects manifested by the bone marrow transplant recipient.

CHAIRMAN UHR: I think the thrust of the discussion is that there have been sufficient advances in the last two decaded, so that the issue of mechanisms underlying allogeneic disease merits further investifation. Whereas many of the clinical situations may be clearly attributable to a GVH reaction, certainly there are some that are not. This was identified as a priority area for investigation since it is pivotal in deciding on a strategy for handling those instances of allogeneic disease that may not be due to the conventional pathogensis, namely, GVHR.

I would like to turn to another issue that was a major one at this conference. The importance of NK cells and nonimmune cells in general in tumor resistance and perhaps other systems has been stressed. I would ask Warner to discuss the heterogeneity of macrophages and NK cells.

WARNER: I think it is fair to say that one of the more exciting issues here has been the strong tendency toward discussing "macrophages" rather than "the macrophage." Several years ago, immunologists used to say "the lymphocyte." That is now obviously quite incorrect, as we recognize distinct subpopulations, principally through the use of surface alloantigenic markers.

In the course of this conference it has become clear that a similar heterogeneity exists within macrophage populations. Many hematologists have stressed this to immunologists for some years, but I guess it took the immunologists their own experience with "immune systems" to start coming around to this view.

At this conference we have heard of distinct subpopulations of macrophages particularly in relation to their effects in various tumor studies. This evidence rests mainly on the basis of specificity of killing different tumor targets. As Henney has pointed out, caution is warranted in interpreting comparative lytic data with different tumor types, since all have their own inherent characteristics about incorporating and releasing chromium label. There is now sufficient ground to say that there are different types of cells that are neither T nor B cells, which nonetheless mediate some form of killing process on various tumor targets.

An alloantigen locus called Mph specifies a macrophage alloantigen and there are many studies with heteroantisera prepared against macrophage subpopulations. The striking advances in characterizing lymphocyte subpopulations by this approach are considered a portent of what to expect with macrophages. Now that we are starting to think about macrophage heterogeniety, it is important to address two major alternatives: do the different types of killing functions displayed by macrophages and NK cells reflect different stages of maturity of one cell lineage type? Alternatively, are these distinctly different and divergent, subpopulations despite precursor–progeny relationships?

Throughout this conference, we have heard of two parallel situations. The studies on NK cells reactive against tumors, and the studies on Hh incompatibility. Throughout our sessions has come the insistent query whether these are facets of the same mechanism. But in posing this proposition, we need to ask the question at two levels. Is the NK cell indeed the effector-type of cell that derives from the M cell and is operative in both mechanisms, the only heterogeneity being with respect to the target affected? At the target level, is it the same *category* of molecule that is being recognized on the cell surface of tumors and stem cells?

At the start of this conference, the terms "antigens" and "immune-response genes" were used in relation to both Hh and NK studies. It may be time now to ascertain whether we are really dealing with a totally different type of recognition system.

From the speed of the interactions in the Hh and NK systems, the recognition event presumably occurs at cell surfaces. Accordingly, there is some type of molecule that is on the surface of both tumor cells and stem cells being recognized. We may eventually define new terms for these components other than immune response, receptors, and antigens.

PARKMAN: What has impressed me at this conference is the nonimmunological aspects of experimental situations that immunologists have been studying. This incidentally includes all the work I have been doing, and the efforts of many others of us as well. More and more I wonder why we are continuing to focus on phenomena such as antibody formation and cell-mediated lympholysis when the action is clearly in the direction of NK cells and other nontraditional systems in natural resistance.

We are going to find 78 or 87 genes in the I region, and they will turn out to have very dubious significance for pressing problems, such as bone marrow transplantation and lymphoma resistance.*

---

*Editors' comment: In the half-century or so of its existence as a discrete discipline, the boundaries of immunology have expanded continuously and, in recent decades, the focus of its concern has shifted profoundly from the descriptive manifestations of immunity at the organismic level to immune mechanisms at the cellular and molecular level. An essentially parallel development was the progressive move, beginning in the 1940s, away from concerns about immunity against infectious diseases to acquired, adaptive, and thymus-dependent immune responses.

Despite its molecular bent, it seems to us that contemporary immunology is no longer so limited or restrictive as to exclude what Parkman has referred to as the "nonimmunological aspects of experimental situations"(such as GVH or marrow rejection). Until recently, however, these varied facets of natural host systems were simply not amenable to investigation, because appropriate techniques had not been developed or concepts formulated. This also reflected fashions in science, which seem particularly to affect immunology, conditioned in large part by a series of major discoveries such as the role of the thymus, T and B cells, cell cooperation, and suppressor cells. As the progression of such major developments preempted immunologic thought for some two decades, the phenomenology of natural resistance, obviously so crucial for vertebrates to successfully cope with the threats of their environment and oncogenesis, remained amorphous and obscure. This conference

GORDON: I have been viewing the conference development from the vantage point of someone relatively new to what would be called conventional cellular immunology. I have been impressed by the many diffenent machanisms that are unique in the field of bone marrow transplantation, such things as NK cells, autocytotoxic cells, and the phenomenon of Hh resistance.

Now, in the conference prospectus, prepared by the organizers, it was stated that one of our ultimate hopes is that we would be able to use bone marrow transplantation to confer upon patients with disease a new pattern of immune reactivity, which would enable them to abrogate that disease state. Elkins has stated that the ultimate irony may be that, in order to prevent some of the unique effector mechanisms that operate in GVHD, we may have to resort to MHC mismatched patients and use techniques such as antiidiotype to control allograft responsiveness. If our goal is to alter the immune reactivity of the host patient, what happens when we deprive the transplanted donor cells of some of the differences in immune reactivity that distinguish it from the host? If we use antiidiotype antibody, we are, to a certain extent, making our donor like the host, in which case we might permit recurrence of the very disease state we are trying to abrogate.

WIGZELL: I don't believe that the absence of reactivity against self-MHC components in the cytolytic sense will endanger the patient. It would be, in effect, giving to the recipient cells that are completely normal despite the absence of reactive clones against MHC of that recipient.

CHAIRMAN UHR: I agree with Wigzell. It seems to me that one ends up with an individual that lacks, in essence, approximately 1–5% of the donor cells that were infused. The same maneuver can be used to eliminate recipient reactivity to donor MHC. One makes a chimera with all of the immune potentialities of the

---

has sought to redress this gross imbalance—especially as methodology, novel experimental situations, and concepts had all finally come into an understandable focus. What emerges from this active interchange is an awareness that experimental and clinical situations, such as resistance to normal and malignant cells, and microbial pathogens, are well within the scope of present-day immunology, especially since they are being explained largely on immunogenetic and immunobiologic concepts.

Noninduced resistance phenomena, all too frequently and erroneously viewed as "nonspecific," in many instances prove to be eminently specific—but involve structures other than the familiar membrane-bound Ig and T cell receptiors. These novel, as yet undefined, recognition structures could emerge as a kind of resonant counterpoint to the classical receptors that have so long dominated immunologic theory and practice.

Each immunologist has his own view of where this remarkable discipline is headed. The extraordinary discoveries so actively discussed and debated during this conference persuade us that the elucidation of the mechanisms operative in these resistance phenomena, functional heterogeneity of macrophages, reactivity to modified self, autocytotoxicity, etc., will, in fact, constitute a major new dimension in the immunology of the 1980s.

donor and host except that there has been eliminated those cells that are alloaggressive to each other from the two populations.

GORDON: My point is that we expect that the Ir potential of the donor would be expressed in the chimeric host, much as the Ir genes of a parent are expressed in an F_1. But I am asking further what value nature places on the ability of the donor cells to react to the MHC gene products of the host. Festenstein's model suggests a selective advantage for allogeneic responsiveness. If we deprive the donor cells of the capacity to respond to the MHC determinants of the host, does that in any way deprive the donor cells, and thus the host, of any selective advantage that could promote a disease state? I am really asking: What price has this kind of deletion-tolerance?

CHAIRMAN UHR: I certainly agree that there are unknown potential dangers in these situations simply because we don't yet know the physiological function of the MHC gene products.

SANFORD: Couldn't one perform a positive selection experiment? The object would be to get rid of reactivity toward a specific MHC product. The cells remaining would still be reactive to a wide variety of antigens—actually to everything else. I should think that this would put some of Gordon's worries to rest.

GORDON: That would not completely satisfy me. If certain disease states show linkage disequilibrium with HLA, to what extent is that a reflection of the price we pay for necessary self tolerance? Is the allograft response only a clinical nuisance and a laboratory curiosity, or does it have biologic significance for both the individual and the species?

WERNET: The Wigzell type of approach would create a selective clonal deletion, I would like to point out that a natural clonal deletion has recently been found in man where of two MHC identical siblings, one did not respond to a defined HLA-D determinant, whereas the other resonded very well to it.
    This phenomenon of natural clonal deletion may be much more common than we know.

O'REILLY: Fetal liver transplantation may also result in clonal deletion, since the fetal liver stem cells will differentiate in the new and allogeneic host. This has actually been done successfully in some six patients. The donor cells will be specifically depleted of the clones capable of effector function in terms of GVHR, and yet they will provide their new host with responsiveness against other allogeneic stimuli.

CHAIRMAN METCALF: Some of the conferees are too young to remember a very spectacular experiment that was done in leukemogenesis, one that I have never been convinced was properly explained. I bring it to your attention, because it might be a very good test system for the function of NK cells.

If one gives C57BL mice split-dose whole-body irradiation, thymic lymphoma develops in about 90% of the mice. A spectacular experiment is to inject normal syngeneic bone marrow into those animals after irradiation, thereby completely preventing leukemia development. At the time, the explanation advanced was that one was promptly supplying an intact immune system that suppressed an activation of a previously latent leukemia virus. It was, in fact, possible to show some elevation of titratable leukemia virus in these irradiated mice. In view of what we now know, that explanation seems rather unlikely. Marrow cell populations are now known to provide unusual cells capable of remarkable functions. Since the irradiation schedule is not in itself lethal, there is no need to inject the entire bone marrow cell population. It is now high time we subfractionate the marrow and determine just which cell is reponsible for this very spectacular antilymphoma effect.

TRENTIN: I believe Kaplan's original explanation of this experiment was that grafted marrow helped overcome some radiation-induced maturation arrest in the thymus. However, in view of what we now know about resistance in C57BL mice, the reseeding with M cells is a more likely explanation. Now, extending this experience a step further, it is possible to repopulate mice that have *no* genetic resistance to marrow transplantation or leukemia, with marrow of mice that *do* possess it and thereby confer this kind of resistance.

The critical experiments with reference to the incidence of spontaneous leukemia in AKR mice have been done by repopulating AKR mice with marrow from another strain that does not produce a prohibitive GVH response, yet reduces the incidence of spontaneous leukemia. So, the message is that there are already in the literature very exciting models for adoptive transfer of this kind of genetic resistance.

TILL: As this conference draws to a close I would like to make a general comment, and that is that almost all of our discussions have been cast in the language of immunology. So, the jargon of "killer cells," "antigen", and "clonal deletion" has come up again and again.

An alternative point of view has been mentioned only occasionally. It is that, when we talk about the phenomena that were the subjects of this conference, we are dealing with physiological regulatory mechanisms. If so, one should be talking also about "regulatory" or "managerial" cells, and as Warner said, "recognition structures," and "networks of regulatory cell interactions."

I would make the fearless prediction that, were this group to reassemble in a couple of years, we would be using the latter language much more than some of the current immunology jargon.

CHAIRMAN UHR: I think that Till has summarized, elegantly, a situation that is becoming apparent to all of us. His comment is an appropiate high point on which to end this discussion.

ABBREVIATIONS

ADCC	antibody-dependent cell-mediated cytotoxicity
AgB	histocompatibility B complex of the rat
BFU-E	erythropoietic burst-forming unit
CD	cellular defined antigens (target determinants in CML)
CFU	colony-forming unit
CFU-C	colony-forming unit generating granulocytes and mononuclear phagocytic cells in culture
CFU-E	colony-forming unit generating erythroid cells in culture
CFU-PM	colony-forming unit from peritoneal cavity generating mononuclear phagocytic cells in culture
CFU-S	pluripotent colony-forming unit generating hemic cells in the spleen of irradiated mice
CML	cell-mediated lympholysis
CMV	cytomegalovirus
Con A	concanavalin A
CSF	colony-stimulating factor
CTL	cytotoxic thymus-derived lymphocyte
DLA	the major canine histocompatibility complex (leukocyte antigens)
DS	dextran sulfate
GVH	graft-versus-host
GVHD	graft-versus-host disease
GVHR	graft-versus-host reaction
H	histocompatibility gene
Hh	hemopoietic-histocompatibility gene
HLA	the major human histocompatibility complex (leukocyte antigens)
HTC	homozygous typing cells
H-2	the major murine histocompatibility complex
Ir	immune response gene
IUdR	5-iodo-2'-deoxyuridine
LD	lymphocyte-defined antigens (stimulator determinants in MLC)
LPS	lipopolysaccharide
Ly	lymphocyte antigens

291

Ly-1,
  Ly-2,
  Ly-3
	lymphocyte antigen systems 1, 2, 3

Ly-1.2	allele 2 of lymphocyte antigen system 1
M cell	marrow-dependent cell (destroyed by ^{89}Sr)
MHC	major histocompatibility complex
MIF	macrophage inhibitory factor
MLC	mixed leukocyte culture
NK	natural killer (cytolytic) cell
PGE	prostaglandin E
PHA	phytohemagglutinin
PLT	primed lymphocyte typing
RES	reticulo-endothelial system
SCID	severe combined immunodeficiency disease
SD	serologically defined antigens (identical or closely associated with CD)
SLC	sperm-lymphocyte mixed culture
Thy-1	thymus alloantigen expressed on murine T lymphocytes
TL	thymus leukemia antigen region of murine chromosome 17
TNP	trinitrophenyl hapten

AUTHOR INDEX

SUBJECT INDEX

A

AKR leukemia, 209–211
AKR lymphoma, 210, 215–223
Alveolar macrophages, 94
Anti-B cell antibody, 257–259
Anti-bone marrow serum, 187, 191, 238
Anti-HLA antibody, 57–59
Anti-idiotype antibody, 78, 254–256
Anti-LyB3 antibody, 257–259
Antilymphoid sera, 241
Anti-NK serum, 179–180, 191
Antispecies sera, 8–9
Antispleen serum, 238, 241
Antithymocyte serum, 52, 54, 238
Aplastic anemia, 49–52, 54, 57–59, 66, 101
Autoimmunity, 85–86, 246–247

B

B cell
  antigens of, 128, 133–134, 135–136,
    138–139
  differentiation of, 20
  in GVHD, 75
  silica and, 110
BCG, 93, 100, 103, 191–195
Besnoitia jellisoni, 103–106
BFU-E, 99
Bone marrow, *see* Marrow

C

Carrageenans, 8–9, 106–108, 187, 238
Cell-mediated lymphocytotoxicity tests, 109,
    141–142, 145–172
CFU-C, 93, 100–102
CFU-E, 98–99
CFU-PM, 93–94, 100
Chimeras, 87–88
Chromium release assay, 54–55, 61–62
CMV, *see* Cytomegalovirus
Colchicine, 193
Colony-stimulating factors, 94–95, 99–100,
    101–102
Cortisone, 189
Corynebacterium parvum, 182, 238
CSF, *see* Colony-stimulating factors
CTL, *see* Cytotoxic T cell
Cyclophosphamide, 238
Cytochalasins, 193
Cytomegalovirus, 67
Cytotoxic T cell
  GVHD and, 69, 75, 78–79, 85–86, 141–142,
    251–252, 268–269
  markers on, 251–252
  NK cells and, 193
Cytoxan, 191

D

Dimethylmyeleran, 23–24
Dog marrow grafts, 50